Vitamins, Herbs, Minerals & Supplements

The Complete Guide

Revised Edition

H. Winter Griffith, M.D.

Technical Consultant:
Cynthia Thomson, M.S., R.D.

Clinical Nutrition Research Specialist, Arizona Cancer Center
University of Arizona Prevention Center

MJF Books

NEW YORK

Notice: The information in this book is true and complete to the best of our knowledge. This book is intended only as an informative guide for those wishing to know more about vitamins, minerals, supplements and medicinal herbs. This book is not intended to replace, countermand or conflict with the advice given to you by your physician. He or she knows your history, symptoms, signs, allergies, general health and the many other variables that challenge his/her judgment in caring for you as a patient. The information in this book is general and is offered with no guarantees on the part of the author, Fisher Books, or Fine Communications, Inc. The author and publisher disclaim all liability in connection with the use of this book.

Published by MJF Books
Fine Communications
Two Lincoln Square
60 West 66th Street
New York, NY 10023

Vitamins, Herbs, Minerals & Supplements: The Complete Guide, Revised Edition
Library of Congress Catalog Card Number 98-67596
ISBN 1-56731-275-6

Copyright © 1988, 1998 Fisher Books

This edition published by arrangement with Fisher Books.
Managing Editor: Sarah Trotta
Assistant Editor: Meg Morris
Editors: Brian Engstrom, Jean Anderson
Copy Editor: Melanie Mallon
Production: Randy Schultz

Manufactured in the United States of America on acid-free paper

MJF Books and the MJF colophon are trademarks of Fine Creative Media, Inc.

10   9   8   7   6   5   4   3   2   1

Contents

About the Author

H. Winter Griffith, M.D., received his medical degree from Emory University in 1953 and spent more than 20 years in private practice. At Florida State University, he established a basic medical science program and also directed the family practice residency program at Tallahassee Memorial Hospital. After moving to the Southwest, he became associate professor of Family and Community Medicine at the University of Arizona College of Medicine. He devoted most of his time to writing medical-information books for general readers.

Dedication

To each of you who wishes to be informed enough to become the most important member of your own healthcare team.

Acknowledgments

Several years ago, Dr. Griffith set a personal goal to translate complicated, technical medical information into easy-to-understand terms that anyone outside the healing professions could use. Four previous books dealing with medications, symptoms, surgery and sports injuries have been major steps toward that goal.

Dr. Griffith remained a student of medicine for 40 years. The need for this book was made clear during his experience as a family doctor, teacher and author, answering questions (or seeking answers) for patients, medical students, nurses and physicians in training.

Special thanks to Sheldon Saul Hendler, M.D., Ph.D., author of *The Complete Guide to the Anti-Aging Nutrients* (Simon & Schuster, 1984; Fireside, 1986) for allowing the use of his material and unique research insights in this book.

Thanks also to everyone else who helped with this book in so many ways, including Brian Engstrom and Jean Anderson, research assistants, and technical consultant Cynthia Thomson, M.S., R.D., who is a registered dietitian with more than 18 years of clinical experience in nutrition. She is currently completing her Ph.D. in Nutritional Sciences at the University of Arizona, where she also works as an investigator on nutritional breast-cancer research trials. She facilitates the Nutritional Medicine Core for the Department of Medicine's program in Integrative Medicine, the first such training program in the United States.

Last but not least, thanks to the authors and publishers of the reference material (listed in the Bibliography) that was so helpful in the preparation of this book.

Vitamins and Minerals

Surveys show that more than half of the U.S. adult population uses dietary supplements of one type or another. In 1996 alone, consumers spent more than $6.5 billion on dietary supplements, according to one New York market-research firm. But even with all the purchases they generate, consumers still ask questions about dietary supplements: Can their claims be trusted? Are they safe? Does the Food and Drug Administration (FDA) approve them?

Many of these questions come in the wake of the 1994 Dietary Supplement Health and Education Act (DSHEA). The Act set up a new framework for FDA regulation of dietary supplements. This legislation created a new office within the National Institutes of Health to coordinate research on dietary supplements, called the Office of Alternative Medicine (OAM). It also provided for an independent dietary-supplements commission to report on the use of claims in dietary-supplement labeling.

The Council for Responsible Nutrition, an organization of manufacturers of dietary supplements and their suppliers, welcomes the change. "Our philosophy has been to maintain consumer access to products and access to information so that consumers can make informed choices," says John Cordaro, the group's president and chief executive officer.

Although the FDA receives numerous questions from consumers, who want to know whether they should use dietary supplements, the agency so far is limited in its ability to respond. Under the provisions of DSHEA, the FDA works under less rigid guidelines for pre-market review of dietary supplements than it does for other products it regulates, such as drugs and many additives used in processed foods. This means consumers and manufacturers, *not* the government, are responsible for checking the safety of dietary supplements and determining the truthfulness of label claims.

Effective in March 1999, the following information must appear on the labels of dietary supplements:

- Statement of identity (for example, "ginseng")
- Net quantity of contents (for example, "60 capsules")

1

- Structure-function claim *and* the message, "This statement has not been evaluated by the Food and Drug Administration. This product is not intended to diagnose, treat, cure or prevent any disease." (A structure-function claim refers to the purpose of or benefit derived from using the product.)
- Directions for use (for example, "Take one capsule daily.")
- Supplement Facts Panel (lists serving size, amount and active ingredient)
- Other ingredients in descending order of predominance and by common name or proprietary blend
- Name and place of business of manufacturer, packer or distributor. This is the address to which to write for more product information

In addition, the American Institute of Nutrition and the American Society for Clinical Nutrition have issued an official statement on vitamin and mineral supplements. This statement was developed jointly with the American Dietetic Association and the National Council against Health Fraud. The American Medical Association's Council on Scientific Affairs reviewed the statement and found it to be consistent with its official statement on dietary supplements.

The statement reads: "Healthy children and adults should obtain adequate nutrient intakes from dietary sources. Meeting nutrient needs by choosing a variety of foods in moderation, rather than by supplementation, reduces the potential risk for both nutrient deficiencies and nutrient excesses. Individual recommendations regarding supplements and diets should come from physicians and registered dietitians."

Supplementation is sometimes necessary in various circumstances. Some of these situations are listed below.

- Women with excessive menstrual bleeding may need iron supplements.
- Pregnant or breastfeeding women have an increased need for certain nutrients, especially iron, folic acid and calcium.
- People with very low calorie intakes frequently consume diets that do not meet their needs for most nutrients.
- Some vegetarians may not receive adequate calcium, iron, zinc and vitamin B-12.
- Newborns are commonly given a single dose of vitamin K to prevent abnormal bleeding. (This is done under the direction of a physician.)
- Certain disorders or diseases and some medications interfere with nutrient intake, digestion, absorption, metabolism or excretion. In addition, expanding scientific research indicates that supplementation with specific nutrients may be beneficial in the prevention of disease. Those who suffer myocardial infarction, for example, may benefit from vitamin-E supplementation.

Nutrients are potentially toxic when ingested in sufficiently large amounts. Safe intake levels vary widely from nutrient to nutrient and may vary with an individual's age and health. In addition, high-dosage vitamin and mineral supplements can interfere with the normal metabolism of other nutrients and with the therapeutic effects of certain drugs. The Recommended Dietary Allowance (RDA) and the Dietary Reference Intake (DRI) represent the best currently available assessments of safe and adequate intakes. They serve as the basis for the Recommended Daily Allowances shown on many product labels, although these are determined by the FDA for labeling purposes and should not be used by individuals as guidelines for their own daily intake. *Recommended Daily Allowances are not the same as Recommended Dietary Allowances.*

Every health professional wants consumers to take proper nutrients and supplements if they need them, but some people abuse these essential substances by taking doses 10 to 20 times the recommended amount or more.

Some people believe if one pill is good, 20 pills must be better. They also believe vitamins, minerals, herbs and supplements are medicine.

As information in this book points out, vitamins, minerals, herbs and supplements can cause side effects, adverse reactions, and interactions with other drugs and nutrients. Many individuals

need to avoid certain substances because of a unique situation, such as pregnancy or age. Others need to be aware that medical conditions, such as heart problems or various disease conditions, can be an indication not to take certain substances.

When deciding whether or not to supplement your diet with vitamins and minerals, remember that too much can be harmful. For example, high doses of vitamin A can cause bone pain and vomiting. High doses of vitamin C can also have toxic effects, including diarrhea and perhaps kidney stones. Too much of this vitamin can interfere with white blood cells' ability to kill bacteria. This can make infections worse rather than clear them up.

Many conditions may also rule out taking some substances. Always be alert to any side effects or interactions you may experience that could put your health in jeopardy. It's up to you to be a "smart" consumer of the vitamins, minerals and supplements your body may need. Get them from the food you eat when you can—supplement with available products when you must.

Vitamins

Vitamins are chemical compounds necessary for growth, health, normal metabolism and physical well-being. Some vitamins are essential parts of *enzymes*—the chemical molecules that catalyze or facilitate the completion of chemical reactions. Other vitamins form essential parts of *hormones*—the chemical substances that promote and protect body health and reproduction. If you're in good health, you need vitamins only in small amounts. They can be found in sufficient quantities in the foods you eat. This assumes you eat a normal, well-balanced diet of foods grown in nutritionally adequate soil.

Traditionally, vitamins have been divided into two categories: *fat-soluble* and *water-soluble.*

Fat-soluble vitamins can be stored in the body. If you take excessive amounts of fat-soluble vitamins, they accumulate to provide needed amounts at a later time. That's the good news. The bad news is, if you take excessive amounts of fat-soluble vitamins, toxic levels can accumulate in storage areas such as the liver. Too much of any fat-soluble vitamin can lead to potentially dangerous, long-term physical problems.

Water-soluble vitamins cannot be stored in the body to any great extent. The daily amount you need must be provided by what you eat over several days.

The amount of vitamins you need increases during illness, following surgery or even as a result of the aging process. In these circumstances, vitamin supplements may be necessary to meet increased needs or prevent a deficiency of select nutrients.

People with special needs for supplements or others at risk of vitamin deficiency are identified and discussed in detail later in this section. See page 10.

Vitamin supplements cannot take the place of good nutrition. Vitamins do not provide energy. Your body needs other substances besides vitamins for adequate nutrition, including carbohydrates, fats, proteins and minerals. Vitamins cannot help maintain a healthy body except in the presence of other nutrients, mainly from food and minerals.

Minerals

Minerals are inorganic chemical elements. They participate in many biochemical and physiological processes necessary for optimum growth, development and health. There is a clear and important distinction between the terms *mineral* and *trace element.* If the body requires more than 100 milligrams of a mineral each day, the substance is labeled *mineral.* If the body requires less than 100 milligrams of a mineral each day, the substance is labeled *trace element.*

Many minerals are essential parts of enzymes. They also participate actively in regulating many physiological functions, including transporting oxygen to each of the body's 60 trillion cells, providing the stimulus for muscles to contract and in many ways guaranteeing normal function of the central nervous system. Minerals are required for growth, maintenance, repair and health of tissues and bones.

Most minerals are widely distributed in foods. *Severe* mineral deficiency is unusual in the Western world. Of all essential minerals, only a few may be deficient in a typical diet. Iron deficiency can be seen in infants, children and pregnant women. Zinc and copper deficiencies are also not uncommon, especially during illness.

Multivitamin/Mineral Preparations

A varied diet will contain all the nutrients you need. For healthy people food is the best, most reliable source of nutrients. If you or your children need supplementation, the best place to start is by taking one of the commercially available multivitamin/mineral preparations. Commercial over-the-counter products usually have a good balance of nutrients. Taking separate products can lead to an imbalance of nutrients, which can lead to an overabundance of one substance at the expense of decreased absorption or effectiveness of another.

Taking separate, individual nutrient supplements will require careful consideration of nutrient-to-nutrient interactions and is more likely to result in excess intake above what may be healthy—in these cases you may want to talk with your doctor, dietitian or pharmacist. The cost tends to be lower if you take a combination product rather than separate products.

Most major pharmaceutical manufacturers supply widely advertised combination products. The brand names are too numerous to list and they change constantly. Your pharmacist, doctor or dietitian should be able to recommend a good source for a superior multivitamin/mineral preparation.

If you study vitamins and minerals, you may find you need supplements for one reason or another. We hope this book provides you with enough information to choose wisely or be able to ask the right questions to find out what is best for you.

Guide to Vitamin, Mineral and Acid Charts

Information in this book is organized in condensed, easy-to-read charts, divided into five main sections: vitamins, minerals, amino acids and nucleic acids, other supplements and medicinal herbs. (Information on the supplement and medicinal-herb sections and charts begins on page 20.) Each substance is described in a multipage format as shown in the sample charts on the following pages. They are arranged alphabetically by the most frequently recognized name—usually a generic name instead of a brand name.

The most common names of substances appear at the top of the chart. For example, vitamin C is frequently called *ascorbic acid.* Both names appear at the top of the chart. Less common names are listed in the first section of the chart, *Basic Information.*

To learn more about any vitamin or mineral, you need to know only one name. Look in the Index for any name you know, page 497. The Index provides a page number for the information you seek about that substance.

The next few pages provide an explanation for each section of a vitamin, mineral, or acid chart. The numbers correspond to the sample chart on pages 8 and 9. This information will help you read and understand the charts that begin on page 28.

1–Generic name

Each chart is titled by the *generic name,* the official chemical name of the substance. If two or more generic names exist, the substance is alphabetized by the most common name, with other names in parentheses at the top of the page or listed under the *Basic Information* section. If a substance has two or more generic names, the Index includes a reference for each name.

A product container may show a generic name, a brand name or both. If the container has no name, ask the pharmacist or health-store attendant for the name.

2–Available from natural sources?

3–Available from synthetic sources?

Many vitamins, minerals and supplements are advertised as

"natural," implying the product is derived from natural sources as opposed to synthetic sources. By definition, minerals are basic chemical substances that can't be manufactured (or synthesized) from other substances. However, many vitamins and supplements are derived from both natural and synthetic sources.

This is confusing to many consumers. Many manufacturers have done everything possible to take financial advantage of that confusion. Advertisers claim natural sources are good and synthetic sources are bad. The truth is, natural and synthetic versions of the same chemical are identical!

Don't pay extra money for *natural* vitamins or supplements. They all have the same effect on your body. The *synthetic* version may be even purer or less contaminated with extraneous materials such as insecticides and fertilizers.

4–Prescription required?

Most vitamins, minerals and supplements are available without prescription. Some formulas with higher dosages to treat specific diseases require a prescription from your doctor. "Yes" means your doctor must prescribe. "No" means you can buy this product without prescription. "Yes, for some" means that certain dosages or forms (such as an injection) require a prescription while others do not.

The information about a generic product is the same, whether it requires a prescription or not. If the generic ingredients are the same, nonprescription products have the same uses, dangers, warnings, precautions, side effects and interactions with other substances that prescription products do.

5–Fat-soluble or water-soluble?

This line applies *only* to vitamins. Fat-soluble vitamins can accumulate in the body and might cause toxic effects in excessive doses, either in a single day or in small, periodic excesses over a long time. Water-soluble vitamins do not accumulate to any great extent in the body. Except under unusual circumstances, the body readily eliminates excess water-soluble accumulation. The dangers of water-soluble vitamins generally depend on the effects of excessive dosages taken over a relatively short period.

6–RDA/DRI and Optimal Intake

This line points you to the page where you'll find information about the substance's Recommended Dietary Allowance (RDA), Dietary Reference Intake (DRI), and Optimal Intake whenever this information is available. Not all substances will have this information for a few possible reasons: Some substances are still under study;

Guide to Vitamin, Mineral and Acid Charts

To find information about a specific vitamin, mineral, or acid, look in the easy-to-read charts starting on page 28. Charts like the sample shown below and on the opposite page appear alphabetically by generic name.

38   BIOTIN

1 —— Biotin (Vitamin H)

Basic Information
2 —— • Available from natural sources? Yes
3 —— • Available from synthetic sources? No
4 —— • Prescription required? No
5 —— • Water-soluble
6 —— • *RDA/DRI and Optimal Intake*, see page XXX

Natural Sources
7 ——

Almonds	Liver
Bananas	Mackerel
Brewer's yeast	Meats
Brown rice	Milk
Bulgur wheat	Mushrooms
Butter	Oat bran
Calf liver	Oatmeal
Cashew nuts	Peanut butter
Cheese	Peanuts
Chicken	Salmon
Clams	Soybeans
Eggs, cooked	Split peas
Green peas	Tuna
Lentils	Walnuts

Benefits
8 ——
• Aids formation of fatty acids
• Facilitates metabolism of amino acids and carbohydrates
• Promotes normal health of sweat glands, nerve tissue, bone marrow, male sex glands, blood cells, skin, hair
• Minimizes symptoms of zinc deficiency

Possible Additional Benefits
9 ——
• May alleviate muscle pain
• May alleviate depression

Who May Benefit from Additional Amounts? **10**

People who consume huge quantities of raw eggs, which contain a compound (avidin) that inhibits biotin. (Cooking eggs destroys this compound and eliminates the problem.)

Deficiency Symptoms **11**

Note: Deficiency is extremely rare.

Babies:
• Dry scaling on scalp and face

Adults:
• Fatigue
• Depression
• Nausea
• Loss of appetite
• Loss of muscular reflexes
• Smooth, pale tongue
• Hair loss
• Increased blood-cholesterol levels
• Anemia
• Conjunctivitis
• Liver enlargement

Usage Information

What this vitamin does: **12**
Biotin is necessary for normal growth, development and health.

Miscellaneous information: **13**
Intestinal bacteria produce all the biotin the body needs, so there is no substantial evidence that normal, healthy adults need dietary supplements of biotin.

14— **Available as:**
- Tablets or capsules: Swallow whole with a full glass of liquid. Don't chew or crush.Take with food or immediately after eating to decrease stomach irritation.
- Biotin is a constituent of many multivitamin/mineral preparations.

STOP Warnings and Precautions

15— **Don't take if you:**
No problems are expected.

16— **Consult your doctor if you:**
No problems are expected.

17— **Over 55:**
No problems are expected.

18— **Pregnancy:**
- No problems are expected.
- Don't take doses greater than DRI.

19— **Breastfeeding:**
- No problems are expected.
- Don't take doses greater than DRI.

20— **Effect on lab tests:**
No expected effects.

21— **Storage:**
- Store in a cool, dry place away from direct light, but don't freeze.
- Store safely out of reach of children.
- Don't store in bathroom medicine cabinet. Heat and moisture may change the action of the vitamin.

Overdose/Toxicity

22— **Signs and symptoms:**
Supplements in amounts suggested by manufacturers on the label are nontoxic.

What to do: ————————**23**
For accidental overdose (such as child taking entire bottle): Dial 911 (emergency), 0 for operator or call your nearest Poison Control Center.

Adverse Reactions or Side Effects ——**24**
None are expected if taken within DRI dosage levels.

Interaction with Medicine, Vitamins or Minerals ——**25**

Interacts with	Combined effect
Long term antibiotics (broad spectrum)	Destroys "friendly" bacteria in intestines that produce biotin. This can lead to significant biotin deficiency.
Sulfonamides	Destroys "friendly" bacteria in intestines that produce biotin. This can lead to significant biotin deficiency.

Interaction with Other Substances ——**26**
Tobacco decreases absorption. Smokers may require supplemental biotin.

Alcohol decreases absorption.

Foods:
Eating large quantities of raw egg whites may cause biotin deficiency. Egg whites contain avidin, which prevents biotin from being absorbed into the body.

Lab Tests to Detect Deficiency ——**27**
None are available, except for experimental purposes.

VITAMINS

some substances are abundantly available in food, so deficiency and excess are rare to non-existent and no guidelines are necessary; some substances are so rare, no guidelines have been established.

7–Natural Sources

This section lists the food and beverage sources from which vitamins, minerals and acids may be obtained. They are listed alphabetically, not in order of the richest sources of the substance. If you want more information about natural sources, many reference works are available at your local library.

8–Benefits

This section consists of *proved benefits,* including body functions the substance maintains or improves. It also lists disease processes and malfunctions the substance cures or improves. These proved benefits have withstood the scrutiny of scientifically controlled studies with results published in medical literature. This medical literature is subjected to review by top authorities in many fields before the material can be published in respected scientific journals.

9–Possible Additional Benefits

Some authors and many newspaper, magazine and television advertisers make unjustified, sometimes outrageous, claims for products. This list contains claims that have *not* withstood the same

scientific scrutiny the *Benefits* section has passed. These claims may be as accurate and as effective as the proven claims, but they haven't been proved with well-controlled studies. Such studies can take years to complete and may be very expensive. Until such studies have been completed, the claims must be listed as possible additional benefits. Do not self-medicate based on these unproven benefits!

10–Who May Benefit from Additional Amounts?

People listed in this category are most likely to need significant care to regain or maintain normal health or are less likely to meet their requirements through diet alone. A summary of groups follows, with a list of reasons why the risk is greater.

Anyone with inadequate dietary intake or increased nutritional needs—Included in this group are people whose energy needs are less than 1,200 calories a day. Fewer than 1,200 calories a day for energy requirements almost never provides enough vitamins and minerals, so supplements are needed. Those most likely to have inadequate dietary intake include

- People of small stature or build who eat only minimal nutrients per day to maintain current weight
- Elderly people with greatly decreased daily activities, particularly aging women

- People who have had limbs amputated
- People with reduced physical activity because of activity-limiting disease, such as coronary-artery disease, intermittent lameness, angina pectoris
- Fad dieters with a dietary imbalance and inadequacy
- People with eating disorders such as anorexia nervosa or bulimia
- Vegetarians

People over 55—People in this age group may have inadequate dietary intake because of difficulty obtaining an adequate diet, or because of disability and depression.

Pregnancy—Pregnant women uniformly need supplementation of folic acid and iron. Sometimes they need other supplements as well. Pregnant women need to increase dietary intake so total body weight increases from 12 to 30 pounds during pregnancy. Many women do not consume enough calories to allow this weight gain and therefore develop a nutritional deficiency. This causes a need for supplementation with a well-rounded, well-balanced preparation containing vitamins and minerals in addition to separate supplementation of folic acid and iron.

Ask your doctor to recommend specific brand names of acceptable multivitamin/mineral preparations. Also seek advice about folic acid and iron.

Breastfeeding women—Breastfeeding women who are healthy and active may need to continue supplementation, especially iron. Consult your doctor.

Most authorities suggest that iron and folic-acid supplements for pregnant and breastfeeding women should be taken as separate products. Iron occasionally causes gastrointestinal side effects that are so uncomfortable to some women that they discontinue the supplements.

Another important nutritional factor with breastfeeding is the need for extra fluids. Fluid deficiency can be as disabling as a nutritional deficiency. Drink at least eight 8-ounce glasses of water a day.

People who abuse alcohol and other drugs—People who consume too much alcohol are likely to develop nutritional deficiencies. Much of the daily caloric intake of these people is the alcohol they consume, which is deficient in nutritional substances. In addition, alcohol abusers have poor food absorption and increased excretion of nutrients because of diarrhea and fluid loss. When the excessive alcohol consumption stops, the nutritional deficiency can be treated with good food and supplements for a while, if liver disease has not already occurred.

Abuse of other drugs frequently leads to decreased appetite and decreased interest in food. Addicts need supplements of both vitamins and minerals.

People with a chronic wasting illness—This group includes people with malignant disease, chronic malabsorption, hyperthyroidism, chronic obstructive pulmonary disease, congestive heart failure, cystic fibrosis and other illnesses. Nutritional risk is increased because these people have greatly increased caloric and nutritional requirements that are difficult to satisfy with food.

People who have recently undergone surgery—Surgery can cause a relative deficiency, even if a person is well nourished before surgery. People who have undergone surgery on the gastrointestinal tract are particularly likely to develop deficiencies during the post-operative period. Supplementation is very helpful. Vitamins and minerals are frequently administered intravenously until the patient can eat. After that, most people benefit from vitamin and mineral supplements for several weeks after the operation.

People with a portion of the gastrointestinal tract removed—These people are likely to develop deficiencies because important nutrient-absorbing parts of the gastrointestinal tract may be absent from the body. A good multivitamin/mineral preparation usually prevents signs and symptoms of deficiencies. People who have had a significant portion of the stomach removed must take Vitamin B-12 supplements for life (usually by injection).

People who must take medicines—Many medications can cause a deficiency of vitamins and minerals. Specific drugs are listed in the *Interaction with*

Medicine, Vitamins or Minerals section of each chart. For example, laxatives, antacids, medicines to treat epilepsy, and oral contraceptives are a few of the medications that can cause a special need for supplementation of certain vitamins and minerals.

People with recent severe burns or injuries—The nutritional requirements for these people is greatly increased. Adequate supplementation can speed healing and recovery. Ask your doctor for specific advice.

11—Deficiency Symptoms

This section contains a list of proven symptoms of deficiency that have withstood the scrutiny of scientifically controlled studies with results published in medical literature.

12—What this substance does

This section includes a brief discussion of the part each substance plays in chemical reactions or combinations that affect growth, development and health maintenance.

13—Miscellaneous information

Information in this section doesn't fit readily into other information blocks on the charts. For example:

✌ Cooking tips to preserve the substance during food preparation ᴥ Time lapse before changes can be expected

ᴥ Information of special interest

If no miscellaneous information exists for a particular substance, this section will be missing.

14–Available as

Vitamins, minerals and acids are often available in different forms. These include injections, tablets, powders, capsules, and other oral forms.

15–Don't take if you

This section lists circumstances when use of this vitamin, mineral or acid may not be safe. In formal medical literature, these circumstances are called *absolute contraindications.*

16–Consult your doctor if you

This section lists conditions under which a vitamin, mineral or acid should be used with caution. In formal medical literature, these circumstances are frequently listed as *relative contraindications.* Using this product under these circumstances may require special consideration on your part and your doctor's. The guiding rule: *The potential benefit must outweigh the possible risk!*

17–Over 55

As a person ages, physical changes occur that require special consideration when using vitamins, minerals and acids. Liver and kidney function usually decreases, metabolism slows and other changes take place. These are expected and must be considered.

Most chemical substances introduced into the body are metabolized or excreted at a rate that depends on kidney and liver functions. In the aging population, smaller doses or longer intervals between doses may be necessary to prevent an unhealthy concentration of vitamins, minerals or acids. These principles are exactly the same for therapeutic medicines and drugs. Toxic effects, severe side effects and adverse reactions occur more frequently and may cause more serious problems in this age group.

18–Pregnancy

Pregnancy creates an increased need for optimal nutrition, which may be difficult to maintain without using some supplemental vitamins and minerals. What you take depends on your age, your present state of nutrition, your state of health and other factors. Work with your doctor to determine what supplements you will need and how much. Don't take any substance without consulting your doctor first!

19–Breastfeeding

Lactating mothers require sound nutrition. Follow your doctor's recommendations about diet, vitamins and minerals during this time. Don't be reluctant to ask questions and challenge your doctor regarding these important topics. But don't take any substance without consulting your doctor first!

20–Effect on lab tests

This section lists lab studies that may be affected when you take vitamins, minerals or supplements. Possible effects include causing a false-positive or false-negative test, resulting in a low result or high result when your actual physical state is the opposite. In general, some tests can be performed accurately only after discontinuing vitamins, minerals or acids for a few days before the test is scheduled.

21–Storage

This section discusses how and where to store vitamins, minerals and acids, with an important reminder: Always store safely away from children!

21–Others

Special warnings and precautions appear here if they don't fit in any other specific information block. This section may contain information about the best time to take the substance, instructions about mixing or diluting, or anything else that is important about this substance. If no additional warnings or precautions exist for a particular substance, this section will be missing, as it is in the sample chart.

22–Signs and symptoms

Symptoms listed here are the ones most likely to develop with toxicity or accidental or deliberate overdose. An overdosed person may not show all symptoms listed and may experience other symptoms not listed. Sometimes signs and symptoms are identical with ones listed as side effects or adverse reactions. The difference is intensity and severity. You must be the judge. Consult a doctor or poison control center if you are in doubt.

23–What to do

If you suspect an overdose or toxicity, whether symptoms are apparent or not, follow instructions in this section. Expanded instructions for *anaphylaxis*— a severe, life-threatening allergic reaction—appear in the Glossary, page 480.

24–Adverse Reactions or Side Effects

Adverse reactions or side effects are symptoms that may occur when you ingest any substance, whether it is food, medicine, vitamin, mineral, herb or supplement. These are effects on the body other than the desired effect for which you take them.

The term *side effect* may include an expected, perhaps unavoidable, effect of a vitamin, mineral or acid. For example, various forms of niacin may cause dramatic dizziness and flushing of the face and neck in

the blush zone in almost everyone who takes a high enough
dose. These symptoms are
harmless, although sometimes
uncomfortable, and have nothing
to do with the intended use or
therapeutic effect of niacin.

The term *adverse effect* is
more significant. These effects
can cause hazards that outweigh
benefits. The "What to do"
column will tell you what to do
for each effect listed.

25–Interaction with Medicine, Vitamins or Minerals

Vitamins, minerals, supplements,
herbs and various medicines may
interact in your body with other
vitamins, minerals, supplements,
herbs and medicines. It doesn't
matter if they are prescription or
nonprescription, natural or
synthetic. Interactions affect
absorption, elimination or distrib-
ution of the substances that
interact with each other.
Sometimes the interaction is
beneficial, but at other times
deadly. You may not be able to
determine from the chart
whether an interaction is good
or bad. Don't guess! Ask your
doctor or pharmacist—some
interactions can kill!

26–Interaction with Other Substances

This list includes possible interactions with food, beverages,
tobacco, cocaine, alcohol and
other substances you may ingest.

27–Lab Tests to Detect Deficiency

Sometimes clinical features—
medical history, signs and
symptoms as interpreted by a
competent professional—are all
that are required to make an
accurate diagnosis of deficiency.
At other times, although clinical
features may suggest a specific
diagnosis, objective proof by a
specific laboratory test adds
confidence. As much data as can
be collected is desirable before
committing to a prolonged,
sometimes expensive, sometimes
hazardous course of treatment.
When lab tests are readily available and reasonable in cost,
doctors can treat their patients
with greater confidence than is
possible without laboratory
confirmation of the diagnosis.
This sections lists many of
those studies.

Note: Analysis of hair
samples to detect deficiencies of
minerals and trace elements,
while easily available commercially, cannot be regarded as a
valid test. Minerals and trace
elements appear in shampoos,
hair-care products and generally
in the environment. In addition,
when nutrition is poor for any
reason, hair growth actually
slows—causing greater concentration of minerals in the hair.
This greater concentration gives
falsely high values. Hair tests are
entirely without value except for
experimental purposes.

Supplements and Medicinal Herbs

Supplements

Supplements are chemical substances that are neither vitamins nor minerals, but they have received notice as nutritional supplements. Many supplements have proven effects in the body but may not yet have proved safe and effective when taken in pill or capsule form to supplement normal food intake. Speculated benefits and claims frequently go beyond what can be proved at present. These include antiaging properties and claims that substances create and preserve health.

People separate into two distinct groups almost immediately when talk turns to supplementation. On one hand, the traditional medical establishment usually cries, "Eat a well-balanced diet, and you will get all the carbohydrates, fat, fiber, protein, vitamins, minerals and micronutrients you need." But hard data now available about our "normal, well-balanced" diet shows we are overfed and undernourished. The majority of experts in the medical field and in nutrition now agree: We consume too many calories, too much fat, too little fiber, too much refined sugar, too much sodium and not enough unrefined carbohydrates, making it difficult to maximize our health through diet.

On the other hand, some view every new supplement or every new promising piece of information about the existing supplements as a miracle that will cure our ills if the overly conservative medical establishment and the FDA will get out of the way. Advertisers are quite successful with this group because many people are easily persuaded that if they take a product, they will be healthier, live longer and look and feel sexier, slimmer and smarter.

Not much is written that takes a middle ground, even though this position probably represents the true status of human nutrition at present. This book *does* take a middle ground! It does not express any personal opinion—only the consensus of the majority of experts, presented as impartially as possible.

Medicinal Herbs

A popular backlash currently exists against conventional medicine as it is practiced today.

The medical profession has brought some negative feelings upon itself. Part of this backlash takes the form of returning to "natural" medicine—specifically to any of the 2,500 herbs that have been used throughout history for medicinal purposes. People self-prescribe these plant materials and believe they are saving time and money by not consulting their physician. Because medicinal herbs are natural and generally unregulated, many people believe they are without hazards. This is not true!

For centuries, people have collected herbs to use for medicinal purposes. Although some are experienced in their use, most of the uses for herbs are based on anecdotal experience rather than scientific study. Some of the most useful medicines, such as digitalis, rauwolfia (used for mental illness and hypertension), cromlyn (used for preventing asthma attacks) and curare (a muscle relaxant), have all come from herbal "folk remedies." Herbs are a potentially invaluable treatment for many ills but will need to undergo standardized scientific study before they are generally accepted for clinical use.

Many medicinal herbs have pharmacological properties that we know are useful. But at the same time they may be harmful or toxic. Medicinal herbs are available in many forms, but most have not been scrutinized for safety and effectiveness by the Food and Drug Administration. It is also important to point out that the most experienced prescribers of herbs are trained Traditional Chinese Medicine (TCM) practitioners who seldom prescribe a single herb but instead claim therapeutic benefits based on herbal combinations.

People have turned to medicinal herbs, believing they are "natural," safe, effective and wonderful. However, experience has taught us any effective medicine can also have uncomfortable side effects, adverse reactions and dangerous potential toxicity, just as many pharmaceuticals do.

Active ingredients of medicinal herbs vary greatly, whether you personally collect plant drugs or buy them. Variable factors include

- Conditions under which the plant was grown (soil conditions, temperature, season)
- Degree of maturity of the plant when it was collected
- Type of drying process
- Type and duration of storage

In conventional medicine, these variables are controlled by manufacturing procedures or government tests or assays to standardize the amount of the active principle and therefore the predictable safety and effectiveness of the material. None of these safeguards currently exist for medicinal herbs except on a voluntary, manufacturer-specific basis.

The Placebo

The *placebo effect* has long been held as an advantage of using medicinal herbs. Many scientists and researchers claim most herbs do not really help people. It is the placebo effect of using these herbs that really heals. The word *placebo* comes from a Latin predecessor meaning "to please" or "to serve." Under a strict interpretation of the term as it is now used, a placebo medication has no pharmacologically or biologically active ingredients. Another interpretation asserts that small amounts could not affect the body, but large amounts of the same substance may.

For centuries, healers have helped people who were ill, no matter what the illness. Many ancient healers used remedies that have no pharmacological effects in the body. But these remedies were not always useless. They frequently proved to be very effective.

Modern studies conclusively prove all remedies help relieve symptoms in some people. In the early 1900s, many patients and physicians believed placebo therapy was quackery. Today, we know this to be untrue. Placebos *can* mimic the effect of almost any active drug. Placebo effects are real and can be a powerful adjuvant to conventional treatments.

How does the placebo effect work? We don't know for certain, but there are different theories. Endorphins—chemicals normally present in the brain—can be activated by exercise, stress, mental exercises and imaging. Once endorphins have been activated, they kill pain the same way narcotics kill pain. Placebo treatment can trigger the production of hormones in the body, such as cortisone and adrenaline. This can affect the way we behave, the way we feel, the way we think. If the placebo can cause production of these chemicals, this may relieve symptoms of many disorders.

Harder to explain is the part that "power of suggestion" may play in the effectiveness of any remedy, whether it is a powerful drug, a supplement, an herb or a placebo. The gentle touch of the healer, the taste and smell of the product, the packaging, the cost—all are factors that have been studied and found to play a part in the placebo effect.

Understanding Common Terms

When you read about medicinal herbs, you will run across the following common terms. They refer to ways in which medicinal herbs can be useful.

Compress—Cloth is soaked in a cool liquid form of an herb, wrung out and applied directly to skin.

Decoction—The herb is boiled 10 to 15 minutes, then allowed to steep.

Extract—A solution resulting from soaking the herb in cold water for 24 hours.

Fomentation—Cloth is soaked in a hot liquid form of an herb, wrung out and applied directly to skin.

Infusion—Tea is prepared by steeping herb in hot water. Infusions can be made from any part of a plant.

Ointment—The powdered form of an herb is mixed with any soft-based salve, such as lanolin, wax or lard.

Poultice—The herb applied to a moistened cloth, then applied directly to skin.

Powder—The useful part of the herb is ground into a powder.

Syrup—The herb is added to brown sugar dissolved in boiling water, then boiled and strained.

Tincture—The powdered herb is added to a 50/50 solution of alcohol and water.

Points to Remember

Precautions apply to all herbal medications. Read the checklist on page 25. Also keep the following in mind:

- Children under age 2 should *not* be given herbal medications.
- Pregnant and lactating women should avoid herbal medicines because of potential damage to the fetus or breastfeeding child.
- Collecting medicinal herbs for yourself is unwise, unless you have received a great deal of training. Correctly identifying plants and knowing how to select, preserve and use them

properly requires a great deal of knowledge and judgment.

The medicinal-herb section of the book, starting on page 185, contains profiles of many of the herbs most generally available and most frequently used in the United States and Canada as well as a number of less common herbs. Some herbs that have been used historically are less commonly used today. In this book, herbs are divided into two sections: "Common Herbs" and "Less Common Herbs."

Labeling

Currently, supplements are regulated under the Dietary Supplement Act of 1994. This act states that supplement labels can only display information related to the structure and function of the supplement and not directly link it to prevention or treatment of disease. The burden of proving false claims or harm remains with the FDA.

In 1998, the FDA Modernization Act of 1997 took effect. According to this law, manufacturers are now permitted to use claims if such claims are based on current, published, authoritative statements from the National Institutes of Health (NIH), Center for Disease Control and Prevention (CDC), the Surgeon General, the Food and Safety Inspection Service and the Agricultural Research Service within the Department of Agriculture.

Guide to Supplement and Medicinal-Herb Charts

The food supplement and medicinal-herb information in this book is organized into condensed, easy-to-read charts. Each supplement and medicinal herb is described on a 1- to 2-page chart, as shown in the sample chart opposite. Charts are arranged alphabetically by the most common name. If you cannot find a name, look for alternate names in the Index or ask your health-product or herbal-medication retailer for alternate names.

Supplement charts and medicinal-herb charts are organized in a similar way. However, not all supplement charts will contain "Biological name" or "Parts used for medicinal purposes" for obvious reasons.

A–Popular name

Each chart is titled by the most popular name. When there is more than one popular name, alternate names are shown in parentheses. If an herb or supplement has several possible names, you'll find the least common listed under *Basic Information.* The Index contains a reference to each name listed. Popular names may vary in different parts of the world.

B–Biological name (genus and species)

This section identifies the medicinal herb by genus and species. These Latin names are commonly used by biologists and plant scientists. They are included to help you make a positive identification. Note: some herbs have more than one biological name and some include so many species, just the genus is listed. The food-supplement charts do not include this information.

C–Parts used for medicinal purposes

Here you'll find what parts of the herb are used to supply the expected effects. Roots, leaves, bark and flowers are commonly used portions of the plant. Sometimes the entire plant is used. Note: The food-supplement charts do not include this information.

D–Chemicals this herb contains

Chemicals and family names of chemically related groups are listed in this section. Chemically related groups include saponins, tannins, volatile oils and others.

Guide to Supplement and Medicinal-Herb Charts

Astragalus   187

A—— Astragalus (Huang-qi, Milk Vetch)

Basic Information

B—— Biological name (genus and species):
Astragalus membranaceous

C—— Parts used for medicinal purposes:
Root

D—— Chemicals this herb contains:
- Asparagine
- Astragalosides
- Calcyosin
- Formononetin
- Kumatakenin
- Sterols

E—— Known Effects
- Stimulates and protects the immune system
- Produces spontaneous sweating

F—— **Miscellaneous information:**
Available as tea, fluid extract, capsules and dried root.

G—— Possible Additional Effects
- May reduce fatigue/weakness
- Potential cold and flu treatment
- May increase stamina
- Potential treatment for immune-deficiency problems (AIDS, cancer)
- May reduce symptoms of chronic fatigue syndrome
- May improve appetite
- May alleviate diarrhea

Warnings and Precautions

H—— **Don't take if you are:**
- Pregnant, think you may be pregnant or plan pregnancy in the near future

Consult your doctor if you: ——————**I**
- Take this herb for any medical problem that doesn't improve in 2 weeks (There may be safer, more effective treatments.)
- Take any medicinal drugs or herbs including aspirin, laxatives, cold and cough remedies, antacids, vitamins, minerals, amino acids, supplements, other prescription or nonprescription drugs

Pregnancy: ————————**J**
Use only on the advice of your physician.

Breastfeeding: ————————**K**
Use only on the advice of your physician.

Infants and children: ————**L**
Treating infants and children under 2 with any herbal preparation is hazardous.

Others: ————————**M**
None.

Storage: ————————**N**
- Store in cool, dry area away from direct light, but don't freeze.
- Store safely out of reach of children.
- Don't store in bathroom medicine cabinet. Heat and moisture may change the action of the herb.

Safe dosage: ————————**O**
Consult your doctor for the appropriate dose for your condition.

Toxicity ————————**P**
Comparative-toxicity rating is not available from standard references.

Adverse Reactions, Side Effects or ————**Q** Overdose Symptoms
None are expected.

E–Known Effects

This section lists identified chemical actions of the medicinal herb or supplement being discussed. These effects have been identified and validated by scientists and researchers through various studies. Some effects may be beneficial; others are harmful.

F–Miscellaneous information

This section contains information that doesn't fit into other information blocks on the chart. If no additional information exists, this section will be missing.

G–Possible Additional Effects

This list contains symptoms or medical problems this drug has been *reported* to treat or improve. These claims may be accurate, but they haven't been proved with well-controlled studies.

H–Don't take if you

Here you'll find circumstances under which the use of this herb or supplement may not be safe. In formal medical literature, these circumstances are listed as *absolute contraindications.*

I–Consult your doctor if you

This section lists conditions in which this herb or supplement should be used with caution. In formal medical literature, these circumstances are called *relative contraindications.* Using an herb or supplement under these circumstances may require special consideration by you and your doctor. The guiding rule: *The potential benefit must outweigh the possible risk!*

J–Pregnancy

As more is learned about effective medications, including herbal medications, the more healthcare workers fear the possible effects of any medicinal product on an unborn child. This fear holds for *all* chemicals that cause changes in the body. That herbal medicines occur naturally does not free them from possibly causing harm. *The best rule to follow is don't take anything during pregnancy if you can avoid it!*

K–Breastfeeding

Although a breastfeeding infant is not as likely to be harmed as an unborn fetus, be cautious. If you take a medicine or an herb during the time you breastfeed, do so *only* under professional supervision.

L–Infants and children

Treating infants and children under 2 years old with any supplement or herbal preparation is hazardous. Dosages, uses and effects of an herb or supplement cannot be gauged easily with a young child. Do not use medicinal herbs or supplements to treat a problem your child may have without first discussing it thoroughly with your doctor.

M–Others

Warnings and precautions appear here if they don't fit into other categories.

N–Storage

This section advises you on how to store supplements and herbs to best preserve them. It also includes a crucial reminder: *Always store any supplement or herb safely away from children!*

O–Safe dosage

Safe dosages of herbs (and many supplements) have not been documented by procedures outlined by the FDA. For these, it is impossible to list a "safe" dosage and have it carry any significance. People who have had experience with herbs are usually qualified to predict safe doses if they know the person's age, medical history and some important facts about his or her current health.

Many reputable distributors of supplements and herb products have recommendations for ranges of safety, but these may vary a great deal from manufacturer to manufacturer, according to age and purity of the product. The most important fact to understand is the more you ingest over a long period of time, the more likely a toxic reaction will occur. Most available herbs and supplements are safe when taken in small doses for short periods of time. Never fall into the trap of thinking "if a little is good, more is better."

This section of the supplement charts also lists the available forms of the substance, even when a safe dosage cannot be recommended. Always follow the manufacturer's instructions and your doctor's advice.

P–Toxicity

This section includes a general, average toxicity rating for each medicinal herb and supplement.

Q–Adverse Reactions, Side Effects or Overdose Symptoms

Adverse reactions or side effects are symptoms that may occur when you ingest any substance, whether it is food, medicine, vitamin, mineral, herb or supplement. These are effects on the body other than the desired effect for which you take them.

The term *adverse effect* means the effects can cause hazards that outweigh benefits.

The term *side effect* may include an expected, perhaps unavoidable, effect of a vitamin, mineral, supplement or medicinal herb. For example, a side effect of horseradish may be nausea. This symptom is harmless although sometimes uncomfortable and has nothing to do with the intended use.

If you suspect an overdose, whether symptoms are present or not, follow instructions in this section.

Warning

Whether you use supplements and medicinal herbs or not is your decision. If you choose to use them, be sure you take them with knowledge and understanding of what they are. Know the supplier, and be sure you know the possible dangers. Consider that self-medication with medicinal herbs or certain supplements may prevent you from receiving better help from more effective medications that have withstood critical scientific investigations.

Checklist for Safer Use of Vitamins, Minerals, Supplements & Medicinal Herbs

The most important caution regarding all vitamins, minerals, supplements and medicinal herbs deals with the amount you take. Despite many popular articles in magazines and newspapers and reports on television, large doses of some of these substances can be hazardous to your health. Don't believe sensational advertisements and take large doses or megadoses. The belief "if a little does good, a lot will do much more" has no place in rational thinking regarding products to protect your health. Stay within safe-dose ranges!

1. Learn all you can about the vitamins, minerals, supplements and medicinal herbs *before* you take them. Information sources include this book, books from your public library, your doctor or your pharmacist.

2. Don't take vitamins, minerals, supplements or medicinal herbs prescribed for someone else, even if your symptoms are the same. At the same time, keep prescription items to yourself. They may be harmful to someone else.

3. Tell your doctor or health-care professional about any symptoms you experience that you suspect may be caused by anything you take.

4. Take vitamins, minerals, supplements and medicinal herbs in good light after you have identified the contents of the container. If you wear glasses, put them on to check and recheck labels.

5. Don't keep medicine by your bedside. You may unknowingly repeat a dose when you are half-asleep or confused.

6. Know the names of all the substances you take.

7. Read labels on medications you take. If the information is incomplete, ask your pharmacist for more details.

8. If the substance is in liquid form, shake it before you take it.

9. Store all vitamins, minerals, supplements and medicinal herbs in cool places away from sunlight and moisture. Bathroom medicine cabinets are usually unacceptable

because they are too warm and humid.

10. If a vitamin, mineral, supplement or medicinal herb requires refrigeration, don't freeze!

11. Obtain a standard measuring spoon from your pharmacy for liquid substances and a graduated dropper to use for liquid preparations for infants and children.

12. Follow manufacturer's or doctor's suggestions regarding diet instructions. Some products work better on a full stomach. Others work best on an empty stomach. Some products work best when you follow a special diet. For example, a low-salt diet enhances effectiveness of any product expected to lower blood pressure.

13. Avoid any substance you know you are allergic to.

14. If you become pregnant while taking any vitamin, mineral, supplement or medicinal herb, tell your physician and discontinue taking it until you have discussed it with him or her. Try to remember the exact dose and the length of time you have taken the substance.

15. Tell any healthcare provider about vitamins, minerals, supplements, medicinal herbs and other substances you take, even if you bought them without a prescription. During an illness or prior to surgery, this information is crucial. Even mention antacids, laxatives, tonics and over-the-counter preparations. Many people believe these products are completely safe and forget to inform doctors, nurses or pharmacists they are using them.

16. Regard all vitamins, minerals, supplements and medicinal herbs as potentially harmful to children. Store them safely away from their reach.

17. Alcohol, marijuana, cocaine, other mood-altering drugs and tobacco can cause life-threatening interactions when mixed with some vitamins, minerals, supplements and medicinal herbs. They can also prevent treatment from being effective or delay your return to good health. Common sense dictates you avoid them, particularly during an illness.

Vitamins

Vitamin is a general term for unrelated organic compounds. Organic compounds all contain the carbon atom. Vitamins occur in small amounts in many foods and are widely dispersed in our food supply.

Vitamins are necessary for normal metabolic functioning of the body. They form a part of enzymes to help complete chemical reactions in the body and are components of hormones. Vitamins may make solutions only in water (water-soluble) or only in fatty liquids (fat-soluble). Without vitamins, life-threatening deficiency diseases can occur, including scurvy from a vitamin-C deficiency, or even pellagra (see Glossary) from a niacin deficiency. Classic deficiency, is rare in the United States due to the abundance of food. Therefore, in recent times, our attention has shifted from treating deficiency to optimizing health through vitamins. Vitamins present in foods are considered *natural* vitamins; those created in a laboratory are considered *synthetic*.

Vitamin A (Beta-carotene, Retinol)

Basic Information

Beta-carotene is a previtamin-A compound found in plants. The body converts beta-carotene to vitamin A.

Retinol comes from animal products such as liver, egg yolk, cheese and milk.

- Available from natural sources? Yes
- Available from synthetic sources? Yes
- Prescription required? No
- Fat-soluble
- *RDA/DRI and Optimal Intake*, see page 476

Natural Sources

Apricots, fresh	Liver
Asparagus	Milk
Broccoli	Mustard greens
Cantaloupe	Pumpkin
Carrots	Spinach
Eggs	Squash, winter
Endive, raw	Sweet potatoes
Kale	Tomatoes
Leaf lettuce	Watermelon

Benefits

- Aids in treatment of some eye disorders, including prevention of night blindness and formation of visual purple in the eye
- Promotes bone growth, teeth development, reproduction
- Helps form and maintain healthy skin, hair, mucous membranes
- Builds body's resistance to respiratory and other infections (including measles in the third world)
- May help treat acne, impetigo, boils, carbuncles and open ulcers when applied externally

Possible Additional Benefits

- May help control glaucoma
- Potential guard against effects of pollution and smog—beta-carotene acts as an antioxidant (see Glossary)
- May speed healing
- Possibly helps remove age spots
- May improve immunity
- May help heal skin lesions, cuts and wounds
- Possible treatment for hyperthyroidism

Who May Benefit from Additional Amounts?

- Anyone with inadequate caloric or nutritional dietary intake or increased nutritional requirements
- Those who abuse alcohol or other drugs
- People with a chronic wasting illness or prolonged fever
- Those under excess stress for long periods
- Anyone who has recently undergone surgery
- People with recent severe burns or injuries
- Malnourished children with impaired immunity

Deficiency Symptoms

- Night blindness
- Lack of tear secretion
- Changes in eyes—eventual blindness if deficiency is severe and untreated
- Susceptibility to infectious diseases, especially respiratory
- Dry, rough skin
- Weight loss
- Poor bone growth
- Weak tooth enamel
- Diarrhea
- Slow growth
- Acne
- Insomnia, fatigue

Usage Information

What this vitamin does:

- Essential for normal function of retina (combines with red pigment of retina—opsin—to form rhodopsin, which is necessary for sight in partial darkness)
- May act as cofactor (see Glossary) in enzyme systems
- Necessary for growth of bone, testicular function, ovarian function, embryonic development, regulation of growth, differentiation of tissues

Miscellaneous information:

- Many months of a vitamin-A-deficient diet are required before symptoms develop. The average person has a 2-year supply of vitamin A stored in the liver.
- Steroids are produced by the adrenal gland and are part of the natural response to stress and immune function. Failure to make these important hormones leaves the immune system in a less-than-ideal state.

Available as:

- Extended-release capsules or tablets: Swallow whole with a full glass of liquid. Don't chew or crush. Take with food or immediately after eating to decrease stomach irritation.
- Oral solution: Dilute in at least 1/2 glass of water or other liquid. Take with or 1 to 1-1/2 hours after meals unless otherwise directed by your doctor.
- Vitamin A is a constituent of many multivitamin/mineral preparations.
- Some forms are available by generic name.

Warnings and Precautions

Don't take if you:

- Are allergic to any preparation containing vitamin A.
- Don't take doses greater than the RDA if you are planning a pregnancy or are pregnant.

Consult your doctor if you have (or are):

- Cystic fibrosis
- Diabetes
- Intestinal disease with diarrhea
- Kidney disease
- Liver disease/liver enlargement
- Overactive thyroid function
- Disease of the pancreas
- Viral hepatitis
- Chronic alcoholism
- Pregnant
- Lactating

Over 55:

- Older people are more likely to be malnourished and need a supplement.
- Dosage must be taken carefully to avoid possible toxicity.

Pregnancy:

- Daily doses of retinol exceeding 5,000IU can produce growth retardation and urinary-tract malformations of the fetus.
- Don't take doses greater than RDA.

VITAMINS

Breastfeeding:
Don't take doses greater than RDA.

Effect on lab tests:
• Chronic vitamin-A toxicity—
  increased blood glucose, blood-urea
  nitrogen, serum calcium, serum
  cholesterol, serum triglycerides
• Poor results on dark-adaptation test
  (see Glossary)
• Poor results on electronystagmogram
  (see Glossary)
• Poor results on electroretinogram
  (see Glossary)

Storage:
• Store in cool, dry place away from
  direct light, but don't freeze.
• Store safely out of reach of children.
• Don't store in bathroom medicine
  cabinet. Heat and moisture may
  change the action of the vitamin.

Others:
• Children are more sensitive to
  vitamin A and are more likely to
  develop toxicity with dosages
  exceeding the RDA.
• Toxicity is slowly reversible on
  withdrawal of vitamin A but may
  persist for several weeks.

Overdose/Toxicity

Signs and symptoms:
Bleeding from gums or sore mouth;
bulging soft spot on head in babies;
sometimes hydrocephaly ("water on
brain"); confusion or unusual excitement; diarrhea; dizziness; double vision;
headache; irritability; dry skin; hair loss;
peeling skin on lips, palms and in
other areas; seizures; vomiting; enlarged
spleen and liver.

Note: Toxicity symptoms usually
appear about 6 hours after ingestion of
overdoses of vitamin A. Symptoms may
also develop gradually if overdose is
milder and over a long period of time.
Overdose does not occur with beta-
carotene, but an excessive amount can
turn skin color to yellow-orange.

What to do:
For symptoms of overdose:
Discontinue vitamin and consult
doctor. Also see *Adverse Reactions or
Side Effects* section below.

For accidental overdose (such as
child taking entire bottle): Dial 911
(emergency), 0 for operator or call
your nearest Poison Control Center.

 Adverse Reactions
or Side Effects

Reaction or effect	What to do
Abdominal pain	Discontinue. Call doctor immediately.
Appetite loss	Discontinue. Call doctor when convenient.
Bone or joint pain	Discontinue. Call doctor immediately.
Discomfort, tiredness or weakness	Discontinue. Call doctor when convenient.
Drying or cracking of skin or lips	Discontinue. Call doctor immediately.
Fever	Discontinue. Call doctor immediately.
Hair loss	Discontinue. Call doctor immediately.
Headache	Discontinue. Call doctor when convenient.
Increase in frequency of urination	Discontinue. Call doctor when convenient.
Increased sensitivity of skin to sunlight	Discontinue. Call doctor when convenient.
Irritability	Discontinue. Call doctor when convenient.
Vomiting	Discontinue. Call doctor immediately.
Yellow-orange patches on soles of feet, palms of hands or skin around nose and lips	Consult doctor. Common with beta-carotene supplementation.

Interaction with Medicine, Vitamins or Minerals

Interacts with	Combined effect
Antacids	Decreases absorption of vitamin A and fat-soluble vitamins D, E and K.
Calcium supplements	Excessive vitamin A may decrease effect of calcium supplementation.
Cholestyramine, colestipol	Decreases absorption of vitamin A.
Mineral oil, neomycin	Decreases absorption of vitamin A.
Olestra-fat substitute	Decreases vitamin-A and beta-carotene absorption.
Oral contraceptives	Increases vitamin-A concentrations.
Retin-A	Used for acne treatment. Retin-A is a vitamin-A analog (see Glossary) and is contraindicated (see Glossary) during pregnancy and lactation.
Vitamin E	Normal amount facilitates absorption, storage in liver and utilization of vitamin A. Excessive dosage may deplete vitamin-A stores in liver. Long-term excess intake of beta-carotene can reduce vitamin-E levels.

Interaction with Other Substances

Tobacco decreases absorption. Smokers may need supplementary vitamin A.

Alcohol abuse interferes with the body's ability to transport and use vitamin A.

Lab Tests to Detect Deficiency

Many months of deficiency are required before lab studies reflect a deficiency.

• Plasma vitamin A and plasma carotene
• Dark-adaptation test
• Electronystagmogram
• Electroretinogram

VITAMINS

Ascorbic Acid (Vitamin C)

Basic Information

• Available from natural sources? Yes
• Available from synthetic sources? Yes
• Prescription required? No
• Water-soluble
• *RDA/DRI and Optimal Intake,* see page 476

Natural Sources

Black currants	Orange juice
Broccoli	Oranges
Brussels sprouts	Papayas
Cabbage	Peppers, sweet and hot
Collards	Potatoes
Grapefruit	Rose hips
Green peppers	Spinach
Guava	Strawberries
Kale	Tangerines
Lemons	Tomatoes
Mangos	Watercress ➜

Benefits

- Promotes healthy capillaries, gums, teeth
- Aids iron absorption
- Helps heal wounds, burns and broken bones
- Prevents and treats scurvy
- Part of treatment for anemia, especially for iron-deficiency anemia
- Part of treatment for urinary-tract infections
- Helps form collagen in connective tissue
- Increases calcium absorption
- Contributes to hemoglobin and red-blood-cell production in bone marrow
- Blocks production of nitrosamines which are thought to be carcinogenic
- Aids adrenal gland function
- Reduces free-radical production

Possible Additional Benefits

- May prevent or reduce symptoms of the common cold and other infections
- May prevent some forms of cancer
- May reduce cholesterol
- Potential protection against heart disease
- Possible blood clot prevention
- May prevent allergies
- May reduce symptoms of arthritis, skin ulcers, allergic reactions
- Possible relief of herpes infections of eyes and genitals
- May prevent periodontal disease
- May reduce toxic effect of alcohol and drugs
- May promote healing of bed sores
- May retard aging
- May improve male fertility

Who May Benefit from Additional Amounts?

- Anyone with inadequate caloric or nutritional dietary intake or increased nutritional requirements
- People more than 55 years old
- Those who abuse alcohol, tobacco or other drugs
- People with a chronic wasting illness, AIDS, acute illness with fever, hyperthyroidism, tuberculosis, cold exposure
- Those under excess stress for long periods
- Anyone who has recently undergone surgery
- Those with a portion of the gastrointestinal tract surgically removed
- People with recent severe burns or injuries
- Those receiving kidney dialysis
- Those who work in a toxic environment
- Anyone with the onset of symptoms of infection

Deficiency Symptoms

- Scurvy: muscle weakness, swollen gums, loss of teeth, tiredness, depression, bleeding under skin, bleeding gums
- Easy bruising
- Swollen or painful joints
- Nosebleeds
- Anemia: weakness, tiredness, paleness
- Frequent infections
- Slow healing of wounds

Usage Information

What this vitamin does:
- Necessary for collagen formation and tissue repair

- Participates in oxidation-reduction reactions (see Glossary)
- Needed for metabolism of phenylalanine, tyrosine, folic acid, iron
- Aids utilization of carbohydrates, synthesis of fats and proteins, preservation of integrity of blood-vessel walls
- Strengthens blood vessels

Miscellaneous information:

Food preparation tips to conserve vitamin C:

- Eat food raw or minimally cooked.
- Shorten cooking time.
- Microwave or steam vegetables in very small amounts of water.
- Avoid leaving food at room temperature for prolonged period.
- Avoid overexposure of food to air and light.

Available as:

- Tablets: Swallow whole with a full glass of liquid. Don't chew or crush. Take with or 1 to 1-1/2 hours after meals unless otherwise directed by your doctor.
- Extended-release capsules or tablets: Swallow whole with a full glass of liquid. Don't chew or crush. Take with food or immediately after eating to decrease stomach irritation.
- Chewable tablets: Chew well before swallowing.
- Effervescent tablets: Allow to dissolve completely in liquid before swallowing.
- Oral solution: Dilute in at least 1/2 glass of water or other liquid. Take with or 1 to 1-1/2 hours after meals unless otherwise directed by your doctor.
- Injectable forms are administered by a doctor or nurse.
- Vitamin C is a constituent of many multivitamin/mineral preparations.

 Warnings and Precautions

Don't take if you:

Are allergic to vitamin C.

Consult your doctor if you have:

- Gout
- Kidney stones
- Sickle-cell anemia
- Iron storage disease

Over 55:

- Needs may be greater because dietary intake tends to be lower.
- Side effects are more likely.

Pregnancy:

- Take prenatal vitamins with vitamin C because of the demands made by bone development, teeth and connective-tissue formation of fetus.
- If mother takes megadoses, newborn may develop deficiency symptoms after birth.
- Don't take doses greater than RDA.

Breastfeeding:

Continue taking prenatal vitamins to support rapid growth of child.

Effect on lab tests:

With megadoses (10 times recommended RDA):

- Blood in stool—possible false-negative test results with large doses
- LDH and SGOT (See Glossary)
- Glucose in urine—depends on method used
- Serum bilirubin—false low level
- Urinary pH—false low level

Storage:

- Store in a cool, dry place away from direct light, but don't freeze.
- Store safely out of reach of children.
- Don't store in bathroom medicine cabinet. Heat and moisture may change the action of the vitamin.

Others:

Very high doses may cause kidney stones, although reported studies do not confirm this.

VITAMINS

Overdose/Toxicity

Signs and symptoms:

Oral forms: flushed face, headache, increased urination, lower abdominal cramps, mild diarrhea, nausea, vomiting. Injectable forms: dizziness and faintness.

What to do:

For symptoms of overdose:
Discontinue vitamin and consult doctor. Also see *Adverse Reactions or Side Effects* section below.

For accidental overdose (such as child taking entire bottle): Dial 911 (emergency), 0 for operator or call your nearest Poison Control Center.

Adverse Reactions or Side Effects

Reaction or effect	What to do
Anemia	Discontinue. Call doctor immediately.
Flushed face	Discontinue. Call doctor when convenient.
Headache	Discontinue. Call doctor when convenient.
Increased frequency of urination	Discontinue. Call doctor when convenient.
Lower abdominal cramps	Seek emergency treatment.
Mild diarrhea	Decrease dose. Call doctor when convenient.
Nausea or vomiting	Seek emergency treatment.
Rebound scurvy-like symptoms	Call doctor when convenient. If you decide to reduce dose, do so gradually to prevent deficiency symptoms.

Interaction with Medicine, Vitamins or Minerals

Interacts with	Combined effect
Aminosalicylic acid (PAS for tuberculosis)	Increases chance of formation of drug crystals in urine. Large doses of vitamin C must be taken to produce this effect.
Anticholinergics	Decreases anticholinergic effect.
Anticoagulants (oral)	Decreases anticoagulant effect.
Aspirin	Decreases vitamin-C effect.
Barbiturates	Decreases vitamin-C effect. Increases barbiturate effect.
Calcium	Assists in absorption of calcium.
Copper	Decreases absorption of copper. Large doses of vitamin C must be taken to produce this effect.
Iron supplements	Increases iron effect.
Quinidine	Decreases quinidine effect.
Salicylates	Decreases vitamin-C effect.
Sulfa drugs	Decreases vitamin-C effect. May cause kidney stones.
Tetracyclines	Decreases vitamin-C effect.

Interaction with Other Substances

Tobacco decreases absorption. Smokers may require supplemental vitamin C.

Alcohol can be more rapidly broken down in body with large doses of vitamin C.

Lab Tests to Detect Deficiency

• Vitamin-C levels in blood plasma
• Measurement of ascorbic-acid level in white blood cells (expensive and used mostly for experimental purposes)

Vitamin B-12

Basic Information

Vitamin B-12 is also called *cyanocobalamin.*

- Available from natural sources? Yes
- Available from synthetic sources? Yes
- Prescription required? Yes, for high doses and injectable forms
- Water-soluble
- *RDA/DRI and Optimal Intake,* see page 476

Natural Sources

Beef	Liverwurst
Beef liver	Mackerel
Blue cheese	Milk
Clams	Oysters
Dairy products	Sardines
Eggs	Snapper
Flounder	Swiss cheese
Herring	

Note: Vitamin B-12 is not found in plant foods.

Benefits

- Promotes normal growth and development
- Treats some types of nerve damage
- Treats pernicious anemia
- Treats and prevents vitamin B-12 deficiencies in people who have had a portion of the stomach or gastrointestinal tract surgically removed
- Prevents vitamin-B-12 deficiency in vegan vegetarians, persons with absorption diseases and elderly with achlorhydria
- Treats Alzheimer's disease

Possible Additional Benefits

- Potential help to those with nervous disorders
- Possibly improves resistance to infection and disease
- May improve memory and the ability to learn
- May increase energy

Who May Benefit from Additional Amounts?

- Strict vegetarians
- Anyone with inadequate caloric or nutritional dietary intake or increased nutritional requirements
- Those who abuse alcohol or other drugs
- People with a chronic wasting illness, AIDS or chronic fever
- Those under excess stress for long periods
- Anyone who has recently undergone surgery
- Those with a portion of the gastrointestinal tract surgically removed
- People with recent severe burns or injuries
- People with pancreas or bowel malignancy

Deficiency Symptoms

Pernicious anemia, with the following symptoms:

- Fatigue, profound
- Weakness, especially in arms and legs
- Irreversible nerve damage

VITAMINS

➡

- Sore tongue
- Nausea, appetite loss, weight loss
- Numbness and tingling in hands and feet
- Difficulty maintaining balance
- Pale lips, tongue and gums
- Shortness of breath
- Depression
- Confusion and dementia/disorientation
- Poor memory
- Bruising

 Usage Information

What this vitamin does:

- Acts as coenzyme (see Glossary) for normal DNA synthesis (see Glossary)
- Promotes normal fat and carbohydrate metabolism and protein syntheses
- Promotes growth, cell development, blood-cell development, manufacture of nerve cell covering, maintenance of normal nervous system function

Miscellaneous information:

There is a very low incidence of vitamin-B-12 toxicity, even with large amounts up to 1,000mcg/day.

Available as:

- Oral and injectable forms: Oral forms are used only as a diet supplement. Only people with portions of the gastrointestinal tract surgically removed or those with pernicious anemia require injections.
- Tablets: Swallow whole with a full glass of liquid. Don't chew or crush. Take with or 1 to 1-1/2 hours after meals unless otherwise directed by your doctor.
- Extended-release capsules or tablets: Swallow whole with a full glass of liquid. Don't chew or crush. Take with food or immediately after eating to decrease stomach irritation.
- Injectable forms are administered by a doctor or nurse.

- Vitamin B-12 is a constituent of many multivitamin/mineral preparations.

 Warnings and Precautions

Don't take if you:

- Are allergic to B-12 given by injection (Allergy to injections produces itching, redness, swelling and, rarely, a blood-pressure drop with loss of consciousness.)
- Have Leber's disease

Consult your doctor if you have:

Anemia of unknown etiology (see Glossary). Folate supplementation can mask B-12 deficiency.

Over 55:

Absorption decreases in elderly with achlorhydria (decrease in hydrochloric acid in stomach).

Pregnancy:

- No problems are expected.
- Don't take doses greater than DRI.

Breastfeeding:

- No problems are expected.
- Don't take doses greater than DRI.

Effect on lab tests:

Tests for serum potassium may show precipitous drop (hypokalemia) within 48 hours after beginning treatment for anemia.

Storage:

- Store in a cool, dry place away from direct light, but don't freeze. Liquid forms should be refrigerated.
- Store safely out of reach of children.
- Don't store in bathroom medicine cabinet. Heat and moisture may change the action of the vitamin.

Others:

The injectable form is the only effective form to treat pernicious anemia or people with portions of the gastrointestinal tract surgically removed. These individuals do not absorb oral forms.

Overdose/Toxicity

Signs and symptoms:
If taken with large doses of vitamin C, vitamin B-12 may cause nosebleed, ear bleeding or dry mouth.

What to do:
For symptoms of overdose:
Discontinue vitamin and consult doctor. Also see *Adverse Reactions or Side Effects* section below.

For accidental overdose: (such as child taking entire bottle): Dial 911 (emergency), 0 for operator or call your nearest Poison Control Center.

Adverse Reactions or Side Effects

Reaction or effect	What to do
Diarrhea (rare)	Discontinue. Call doctor immediately.
Itching skin after injections (rare)	Seek emergency treatment.

Interaction with Medicine, Vitamins or Minerals

Interacts with	Combined effect
Aminosalicylates	Reduces absorption of vitamin B-12.
Antibiotics	May cause false low test results for vitamin B-12.

Chloramphenicol	May prevent therapeutic response when vitamin B-12 is used to treat anemia.
Cholestyramine	Reduces absorption of vitamin B-12.
Colchicine	Reduces absorption of vitamin B-12.
Epoetin	Reduces absorption of vitamin B-12.
Folic acid	Large doses mask deficiency of vitamin B-12.
Neomycin (oral forms)	Reduces absorption of vitamin B-12.
Potassium (extended-release forms)	Reduces absorption of vitamin B-12. May increase need for vitamin B-12.

Interaction with Other Substances

Tobacco decreases absorption. Smokers may require supplemental vitamin B-12.

Alcohol in excessive amounts for long periods may lead to vitamin B-12 deficiency.

Lab Tests to Detect Deficiency

• Serum vitamin B-12, a radioactive study usually performed with serum-folic-acid test, called the *Schilling test*
• Reticulocyte count

VITAMINS

Biotin (Vitamin H)

Basic Information

- Available from natural sources? Yes
- Available from synthetic sources? No
- Prescription required? No
- Water-soluble
- *RDA/DRI and Optimal Intake,* see page 476

Natural Sources

Almonds	Liver
Bananas	Mackerel
Brewer's yeast	Meats
Brown rice	Milk
Bulgur wheat	Mushrooms
Butter	Oat bran
Calf liver	Oatmeal
Cashew nuts	Peanut butter
Cheese	Peanuts
Chicken	Salmon
Clams	Soybeans
Eggs, cooked	Split peas
Green peas	Tuna
Lentils	Walnuts

Benefits

- Aids formation of fatty acids
- Facilitates metabolism of amino acids and carbohydrates
- Promotes normal health of sweat glands, nerve tissue, bone marrow, male sex glands, blood cells, skin, hair
- Minimizes symptoms of zinc deficiency

Possible Additional Benefits

- May alleviate muscle pain
- May alleviate depression

Who May Benefit from Additional Amounts?

People who consume huge quantities of raw eggs, which contain a compound (avidin) that inhibits biotin. (Cooking eggs destroys this compound and eliminates the problem.)

Deficiency Symptoms

Note: Deficiency is extremely rare.

Babies:
Dry scaling on scalp and face

Adults:
- Fatigue
- Depression
- Nausea
- Loss of appetite
- Loss of muscular reflexes
- Smooth, pale tongue
- Hair loss
- Increased blood-cholesterol levels
- Anemia
- Conjunctivitis
- Liver enlargement

Usage Information

What this vitamin does:
Biotin is necessary for normal growth, development and health.

Miscellaneous information:
Intestinal bacteria produce all the biotin the body needs, so there is no substantial evidence that normal, healthy adults need dietary supplements of biotin.

Available as:
- Tablets or capsules: Swallow whole with a full glass of liquid. Don't chew or crush. Take with food or immediately after eating to decrease stomach irritation.
- Biotin is a constituent of many multivitamin/mineral preparations.

 ## Warnings and Precautions

Don't take if you:
No problems are expected.

Consult your doctor if you:
No problems are expected.

Over 55:
No problems are expected.

Pregnancy:
- No problems are expected.
- Don't take doses greater than DRI.

Breastfeeding:
- No problems are expected.
- Don't take doses greater than DRI.

Effect on lab tests:
No expected effects.

Storage:
- Store in a cool, dry place away from direct light, but don't freeze.
- Store safely out of reach of children.
- Don't store in bathroom medicine cabinet. Heat and moisture may change the action of the vitamin.

 ## Overdose/Toxicity

Signs and symptoms:
Supplements in amounts suggested by manufacturers on the label are nontoxic.

What to do:
For accidental overdose (such as child taking entire bottle): Dial 911 (emergency), 0 for operator or call your nearest Poison Control Center.

 ## Adverse Reactions or Side Effects

None are expected if taken within DRI dosage levels.

 ## Interaction with Medicine, Vitamins or Minerals

Interacts with	Combined effect
Long term antibiotics (broad spectrum)	Destroys "friendly" bacteria in intestines that produce biotin. This can lead to significant biotin deficiency.
Sulfonamides	Destroys "friendly" bacteria in intestines that produce biotin. This can lead to significant biotin deficiency.

 ## Interaction with Other Substances

Tobacco decreases absorption. Smokers may require supplemental biotin.

Alcohol decreases absorption.

Foods:
Eating large quantities of raw egg whites may cause biotin deficiency. Egg whites contain avidin, which prevents biotin from being absorbed into the body.

 ## Lab Tests to Detect Deficiency

None are available, except for experimental purposes.

Choline

 Basic Information

- Choline is a precursor for acetylcholine.
- Available from natural sources? Yes
- Available from synthetic sources? Yes
- Prescription required? No
- DRI information, see page 476

 Natural Sources

Breast milk	Kale
Cabbage	Lentils
Calf liver	Oatmeal
Cauliflower	Peanuts
Egg yolk	Soybeans
Garbanzo beans	Soy lecithin
(chickpeas)	Wheat germ

 Benefits

- Maintains cell membrane integrity
- Choline is a component of lecithin, a structural component of cell walls
- Acetylcholine functions as a neurotransmitter

 Possible Additional Benefits

- May prevent some diseases of the nervous system, such as Alzheimer's disease, Huntington's disease and tardive dyskinesia (involuntary, abnormal facial movements including grimacing, sticking out tongue and sucking movements)
- May reduce symptoms of Alzheimer's disease
- May reduce liver damage caused by alcoholism and hepatitis
- May lower cholesterol level in human serum

 Who May Benefit From Additional Intake?

No one

 Deficiency Symptoms

- Fatty deposition in liver
- Hemorrhagic kidney disease

 Usage Information

What this supplement does:

Choline is involved in production of acetylcholine. Acetylcholine must be present in the body for proper function of the nervous system, including mood, behavior, orientation, personality traits, judgment.

Miscellaneous information:

- The major source for choline is lecithin. It is used as a thickener in several foods, including mayonnaise, margarine, ice cream.
- Humans can synthesize choline from ethanolamine and methyl groups derived from methionine.

Available as:

Capsules: Swallow whole with full glass of liquid. Don't chew or crush. Take with or 1 to 1-1/2 hours after meals unless otherwise directed by your doctor.

 Warnings and Precautions

Don't take if you:

Are healthy and eat a well-balanced diet.

Consult your doctor if you have:
Plans to use choline to treat Alzheimer's disease with lecithin/choline.

Over 55:
Don't take if you are healthy.

Pregnancy:
Don't take if you are healthy. Check with your doctor if you have any questions.

Breastfeeding:
Don't take if you are healthy. Check with your doctor if you have any questions.

Effect on lab tests:
May cause inaccurate results in choline/sphingomyelin test as part of examination of amniotic fluid.

Storage:
• Store in cool, dry place away from direct light, but don't freeze.
• Store safely out of reach of children.
• Don't store in bathroom medicine cabinet. Heat and moisture may change the action of the supplement.

Others:
Don't take more than 1 gram per day.

Overdose/Toxicity

Signs and symptoms:
Nausea, vomiting, dizziness.

What to do:
For symptoms of overdosage:
Discontinue supplement and consult doctor. Also see *Adverse Reactions or Side Effects* section below.

For accidental overdosage (such as child taking entire bottle): Dial 911 (emergency), 0 for operator or call your nearest Poison Control Center.

Adverse Reactions or Side Effects

Reaction or effect	What to do
"Fishy" body odor	Discontinue. Call doctor when convenient.

Interaction with Medicine, Vitamins or Minerals

Interacts with	Combined effect
Methotrexate	Decreases choline absorption.
Nicotinic acid (nicotinamide, vitamin B-3)	Decreases choline effectiveness.
Phenobarbital	Decreases choline absorption.

Interaction with Other Substances

None are known.

Lab Tests to Detect Deficiency

Assessed by measuring serum-alanine amino-transferase levels

VITAMINS

Vitamin D

 ## Basic Information

Vitamin D is also called *cholecalciferol* or *sunshine vitamin.*

- Available from natural sources? Yes
- Available from synthetic sources? Yes
- Prescription required? No
- Fat-soluble
- *RDA/DRI and Optimal Intake,* see page 476

 ## Natural Sources

Cod-liver oil	Salmon
Egg substitutes	Sardines
Halibut-liver oil	Sunlight
Herring	Tuna
Mackerel	Vitamin-D-fortified milk

 ## Benefits

- Regulates growth, hardening and repair of bone by controlling absorption of calcium and phosphorus from small intestine
- Prevents rickets
- Treats hypocalcemia (low blood calcium) in those with kidney disease
- Treats post-operative muscle contractions
- Works with calcium to control bone formation
- Promotes normal growth and development of infants and children
- Promotes strong bones and teeth

 ## Possible Additional Benefits

- May reduce risk of breast or colon cancer
- Possible treatment for aging symptoms
- May treat vitamin-D malabsorption in those with cystic fibrosis

 ## Who May Benefit from Additional Amounts?

- Children who live in sunshine-deficient areas
- Anyone with inadequate caloric or nutritional dietary intake or increased nutritional requirements
- People more than 55 years old with limited sun exposure (for example, people who are institutionalized, use sunscreen or live in an area of limited sun exposure)
- Pregnant or breastfeeding women
- Those who abuse alcohol or other drugs
- People with a chronic wasting illness
- Those under excess stress for long periods
- Anyone who has recently undergone surgery
- Those with a portion of the gastrointestinal tract surgically removed
- People with recent severe burns or injuries
- Dark-skinned individuals
- Anyone with a liver impairment such as cirrhosis or obstructive jaundice (consult doctor)
- Breastfed babies
- Vegan vegetarians with limited sun exposure
- Those with cystic fibrosis

Deficiency Symptoms

- Rickets (a childhood deficiency disease): bent, bowed legs; malformations of joints or bones, late tooth development, weak muscles, listlessness
- Osteomalacia (adult rickets): pain in ribs, lower spine, pelvis and legs; muscle weakness and spasm; brittle, easily broken bones

 Usage Information

What this vitamin does:

- Absorbs and uses calcium and phosphorus to make bone
- Essential for normal growth and development

Available as:

- Extended-release capsules or tablets: Swallow whole with a full glass of liquid. Don't chew or crush. Take with food or immediately after eating to decrease stomach irritation.
- Oral solution: Dilute in at least 1/2 glass of water or other liquid. Take with or 1 to 1-1/2 hours after meals unless otherwise directed by your doctor.
- Put liquid vitamin D directly into mouth or mix with cereal, fruit juice or food.
- Vitamin D is a constituent of many multivitamin/mineral preparations.
- Some forms are available by generic name.

 Warnings and Precautions

Don't take if you:

Are allergic to vitamin D, ergocalciferol or any vitamin-D derivative.

Consult your doctor if you have:

- Any plans to become pregnant while taking vitamin D
- Epilepsy
- Heart or blood-vessel disease
- Kidney, liver or pancreatic disease
- Chronic diarrhea
- Intestinal problems
- Sarcoidosis

Over 55:

Adverse reactions and side effects are more likely. Supplements may be necessary.

Pregnancy:

- Taking too much during pregnancy may cause abnormalities in the fetus. Consult doctor before taking a supplement to ensure correct dosage.
- Don't take doses greater than DRI.

Breastfeeding:

- It is important to receive the correct amount so enough vitamin D is available for normal growth and development of baby. Consult doctor about supplements.
- Don't take doses greater than DRI.

Effect on lab tests:

- May decrease serum alkaline phosphatase
- May increase levels of calcium, cholesterol and phosphate in test results
- May increase level of magnesium in test results
- May increase amounts of calcium and phosphorus in urine

Storage:

- Store in a cool, dry place away from direct light, but don't freeze. Avoid overexposure to air.
- Store safely out of reach of children.
- Don't store in bathroom medicine cabinet. Heat and moisture may change the action of the vitamin.

Others:

- Absence of sunlight prevents natural formation of vitamin D by skin. →

VITAMINS

Sunshine provides sufficient amounts of vitamin D for people who live in sunny climates. Those who live in northern areas with fewer days of sunshine and extended periods of cloud cover and darkness must depend on dietary sources for vitamin D.

• Avoid doses greater than DRI.

Overdose/Toxicity

Signs and symptoms:
High blood pressure, irregular heartbeat, nausea, weight loss, seizures, abdominal pain, appetite loss, mental- and physical-growth retardation, premature hardening of arteries, kidney damage.

What to do:

For symptoms of overdose:
Discontinue vitamin and consult doctor. Also see *Adverse Reactions or Side Effects* section below.

For accidental overdose (such as child taking entire bottle): Dial 911 (emergency), 0 for operator or call your nearest Poison Control Center.

For toxic symptoms: Discontinue vitamin and seek immediate medical help. Hospitalization may be necessary.

Adverse Reactions or Side Effects

Reaction or effect	What to do
Appetite loss	Discontinue. Call doctor when convenient.
Constipation	Discontinue. Call doctor when convenient.
Diarrhea	Discontinue. Call doctor immediately.
Dry mouth	Discontinue. Call doctor when convenient.
Headache	Discontinue. Call doctor immediately.
Increased thirst	Discontinue. Call doctor when convenient.
Mental confusion	Discontinue. Call doctor immediately.
Metallic taste	Discontinue. Call doctor when convenient.
Nausea or vomiting	Discontinue. Call doctor immediately.
Unusual tiredness	Discontinue. Call doctor when convenient.

Interaction with Medicine, Vitamins or Minerals

Interacts with	Combined effect
Antacids with aluminum	Decreases absorption of vitamin D and fat-soluble vitamins A, E and K.
Antacids with magnesium	May cause too much magnesium in blood, especially in people with kidney failure.
Anticonvulsants	May reduce effect of vitamin D from natural sources and require supplements to prevent loss of strength in bones.
Barbiturates	May reduce effect of vitamin D from natural sources and require supplements to prevent loss of strength in bones.
Calcitonin	Reduces effect of calcitonin when treating hypercalcemia.
Calcium (high doses)	Increases risk of hypercalcemia.
Cholestyramine	Impairs absorption of vitamin D. May need supplements.
Colestipol	Impairs absorption of vitamin D. May need supplements.
Cortisone	Decreases absorption of vitamin D.
Digitalis preparations	Increases risk of heartbeat irregularities.

Diuretics, thiazide	Increases risk of hypercalcemia.
Hydantoin	May reduce effect of vitamin D from natural sources and require supplements to prevent loss of strength in bones.
Mineral oil	Increases absorption of vitamin D. May need supplements.
Phosphorus-containing medicines	Increases risk of too much phosphorus in blood.
Primidone	May reduce effect of vitamin D from natural sources and require supplements to prevent loss of strength in bones.
Vitamin-D derivatives, such as calciferol, calcitrol, dihydrotachysterol, ergocalciferol	Additive effects may increase potential for toxicity.

Interaction with Other Substances

Alcohol abuse depletes liver stores of vitamin D.

Olestra fat substitute can decrease absorption of vitamin D.

Lab Tests to Detect Deficiency

- Reduced levels of vitamin-D forms in blood
- Decreased serum phosphate and calcium, increased alkaline phosphatase, urinary hydroxyproline, parathyroid hormone (PTH) levels
- Bone X-ray

VITAMINS

Vitamin E

Basic Information

Vitamin E is also called *alpha-tocopherol.*

D alpha-tocopherol is the most absorbable.

- Available from natural sources? Yes
- Available from synthetic sources? Yes
- Prescription required? No, except for injectable forms
- Fat-soluble
- *RDA/DRI and Optimal Intake,* see page 476

Natural Sources

Almonds	Fortified cereals
Asparagus	Hazelnuts (filberts)
Avocados	Peanuts/Peanut oil
Brazil nuts	Safflower nuts/oil
Broccoli	Soybean oil
Canola oil	Spinach
Corn	Sunflower seeds
Corn oil/margarine	Walnuts
Cottonseed oil	Wheat germ
	Wheat germ oil

Benefits

- Promotes normal growth and development

➡

- Treats and prevents vitamin-E deficiency in premature or low-birthweight infants
- Acts as anti-blood clotting agent
- Promotes normal red-blood-cell formation
- Promotes vitamin-C recycling
- Reduces risk of fatal first myocardial infarction in men
- Protects against prostate cancer
- Improves immunity—especially in vitamin-E deficient people
- Antioxidant (see Glossary) for cancer, heart disease, tissue, free radicals in the body

 ## Possible Additional Benefits

- May reduce symptoms of fibrocystic disease of breast
- May reduce circulatory problems of lower extremities
- Possible coronary artery heart disease prevention
- Potentially enhances sexual performance
- May improve muscle strength and stamina
- May promote healing of burns and wounds
- May retard aging
- Possible relief from menopausal symptoms
- Potential treatment for bee stings, diaper rash
- May decrease scar formation
- May improve athletic performance
- Possible acne treatment
- May prevent eye and lung problems in low-birthweight or premature infants
- May treat skin disorders associated with lupus
- Possibly reduces blood glucose levels in some diabetics
- May protect against macular degeneration, cataracts

 # Who May Benefit from Additional Amounts?

- Anyone with inadequate caloric or nutritional dietary intake or increased nutritional requirements
- People more than 55 years old
- Those who abuse alcohol or other drugs
- People who have a chronic wasting illness
- Those under excess stress for long periods
- Anyone who has recently undergone surgery
- Those with liver, gallbladder or pancreatic disease
- People with recent severe burns or injuries
- People with hyperthyroidism
- Anyone at risk for myocardial infarction
- People with cystic fibrosis
- People with celiac disease

 ## Deficiency Symptoms

Premature infants and children:
- Irritability
- Edema
- Hemolytic anemia

Adults:
- Lethargy
- Apathy
- Inability to concentrate
- Nerve dysfunction

 ## Usage Information

What this vitamin does:
- Prevents a chemical reaction called *oxidation* (see Glossary)—excessive oxidation can sometimes cause harmful effects
- Acts as a cofactor (see Glossary) in several enzyme systems

Miscellaneous information:

- Vitamin E is a constituent of many skin ointments, salves and creams. Claims for beneficial effects have not been confirmed, but topical application probably does not cause harm.
- Several weeks of treatment may be necessary before symptoms caused by a deficiency will improve.
- Freezing may destroy vitamin E.
- Extreme heat causes vitamin E to break down. Avoid deep-fat frying foods that are natural sources of vitamin E.
- Vitamin E functions as an antioxidant (see Glossary), prevents enzyme action of peroxidase on unsaturated bonds of cell membranes and protects red blood cells from disintegrating.

Available as:

- Tablets or capsules: Swallow whole with a full glass of liquid. Don't chew or crush. Take with food or immediately after eating to decrease stomach irritation.
- Drops: Dilute dose in beverage before swallowing, or squirt directly into mouth.
- Vitamin E is a constituent of many multivitamin/mineral preparations.

 ## Warnings and Precautions

Don't take if you:
- Are allergic to vitamin E
- Are taking coumadin

Consult your doctor if you have:
- Iron-deficiency anemia
- Bleeding or clotting problems
- Cystic fibrosis
- Intestinal problems
- Liver disease
- Overactive thyroid
- Low-birthweight baby (supplementation appears to increase immune function)

Over 55:
No problems are expected.

Pregnancy:
- No problems are expected, except with doses greater than RDA.
- Low-birthweight babies are at risk for vitamin-E deficiency.

Breastfeeding:
No problems are expected.

Effect on lab tests:
Serum cholesterol and serum triglycerides may register high if you take large doses of vitamin E.

Storage:
- Store in a cool, dry area away from direct light, but don't freeze.
- Store safely out of reach of children.
- Don't store in bathroom medicine cabinet. Heat and moisture may change the action of the vitamin.

Others:
Beware of doses greater than RDA.

 ## Overdose/Toxicity

Signs and symptoms:
High doses deplete vitamin-A stores in body. Very high doses (over 1,000IU/day) may cause nausea; flatulence; headache; fainting; diarrhea; tendency to bleed; altered immunity; impaired sex functions; increased risk of blood clots; altered metabolism of thyroid, pituitary and adrenal hormones.

What to do:

For accidental overdose (such as a child taking entire bottle): Dial 911 (emergency), 0 for operator or call your nearest Poison Control Center.

For symptoms of toxicity:
Discontinue vitamin and consult doctor. Also see *Adverse Reactions or Side Effects* section below.

→

Adverse Reactions or Side Effects

Reaction or effect	What to do
Abdominal pain	Discontinue. Call doctor immediately.
Breast enlargement	Discontinue. Call doctor when convenient.
Diarrhea	Discontinue. Call doctor immediately.
Dizziness	Discontinue. Call doctor when convenient.
Flu-like symptoms	Discontinue. Call doctor immediately.
Headache	Discontinue. Call doctor when convenient.
Nausea	Discontinue. Call doctor immediately.
Tiredness or weakness	Discontinue. Call doctor when convenient.
Vision blurred	Discontinue. Call doctor immediately.

 Interaction with Medicine, Vitamins or Minerals

Interacts with	Combined effect
Antacids	Decreases vitamin-E absorption.
Anticoagulants, coumadin- or indandione-type	May increase spontaneous or hidden bleeding.
Aspirin (long-term use)	May reduce blood clotting to greater extent than desired to decrease cardiac disease.
Cholestyramine	May decrease absorption of vitamin E.
Colestipol	May decrease absorption of vitamin E.
Iron supplements	Decreases effect of iron with iron-deficiency anemia. Decreases vitamin-E effect in healthy people.
Mineral oil	May decrease absorption of vitamin E.
Sucralfate	May decrease absorption of vitamin E.
Vitamin A	Facilitates absorption, storage and utilization of vitamin A. Reduces potential toxicity of vitamin A. Excessive doses of vitamin E cause vitamin-A depletion.

 Interaction with Other Substances

Tobacco decreases absorption. Smokers may require supplemental vitamin E.

Alcohol abuse depletes vitamin-E stores in tissue.

Olestra fat substitute reduces absorption of vitamin E.

 Lab Tests to Detect Deficiency

- Blood tocopherol level
- Excess creatine in urine to indicate muscle breakdown
- Red-blood-cell fragility test

Folic Acid (Vitamin B-9, Folate)

Basic Information

Folic acid is also called *pteroylglutamic acid* and *folacin.*

Folate comes from dietary sources.

Folic acid comes from supplements.

- Available from natural sources? Yes
- Available from synthetic sources? Yes
- Prescription required? No
- Water-soluble
- *RDA/DRI and Optimal Intake,* see page 476

Natural Sources

Asparagus	Citrus fruits/juices
Avocados	Endive
Bananas	Fortified grain products
Beans	Garbanzo beans
Beets	(chickpeas)
Brewer's yeast	Green, leafy
Brussels sprouts	vegetables
Cabbage	Lentils
Calf liver	Sprouts
Cantaloupe	Wheat germ

Benefits

- Promotes normal red-blood-cell formation
- Maintains nervous system, intestinal tract, sex organs, white blood cells, normal patterns of growth
- Regulates embryonic and fetal development of nerve cells and prevents neural-tube defects
- Promotes normal growth and development
- Treats anemias due to folic-acid deficiency occurring from alcoholism, liver disease, hemolytic anemia, sprue, pregnancy, breastfeeding, oral-contraceptive use
- Aids metabolism of amino acids and protein synthesis (RNA, DNA)

Possible Additional Benefits

B-9 may reduce cervical dysplasia.

Who May Benefit from Additional Amounts?

- Anyone with inadequate caloric or nutritional dietary intake or increased nutritional requirements
- People more than 55 years old with inadequate dietary intake
- Pregnant or breastfeeding women
- Women who use oral contraceptives
- Those who abuse alcohol or other drugs
- People with a chronic wasting illness, AIDS/HIV
- Those under excess stress for long periods
- Those with a portion of the gastrointestinal tract surgically removed
- People with recent severe burns or injuries
- Women capable of becoming pregnant

Deficiency Symptoms

- Megaloblastic anemia, in which red blood cells are large and uneven in size

VITAMINS

→

- Irritability
- Weakness
- Lack of energy
- Loss of appetite
- Paleness
- Sore, red tongue
- Mild mental symptoms, such as forgetfulness and confusion
- Diarrhea

 ## Usage Information

What this vitamin does:
- Acts as coenzyme (see Glossary) for normal DNA synthesis
- Functions as part of coenzyme in amino acid and nucleoprotein synthesis
- Promotes normal red-blood-cell formation

Miscellaneous information:
- Cooking vegetables causes loss of some folate content.
- In January 1998 the USRDA began a fortification program to increase folate content of grain- and flour-containing products.

Available as:
- Tablets: Swallow whole with a full glass of liquid. Don't chew or crush. Take with or 1 to 1-1/2 hours after meals unless otherwise directed by your doctor.

 ## Warnings and Precautions

Don't take if you:
- Have pernicious anemia (Folic acid will make the blood appear normal, but neurological problems may progress and be irreversible.)
- Take anticonvulsant medication

Consult your doctor if you:
- Have anemia
- Are taking methotrexate

Over 55:
No problems are expected.

Pregnancy:
- No problems are expected.
- Don't take doses greater than DRI.

Breastfeeding:
- No problems are expected.
- Don't take doses greater than DRI.

Effect on lab tests:
May cause false low results in tests for vitamin B-12.

Storage:
- Store in a cool, dry place away from direct light, but don't freeze.
- Store safely out of reach of children.
- Don't store in bathroom medicine cabinet. Heat and moisture may change the action of the vitamin.

Others:
Renal dialysis reduces blood folate. Patients on dialysis should increase intake to more than 400mg per day.

 ## Overdose/Toxicity

Signs and symptoms:
Prolonged use of high doses can produce damaging folacin crystals in the kidney. Doses over 1,500mcg/day can cause appetite loss, nausea, flatulence, abdominal distension and may obscure existence of pernicious anemia.

What to do:

For symptoms of overdose:
Discontinue vitamin and consult doctor. Also see *Adverse Reactions or Side Effects* section below.

For accidental overdose (such as child taking entire bottle): Dial 911 (emergency), 0 for operator or call your nearest Poison Control Center.

Adverse Reactions or Side Effects

Reaction or effect	What to do
Bright-yellow urine (always)	Nothing.
Diarrhea	Discontinue. Call doctor.
Fever	Discontinue. Call doctor immediately.
Shortness of breath due to anemia	Discontinue. Call doctor immediately.
Skin rash	Discontinue. Call doctor when convenient.

Interaction with Medicine, Vitamins or Minerals

Interacts with	Combined effect
Analgesics	Decreases effect of folic acid.
Antacids containing aluminum or magnesium	Prolonged use may decrease absorption of folic acid. Take folic acid two hours before taking an antacid.
Antibiotics	May cause false low results in tests for serum folic acid.
Anticonvulsants	Decreases effect of folic acid and anticonvulsant.
Chloramphenicol	Produces folic-acid deficiency.
Cortisone drugs	Decreases effect of folic acid.
Epoetin	Decreases effect of folic acid.
Methotrexate	Decreases effect of folic acid. Methotrexate is a folate antagonist (see Glossary).
Oral contraceptives	Those who take oral contraceptives may require additional folic acid or dietary folate.

Phenytoin	Decreases phenytoin effect. Patients taking phenytoin should avoid taking folic acid.
Pyrimethamine	Decreases effect of folic acid and interferes with effectiveness of pyrimethamine. Avoid this combination
Quinine	Decreases effect of folic acid.
Sulfasalazine and other sulfa drugs	Decreases effect of folic acid.
Triamterene	Decreases effect of folic acid.
Trimethoprim	Decreases effect of folic acid.

Interaction with Other Substances

Tobacco decreases absorption. Smokers may require supplemental folic acid.

Alcohol abuse makes deficiency more likely. Alcoholism is the principal cause of folic-acid deficiency.

Lab Tests to Detect Deficiency

- Serum folate
- Blood cells showing macrocytic anemia coupled with normal levels of B-12 in blood
- Red-blood-cell (RBC) folate

VITAMINS

Niacin (Vitamin B-3)

Basic Information

- Available from natural sources? Yes
- Available from synthetic sources? Yes
- Prescription required? Yes, for high doses used for cholesterol reduction
- Water-soluble
- *RDA/DRI and Optimal Intake*, see page 476

Natural Sources

Beef liver	Peanuts
Brewer's yeast	Pork/ham
Chicken,	Potatoes
white meat	Salmon
Dried beans/peas	Soybeans
Fortified cereals	Swordfish
Halibut	Tuna
Peanut butter	Turkey

Benefits

- Treats pellagra (see Glossary)
- Corrects niacin deficiency
- Reduces cholesterol and triglycerides in blood
- Dilates blood vessels if taken in doses larger than 75mg (consult doctor)
- Treats vertigo (dizziness) and ringing in ears

Possible Additional Benefits

- May reduce risk of heart attacks
- May reduce depression
- May reduce migraine headaches
- Potentially improves poor digestion

Who May Benefit from Additional Amounts?

- Anyone with inadequate caloric or nutritional dietary intake or increased nutritional requirements
- People more than 55 years old with poor dietary intake
- Pregnant or breastfeeding women
- Those who abuse alcohol or other drugs
- People with a chronic wasting illness, including malignancies, pancreatic insufficiency, cirrhosis of the liver, sprue
- People with recent severe burns or injuries
- Infants born with errors of metabolism (congenital disorders due to chromosome abnormalities)

Deficiency Symptoms

Early symptoms:
- Delirium
- General fatigue/lethargy
- Loss of appetite
- Headaches
- Swollen, red tongue
- Skin lesions, including rashes, dry scaly skin, wrinkles, coarse skin texture
- Indigestion
- Dermatitis/dark pigmentation
- Diarrhea
- Irritability
- Dizziness

Late symptoms of severe deficiency, called *pellagra:*
- Dementia
- Death

Usage Information

What this vitamin does:
- Aids in release of energy from foods
- Helps synthesize DNA
- Becomes component of two coenzymes (see Glossary), NAD and NADP, which are both necessary for utilization of fats, tissue respiration and production of sugars

Miscellaneous information:
- The body manufactures niacin from tryptophan, an amino acid.
- Vitamin B-6 is needed to convert tryptophan to niacin.
- Long-term, high-dose leucine supplementation can cause tryptophan and niacin deficiency.

Available as:
- Tablets or capsules: Swallow whole with a full glass of liquid. Don't chew or crush. Take with or 1 to 1-1/2 hours after meals unless otherwise directed by your doctor.
- Extended-release capsules or tablets: Swallow whole with a full glass of liquid. Don't chew or crush. Take with food or immediately after eating to decrease stomach irritation.
- Oral solution: Dilute in at least 1/2 glass of water or other liquid. Take with or 1 to 1-1/2 hours after meals unless otherwise directed by your doctor.
- Injectable forms are administered by a doctor or nurse.
- Niacin is a constituent of most multivitamin/mineral preparations.
- Some forms are available by generic name.

 ## Warnings and Precautions

Don't take if you:
- Are allergic to niacin or any niacin-containing vitamin mixtures
- Have impaired liver function
- Have an active peptic ulcer

Consult your doctor if you have:
- Diabetes
- Gout
- Gallbladder or liver disease
- Arterial bleeding
- Glaucoma

Over 55:
Response to niacin cannot be predicted. Dose must be individualized.

Pregnancy:
Risk to fetus with high doses outweighs benefits. Do not use.

Breastfeeding:
- Studies are inconclusive. Consult doctor about supplements.
- Don't take doses greater than DRI.

Effect on lab tests:
- Urinary catecholamine concentration may falsely elevate results.
- Urine glucose (using Benedict's reagent) may produce false-positive reactions.
- Niacin can elevate blood sugar and falsely increase growth-hormone level in blood.
- Large daily doses may elevate blood uric acid.

Storage:
- Store in a cool, dry place away from direct light, but don't freeze.
- Store safely out of reach of children.
- Don't store in bathroom medicine cabinet. Heat and moisture may change the action of the vitamin.

VITAMINS

Others:
High dosages over long periods may cause liver damage or aggravate a stomach ulcer.

Overdose/Toxicity

Signs and symptoms:
Body flush, nausea, diarrhea, weakness, lightheadedness, headache, fainting, high blood sugar, high uric acid, heart-rhythm disturbances, jaundice.

What to do:
For symptoms of overdose:
Discontinue vitamin and consult doctor. Also see *Adverse Reactions or Side Effects* section below.

For accidental overdose (such as child taking entire bottle): Dial 911 (emergency), 0 for operator or call your nearest Poison Control Center.

Adverse Reactions or Side Effects

Reaction or effect	What to do
Abdominal pain	Discontinue. Call doctor immediately.
Darkening of urine	Nothing.
Diarrhea	Discontinue. Call doctor when convenient.
Faintness	Discontinue. Call doctor immediately.
Headache	Discontinue. Call doctor when convenient.
"Hot" feeling, with skin flushed in blush zone (always)	Nothing.
Jaundice (yellow skin and eyes)	Discontinue. Call doctor immediately.
Nausea or vomiting	Discontinue. Call doctor immediately.
Skin dryness	Discontinue. Call doctor when convenient.

Interaction with Medicine, Vitamins or Minerals

Interacts with	Combined effect
Antidiabetics	Decreases antidiabetic effect.
Beta-adrenergic blockers	Lowers blood pressure to extremely low level.
Chenodiol	Decreases chenodiol effect.
Guanethidine	Increases guanethidine effect.
HMG-CoA reductase inhibitors	Increases risk of rhabdomyolysis and renal failure.
Isoniazid	Decreases niacin effect.
Mecamylamine	Lowers blood pressure to extremely low level.
Pargyline	Lowers blood pressure to extremely low level.
Ursodiol	Decreases ursodiol effect.

Interaction with Other Substances

Tobacco decreases absorption. Smokers may require supplemental niacin.

Alcohol may cause extremely low blood pressure. Use caution.

Lab Tests to Detect Deficiency

- Urinary N-1 methylnicotinamide
- Urinary 2-pyridone/N-1 methylnicotinamide—test results not always conclusive

Pantothenic Acid (Vitamin B-5)

Basic Information

- Available from natural sources? Yes
- Available from synthetic sources? Yes
- Prescription required? No
- Water-soluble
- *RDA/DRI and Optimal Intake,* see page 476

Natural Sources

Avocados	Meats, all kinds
Bananas	Milk
Blue cheese	Oranges
Broccoli	Peanut butter
Chicken	Peanuts
Collard greens	Peas
Eggs	Soybeans
Lentils	Sunflower seeds
Liver	Wheat germ
Lobster	Whole-grain products

Benefits

- Promotes normal growth and development
- Aids release of energy from foods
- Helps synthesize numerous body materials

Possible Additional Benefits

- May stimulate wound healing in animals
- May alleviate stress
- May reduce fatigue

Who May Benefit from Additional Amounts?

- Anyone with inadequate caloric or nutritional dietary intake or increased nutritional requirements
- People more than 55 years old with vitamin-B deficiencies
- Pregnant or breastfeeding women
- Those who abuse alcohol or other drugs
- People with a chronic wasting illness, including sprue, celiac disease, regional enteritis
- Those under excess stress for long periods
- Anyone who has recently undergone surgery
- Athletes and workers who participate in vigorous physical activities

Deficiency Symptoms

No proven symptoms exist for pantothenic acid alone. However, lack of one B vitamin usually means lack of other B nutrients. Pantothenic acid is usually given with other B vitamins if there are symptoms of any vitamin-B deficiency, including excessive fatigue, sleep disturbances, loss of appetite, nausea or dermatitis.

Usage Information

What this vitamin does:

Vitamin B-5 is converted to a coenzyme (see Glossary) in energy metabolism of carbohydrates, protein and fat.

VITAMINS

➜

Available as:

- Tablets: Swallow whole with a full glass of liquid. Don't chew or crush. Take with or 1 to 1-1/2 hours after meals unless otherwise directed by your doctor.
- Vitamin B-5 is a constituent of many multivitamin/mineral preparations and B-complex vitamins.

Warnings and Precautions

Don't take if you are:
- Allergic to pantothenic acid
- Taking levodopa for Parkinson's disease

Consult your doctor if you have:
Hemophilia.

Over 55:
No problems are expected.

Pregnancy:
Don't exceed recommended dose.

Breastfeeding:
Don't exceed recommended dose.

Effect on lab tests:
No expected effects.

Storage:
- Store in a cool, dry place away from direct light, but don't freeze.
- Store safely out of reach of children.
- Don't store in bathroom medicine cabinet. Heat and moisture may change the action of the vitamin.

Others:
Avoid doses greater than five times the DRI.

Overdose/Toxicity

What to do:
For symptoms of overdose:
Discontinue vitamin and consult doctor. Also see *Adverse Reactions or Side Effects* section below.

For accidental overdose (such as child taking entire bottle): Dial 911 (emergency), 0 for operator or call your nearest Poison Control Center.

Adverse Reactions or Side Effects

Reaction or effect	What to do
Diarrhea	Discontinue or reduce close to DRI levels.

Interaction with Medicine, Vitamins or Minerals

Interacts with	Combined effect
Levodopa	Small amounts of pantothenic acid nullify levodopa's effect. Carbidopa-levodopa combination is not affected by this interaction.

Interaction with Other Substances

Tobacco decreases absorption. Smokers may require supplemental pantothenic acid.

Lab Tests to Detect Deficiency

Methods are limited and expensive. Tests are used only for research at present. Methods are available to measure blood levels and levels in 24-hour urine collections.

Phytonadione (Vitamin K)

Basic Information

Phytonadione and menadiol are forms of vitamin K.

- Available from natural sources? Yes
- Available from synthetic sources? Yes
- Prescription required? Yes
- Fat-soluble
- *RDA/DRI and Optimal Intake,* see page 476

Natural Sources

Alfalfa	Green, leafy lettuce
Asparagus	Liver
Broccoli	Seaweed
Brussels sprouts	Spinach
Cabbage	Turnip greens
Cheddar cheese	

Benefits

- Promotes normal growth and development
- Prevents hemorrhagic disease of the newborn
- Treats bleeding disorders due to vitamin-K deficiency
- Regulates normal blood clotting
- Promotes bone health

Possible Additional Benefits

None are known.

Who May Benefit from Additional Amounts?

- Those with a portion of the gastrointestinal tract surgically removed
- All newborns
- Anyone taking long-term antibiotics that may destroy normal "friendly" bacteria in the intestinal tract
- People who do not have enough bile to absorb fats (replacement must be given by injection or in water-soluble form)
- Infants who are breastfed or fed with milk-substitute formula
- People on mineral oil (for constipation)

Deficiency Symptoms

Infants:
- Failure to grow and develop normally
- Hemorrhagic disease of the newborn characterized by vomiting blood and bleeding from intestine, umbilical cord, circumcision site (symptoms begin 2 or 3 days after birth)

Adults:

Abnormal blood clotting that can lead to

- nosebleeds
- blood in urine
- stomach bleeding
- bleeding from capillaries or skin, causing spontaneous black-and-blue marks
- prolonged clotting time (a laboratory test)

VITAMINS

Usage Information

What this vitamin does:

Promotes production of active prothrombin (factor II), proconvertin (factor VII) and other factors necessary for normal blood clotting.

Miscellaneous information:

• Very little vitamin K is lost from processing or cooking foods.
• When a severe bleeding disorder exists due to a vitamin-K deficiency, fresh whole blood may be needed during severe bleeding episodes.

Available as:

• Tablets: Swallow whole with a full glass of liquid. Don't chew or crush. Take with or 1 to 1-1/2 hours after meals unless otherwise directed by your doctor.
• Injectable forms are administered by a doctor or nurse.
• Water-soluble tablets and liquids are also available.

Note: Vitamin K is not usually included in most multivitamin/mineral preparations.

Warnings and Precautions

Don't take if you:

• Are allergic to vitamin K
• Have a G6PD deficiency (see Glossary)
• Have liver disease

Consult your doctor if you have:

• Cystic fibrosis
• Prolonged diarrhea
• Prolonged intestinal problems
• Taken any other medicines
• Plans for surgery (including dental surgery) in the near future

Over 55:
• No problems are expected.
• Don't take doses greater than RDA.

Pregnancy:
• No studies are available in humans. Avoid if possible.
• Don't take doses greater than RDA.

Breastfeeding:
Don't take doses greater than RDA.

Effect on lab tests:
Changes prothrombin times.

Storage:
• Store in a cool, dry place away from direct light, but don't freeze.
• Store safely out of reach of children.
• Don't store in bathroom medicine cabinet. Heat and moisture may change the action of the vitamin.

Others:
• Avoid overdosage. Vitamin K is a fat-soluble vitamin. Excess intake can lead to impaired liver function.
• Tell any dentist or doctor who plans surgery that you take vitamin K.

Overdose/Toxicity

Signs and symptoms:
Brain damage in infants and impaired liver function in infants and adults who take large doses.

What to do:

For symptoms of overdose:
Discontinue vitamin and consult doctor. Also see *Adverse Reactions or Side Effects* section below.

For accidental overdose (such as child taking entire bottle): Dial 911 (emergency), 0 for operator or call your nearest Poison Control Center.

Adverse Reactions or Side Effects

Reaction or effect	What to do
Hemolytic anemia in infants	Seek emergency treatment.
Hyperbilirubinemia (too much bilirubin in the blood) in newborns or infants given too much vitamin K, marked by jaundice (yellow skin and eyes)	Seek emergency treatment.

Allergic reactions, including:

Face flushing	Discontinue. Call doctor immediately.
Gastrointestinal upset	Discontinue. Call doctor immediately.
Rash	Discontinue. Call doctor immediately.
Redness, pain or swelling at injection site	Discontinue. Call doctor immediately.
Skin itching	Seek emergency treatment.

Interaction with Medicine, Vitamins or Minerals

Interacts with	Combined effect
Antacids (long-term use)	Large amounts may interfere with vitamin-K effect.
Antibiotics, broad spectrum (long-term use)	Causes vitamin-K deficiency.
Anticoagulants (oral)	Decreases anticoagulant effect.
Cholestyramine	Decreases vitamin-K absorption.
Colestipol	Decreases vitamin-K absorption.
Coumarin (isolated from sweet clover)	Decreases vitamin-K effect.
Dactinomycin	May decrease vitamin-K effect.
Hemolytics	Increases potential for toxic side effects.
Mineral oil (long-term use)	Causes vitamin-K deficiency.
Primaquine	Increases potential for toxic side effects.
Quinidine	Causes vitamin-K deficiency.
Salicylates	Increases need for vitamin K when administered over long time.
Sucralfate	Decreases vitamin-K effect.
Sulfa drugs	Causes vitamin-K deficiency.

Interaction with Other Substances

None are known.

Lab Tests to Detect Deficiency

• Prothrombin time
• Serum prothrombin
• Serum vitamin K

VITAMINS

Pyridoxine (Vitamin B-6)

 Basic Information

Pyridoxine is also called *pyridoxal phosphate.*

- Available from natural sources? Yes
- Available from synthetic sources? Yes
- Prescription required? No
- Water-soluble
- *RDA/DRI and Optimal Intake,* see page 476

 Natural Sources

Avocados	Lentils
Bananas	Potatoes
Beef liver	Salmon
Chicken	Shrimp
Fortified cereals	Soybeans
Ground beef	Sunflower seeds
Ham	Tuna
Hazelnuts (filberts)	Wheat germ

 Benefits

- Participates actively in many chemical reactions of proteins and amino acids
- Helps normal function of brain
- Promotes normal red-blood-cell formation
- Helps in energy production
- Acts as coenzyme (see Glossary) in carbohydrate, protein and fat metabolism
- Treats some forms of anemia
- Treats cycloserine and isoniazid poisoning
- Maintains normal homocysteine levels
- Acts as a tranquilizer

 Possible Additional Benefits

- May promote normal nerve and muscle function
- May lower blood cholesterol
- May reduce inflammation associated with arthritis and carpal-tunnel syndrome
- Possible arteriosclerosis prevention in people with high homocysteine levels
- May reduce symptoms of premenstrual syndrome
- Potential asthmatic symptom reduction
- May promote ease in sleep by increasing serotonin

 Who May Benefit from Additional Amounts?

- Anyone with inadequate caloric or nutritional dietary intake or increased nutritional requirements
- Pregnant or breastfeeding women
- Those who abuse alcohol or other drugs
- People with a chronic wasting illness
- Those under excess stress for long periods
- Women taking oral contraceptives or estrogen
- People with hyperthyroidism
- People with elevated homocysteine levels

Deficiency Symptoms

Symptoms of vitamin-B-6 deficiency are nonspecific and hard to reproduce experimentally.

- Weakness
- Mental confusion
- Irritability
- Nervousness
- Insomnia
- Poor walking coordination
- Hyperactivity
- Abnormal electroencephalogram
- Anemia
- Skin lesions
- Tongue discoloration
- Muscle twitching

 Usage Information

What this vitamin does:
- Acts as coenzyme (see Glossary) for metabolic functions affecting protein, carbohydrates and fat utilization
- Promotes conversion of tryptophan to niacin or serotonin

Miscellaneous information:
Avoid cooking foods that contain vitamin B-6 in large amounts of water.

Available as:
- Tablets: Swallow whole with a full glass of liquid. Don't chew or crush. Take with or 1 to 1-1/2 hours after meals unless otherwise directed by your doctor.
- Extended-release capsules or tablets: Swallow whole with a full glass of liquid. Don't chew or crush. Take with food or immediately after eating to decrease stomach irritation.
- Vitamin B-6 is a constituent of many multivitamin/mineral preparations and B-complex vitamins.

 Warnings and Precautions

Don't take if you:
Are allergic to vitamin B-6.

Consult your doctor if you have:
- Been under severe stress with illness, burns, an accident, recent surgery
- Intestinal problems
- Liver disease
- Overactive thyroid
- Sickle-cell disease

Over 55:
Are more likely to have marginal deficiency.

Pregnancy:
Don't take doses greater than DRI. Large doses can cause pyridoxine dependency syndrome in the child.

Breastfeeding:
Megadoses (greater than DRI) can cause dangerous side effects in the infant.

Effect on lab tests:
May produce false-positive results in urobilinogen determinations using Ehrlich's reagent.

Storage:
- Store in a cool, dry place away from direct light, but don't freeze.
- Store safely out of reach of children.
- Don't store in bathroom medicine cabinet. Heat and moisture may change the action of the vitamin.

Others:
Regular B-6 supplements are recommended if you take chloramphenicol, cycloserine, ethionamide, hydralazine, immunosuppressants, isoniazid or penicillamine. These decrease pyridoxine absorption and can cause anemia or tingling and numbness in hands and feet.

VITAMINS

Overdose/Toxicity

- B-6 is toxic at high doses (100-250 times RDA), causing reversible nerve damage.
- Excess can cause increased oxalate in urine, leading to stone formation.

Signs and symptoms:
Clumsiness, numbness in hands and feet.

What to do:
For symptoms of overdose:
Discontinue vitamin and consult doctor. Also see *Adverse Reactions or Side Effects* section below.

For accidental overdose (such as child taking entire bottle): Dial 911 (emergency), 0 for operator or call your nearest Poison Control Center.

 Adverse Reactions or Side Effects

Reaction or effect	What to do
Depression when taken with oral contraceptive pills	Discontinue pyridoxine. Call doctor when convenient.
Doses of 200mg/day can produce dependency, causing need to continue to take high doses (undesirable)	Discontinue doses greater than DRI gradually.
Large doses (2 to 6 g/day) taken for several months are reported to cause severe sensory neuropathy (see Glossary) with unsteady gait, numb feet and hands, clumsiness	Discontinue doses greater than DRI. Call doctor immediately.

 Interaction with Medicine, Vitamins or Minerals

Interacts with	Combined effect
Chloramphenicol, cycloserine, ethionamide, hydralazine, isoniazid, penicillamine, and immuno-suppressants (such as ACTH, adreno-corticoids, azathioprine, chlorambucil, cyclophosphamide, cyclosporine, mercaptopurine)	May increase excretion of pyridoxine and cause anemia or peripheral neuritis, which includes pain and numbness and coldness in feet and fingertips. If you take these medicines, you may need increased pyridoxine. Consult your doctor.
Estrogen or oral contraceptives	May increase requirements of pyridoxine and cause depression. Consult doctor.
Levodopa	Prevents levodopa from controlling symptoms of Parkinson's disease. This problem does not occur with carbidopa-levodopa combination.
Phenytoin	Large doses of B-6 hasten breakdown of phenytoin.

 Interaction with Other Substances

Tobacco decreases absorption. Smokers may require supplemental vitamin B-6.

 Lab Tests to Detect Deficiency

- Pyridoxine level in blood
- Xanthurenic-acid level in urine

Riboflavin (Vitamin B-2)

Basic Information

- Available from natural sources? Yes
- Available from synthetic sources? Yes
- Prescription required? No
- Water-soluble
- *RDA/DRI and Optimal Intake,* see page 476

Natural Sources

Bananas	Ham
Beef liver	Mixed vegetables
Dairy products	Pork
Eggs	Tuna
Enriched breads	Wheat germ
Fortified cereals	

Benefits

- Aids release of energy from food
- Maintains healthy mucous membranes lining respiratory, digestive, circulatory and excretory tracts when used in conjunction with vitamin A
- Preserves integrity of nervous system, skin, eyes
- Promotes normal growth and development
- Activates vitamin B-6
- Essential for conversion of tryptophan to niacin

Possible Additional Benefits

- May increase body growth during normal developmental stages
- Possible treatment for cheilitis

Who May Benefit from Additional Amounts?

- Anyone with inadequate caloric or nutritional dietary intake or increased nutritional requirements
- Pregnant or breastfeeding women
- Those who abuse alcohol or other drugs
- People with a chronic wasting illness
- Those under excess stress for long periods
- Anyone who has recently undergone surgery
- Athletes and workers who participate in vigorous physical activities
- People who have hyperthyroidism

Deficiency Symptoms

- Cracks and sores in corners of mouth
- Inflammation of tongue and lips
- Eyes overly sensitive to light and easily tired
- Itching and scaling of skin around nose, mouth, scrotum, forehead, ears, scalp
- Trembling
- Insomnia

Usage Information

What this vitamin does:

- Acts as component in two coenzymes (see Glossary)—flavin mononucleotide and flavin adenine dinucleotide—needed for normal tissue respiration
- Activates pyridoxine
- Works in conjunction with other B vitamins

V I T A M I N S

→

Miscellaneous information:

- A balanced diet prevents deficiency without supplements.
- Large doses may produce dark yellow urine.
- Processing food may decrease quantity of vitamin B-2.
- Mixing with baking soda destroys riboflavin.
- Exposure to sunlight destroys riboflavin. Store milk in colored plastic jugs or cardboard containers.

Available as:

- Tablets: Swallow whole with a full glass of liquid. Don't chew or crush. Take with food or immediately after eating to decrease stomach irritation.
- Riboflavin is a constituent of many multivitamin/mineral preparations and B-complex vitamins.

 Warnings and Precautions

Don't take if you:

- Are allergic to any B vitamin
- Have chronic kidney failure

Consult your doctor if you are:
Pregnant or planning a pregnancy.

Over 55:
Have a greater need for vitamin B-2.

Pregnancy:
Don't take doses greater than DRI.

Breastfeeding:
Don't take doses greater than DRI.

Effect on lab tests:

- Urinary catecholamine concentration may show false elevation.
- Urobilinogen determinations (Ehrlich's) may produce false-positive results.

Storage:

- Store in a cool, dry place away from direct light, but don't freeze.
- Store safely out of reach of children.
- Don't store in bathroom medicine cabinet. Heat and moisture may change the action of the vitamin.

 Overdose/Toxicity

Vitamin B-2 is unlikely to cause toxic symptoms in healthy people with normal kidney function.

Signs and symptoms:
None expected.

What to do:
For accidental overdose (such as child taking entire bottle): Dial 911 (emergency), 0 for operator or call your nearest Poison Control Center.

 Adverse Reactions or Side Effects

Reaction or effect	What to do
Yellow urine (with large doses)	No action is necessary.

 Interaction with Medicine, Vitamins or Minerals

Interacts with	Combined effect
Antidepressants (tricyclic)	Decreases B-2 effect.
Phenothiazines	Decreases B-2 effect.
Probenecid	Decreases B-2 effect.

 Interaction with Other Substances

Tobacco decreases absorption. Smokers may require supplemental vitamin B-2.

Alcohol prevents uptake and absorption of vitamin B-2.

 Lab Tests to Detect Deficiency

- Serum riboflavin
- Erythrocyte riboflavin
- Glutathione reductase

Thiamine (Vitamin B-1)

 ## Basic Information

- Available from natural sources? Yes
- Available from synthetic sources? Yes
- Prescription required? Yes, for injectable forms
- Water-soluble
- *RDA/DRI and Optimal Intake,* see page 476

 ## Natural Sources

Baked potato	Orange juice
Beef kidney/liver	Oranges
Brewer's yeast	Oysters
Flour, rye and	Peanuts
whole-grain	Peas
Garbanzo beans	Raisins
(chickpeas),	Rice, brown
dried	and raw
Ham	Wheat germ
Kidney beans,	Whole-grain
dried	products
Navy beans, dried	

 ## Benefits

- Keeps mucous membranes healthy
- Maintains normal function of nervous system, muscles, heart
- Aids in treatment of herpes zoster
- Promotes normal growth and development
- Treats beriberi (thiamine-deficiency disease)
- Replaces deficiency caused by alcoholism, cirrhosis, overactive thyroid, infection, breastfeeding, absorption diseases, pregnancy, prolonged diarrhea, burns

 ## Possible Additional Benefits

- May reduce depression
- May reduce fatigue
- May reduce motion sickness
- May improve appetite and mental alertness

 ## Who May Benefit from Additional Amounts?

- People who abuse alcohol or other drugs (Alcoholics need more thiamine. Thiamine accelerates metabolism, using extra carbohydrates and calories from alcohol.)
- Anyone with inadequate caloric or nutritional dietary intake or increased nutritional requirements
- People over 55 years old
- Pregnant or breastfeeding women
- People with a chronic wasting illness, especially diabetes
- Those under excess stress for long periods
- Anyone who has recently undergone surgery
- People with liver disease, overactive thyroid, prolonged diarrhea

 ## Deficiency Symptoms

Normal deficiency:

- Loss of appetite
- Fatigue
- Nausea
- Mental problems, such as rolling of eyeballs, depression, memory loss, difficulty concentrating and dealing

VITAMINS

→

with details, personality changes, rapid heartbeat
- Gastrointestinal disorders
- Tender, atrophied muscles
- Wernicke's encephalopathy

Gross deficiency:
- Leads eventually to beriberi, which is rare except in severely ill alcoholics
- Pain or tingling in arms or legs
- Decreased reflex activity
- Fluid accumulation in arms and legs
- Heart enlargement
- Constipation
- Nausea
- Vomiting

Usage Information

What this vitamin does:
Thiamine functions in combination with adenosine triphosphate to form coenzyme (see Glossary) necessary for converting carbohydrates into energy in muscles and nervous system.

Miscellaneous information:
- Cook foods in minimum amount of water or steam.
- Avoid high cooking temperatures and long heat exposure.
- Avoid using baking soda when you take thiamine unless it is used as a leavening agent in baked products.
- Thiamine is stable when frozen and stored.
- A balanced diet should provide enough thiamine for healthy people to make supplementation unnecessary. The best dietary sources of thiamine are whole-grain cereals and meat.

Available as:
- Tablets: Swallow whole with a full glass of liquid. Don't chew or crush. Take with or 1 to 1-1/2 hours after meals unless otherwise directed by your doctor.

- Liquid: Dilute in at least 1/2 glass of water or other liquid. Take with or 1 to 1-1/2 hours after meals unless otherwise directed by your doctor.
- Injectable forms are administered by a doctor or nurse.
- Available as part of B complex.

Warnings and Precautions

Don't take if you:
Are allergic to any B vitamin.

Consult your doctor if you have:
Liver or kidney disease.

Over 55:
No problems are expected.

Pregnancy:
Don't take doses greater than DRI.

Breastfeeding:
Don't take doses greater than DRI.

Effect on lab tests:
Interferes with results of serum theophyline and may produce false-positive results in tests for uric acid or urobilinogen.

Storage:
- Store in a cool, dry place away from direct light, but don't freeze.
- Store safely out of reach of children.
- Don't store in bathroom medicine cabinet. Heat and moisture may change the action of the vitamin.

Others:
Most excess thiamine is excreted in urine if kidney function is normal.

Overdose/Toxicity

Signs and symptoms:
Occasionally large doses of vitamin B-1 have caused hypersensitive reactions resembling anaphylactic shock. Several hundred milligrams may cause drowsiness in some people.

What to do:
For symptoms of overdose:
Discontinue vitamin and consult doctor. Also see *Adverse Reactions or Side Effects* section below.

For accidental overdose (such as child taking entire bottle): Dial 911 (emergency), 0 for operator or call your nearest Poison Control Center.

Adverse Reactions or Side Effects

Reaction or effect	What to do
Skin rash or itching (rare)	Discontinue. Call doctor immediately.
Swelling in facial area	Discontinue. Call doctor immediately.
Wheezing (more likely after intravenous dose)	Seek emergency treatment.

Interaction with Medicine, Vitamins or Minerals

Interacts with	Combined effect
Antibiotics or sulfa drugs	Decreases thiamine levels.
Drugs used to relax muscles during surgery	Produces excessive muscle relaxation. Tell your doctor before surgery if you are taking supplements.

Oral contraceptives	Decreases thiamine levels.
Wernicke's encephalopathy treatment	Take thiamine before taking glucose.

Interaction with Other Substances

Tobacco decreases absorption. Smokers may require supplemental vitamin B-1.

Alcohol reduces intestinal absorption of vitamin B-1, which is necessary to metabolize alcohol.

Beverages:
Carbonates and citrates (additives listed on many beverage labels) decrease thiamine effect.

Foods:
Carbonates and citrates (additives listed on many food labels) decrease thiamine effect.

Lab Tests to Detect Deficiency

- Transketolase function study on red blood cells
- Pyruvic-acid blood level
- 24-hour urine collection

VITAMINS

Minerals

Many minerals are essential parts of *enzymes.* They also actively participate in regulating many physiological functions: transporting oxygen to each of the body's cells, providing sparks to make muscles contract and participating in many ways to guarantee normal function of the central nervous system. Minerals are required for growth, maintenance, repair and health of tissues and bones.

Most minerals are widely distributed in foods. *Severe* mineral deficiency is unusual in the United States and Canada. As with vitamins, certain groups may be more likely to have a deficiency than others. For example: pregnant women and children are at higher risk for iron deficiency, elderly persons are more at risk for zinc deficiency, and calcium requirements are increased for those at risk for osteoporosis.

MINERALS

Arsenic

 ## Basic Information

This metallic element is extremely poisonous.

- Available from natural sources? Yes
- Available from synthetic sources? No
- Prescription required? Yes, for some forms

 ## Natural Sources

Breads   Meats
Cereals   Starchy vegetables
Fish

 ## Benefits

- Arsenic is thought to be essential in trace amounts, but the benefits of this mineral are unknown.
- Arsenic is used in homeopathic treatment for some digestive problems that include burning pain and symptoms of dehydration.

 ## Possible Additional Benefits

Arsenic may help metabolize methionine.

 ## Who May Benefit from Additional Amounts?

Most individuals get an adequate amount from their diet.

 ## Deficiency Symptoms

No proven symptoms exist.

 ## Usage Information

What this mineral does:
- The exact function of arsenic is unclear, but it may aid in methionine metabolism.
- Toxicity occurs in doses larger than 250mcg a day. Most diets contain about 140mcg a day.

Available as:
Arsenicum album (Ars alb) a dilute form of arsenic is sometimes used to treat digestive problems. It is available as a liquid or tablet.

 ## Warnings and Precautions

Over 55:
Older persons may have a higher risk of excess arsenic due to decreased liver or kidney function.

Pregnancy: **Breastfeeding:**
Do not take.   Do not take.

Effect on lab tests:
Unknown.

Storage:
- Store safely out of reach of children.
- Store in a cool, dry place away from direct light, but don't freeze.
- Don't store in bathroom medicine cabinet. Heat and moisture may change the action of the mineral.

 ## Overdose/Toxicity

Signs and symptoms:
- Chronic symptoms include head-aches, convulsion, confusion, drowsiness and change in color of fingernails.

- Acute symptoms include vomiting, diarrhea, blood in urine, muscle cramps, fatigue, weakness, hair loss and dermatitis.
- Coma and death are possible when toxic arsenic levels accumulate.
- Lungs, skin, kidneys and liver are most affected by toxicity.
- Many types of cancer have been linked to arsenic exposure.

What to do:

For symptoms of overdose:
Discontinue mineral and consult doctor immediately. Also see *Adverse Reactions or Side Effects* section below.

For accidental overdose (such as child taking entire bottle): Dial 911 (emergency), 0 for operator or call your nearest Poison Control Center.

Adverse Reactions or Side Effects

Reaction or effect	What to do
Headaches	Discontinue. Call doctor immediately
Confusion	Discontinue. Call doctor immediately
Drowsiness	Discontinue. Call doctor immediately
Change in fingernail color	Discontinue. Call doctor immediately
Nausea	Discontinue. Call doctor immediately
Diarrhea	Discontinue. Call doctor immediately
Cramps	Discontinue. Call doctor immediately
Blood in urine	Discontinue. Call doctor immediately
Hair loss	Discontinue. Call doctor immediately
Dermatitis	Discontinue. Call doctor immediately

Interaction with Medicine, Vitamins or Minerals

Interacts with	Combined Effect
Dimercaprol	Treats arsenic toxicity, especially in the first 24 hours after exposure.
Vitamin C	Defends (somewhat) against arsenic toxicity.

Lab Tests to Detect Deficiency

Deficiency is determined by hair or blood tests.

M I N E R A L S

Boron

Basic Information

Boron is found in high concentrations in the parathyroid glands.

- Available from natural sources? Yes
- Available from synthetic sources? No
- Prescription required? No

Natural Sources

Apples	Drinking Water	Leafy vegetables
Beer	(in certain areas)	Legumes
Carrots	Grains	Nuts
Cider	Grapes	Pears

Benefits

- Important for preservation and development of bone
- Inhibits osteoporosis by halting demineralization (see Glossary) of bones
- Increases calcium absorption and metabolism
- Promotes normal growth and development

→

Possible Additional Benefits

- May help treat osteoarthritis
- May improve immune system by boosting production of infection-fighting antibodies
- May treat arthritis pain and stiffness
- May reduce hypertension

Who May Benefit from Additional Amounts?

Individuals at high risk for developing osteoporosis

Deficiency Symptoms

Poor bone development

Usage Information

What this mineral does:
- Necessary element for plants
- Important for mineral and energy metabolism
- Regulates hormones
- Important for bone growth and maintenance
- Contributes to health of cell membranes
- Aids some enzyme reactions

Miscellaneous Information:
Boric acid is commonly used as an eye wash and antiseptic for the skin.

Available as:
- Individual supplement
- A constituent of some multivitamins

Warnings and Precautions

Consult your doctor if you have:
- Osteoporosis
- Hypercalcemia

Pregnancy:
Consult your doctor.

Breastfeeding:
Consult your doctor.

Storage:
- Store safely out of reach of children.
- Store in a cool, dry place away from direct light, but don't freeze.
- Don't store in bathroom medicine cabinet. Heat and moisture may change the action of the mineral.

Overdose/Toxicity

Signs and symptoms:
Nausea, vomiting, hair loss, skin rash, lethargy, headache, diarrhea, hypothermia, restlessness, kidney damage, circulatory collapse and shock leading to death.

What to do:
For symptoms of overdose:
Discontinue mineral and consult doctor immediately. Also see *Adverse Reactions or Side Effects* section below.

For accidental overdose (such as child taking entire bottle): Dial 911 (emergency), 0 for operator or call your nearest Poison Control Center.

Adverse Reactions or Side Effects

Reaction or effect	What to do
Appetite loss	Discontinue. Call doctor when convenient.
Nausea	Discontinue. Call doctor when convenient.
Weight loss	Discontinue. Call doctor when convenient.

Interaction with Medicine, Vitamins or Minerals

Interacts with	Combined effect
Calcium	Aids metabolism of calcium.
Magnesium	Aids metabolism of magnesium.
Phosphorus	Aids metabolism of phosphorus.

Lab Tests to Detect Deficiency

None are available.

Calcium

Basic Information

Calcium citrate and *calcium gluconate* are common forms of calcium supplements.

- Available from natural sources? Yes
- Available from synthetic sources? Yes
- Prescription required? Yes, for some forms
- *RDA/DRI and Optimal Intake,* see page 476

Natural Sources

Almonds	Kelp
Brazil nuts	Milk
Broccoli	Pudding
Calcium-fortified cereal, rice, juice	Salmon, canned
	Sardines, canned
Caviar	Tofu
Cheese	Turnip greens
Cottage cheese	Yogurt

Benefits

- Helps prevent osteoporosis
- Treats calcium depletion in people with hypoparathyroidism, osteomalacia, rickets
- Used medically to treat tetany (severe muscle spasms) caused by sensitivity reactions, cardiac arrest, lead poisoning
- Used medically as an antidote to magnesium poisoning
- Prevents muscle or leg cramps in some people
- Promotes normal growth and development
- Builds bones and teeth
- Maintains bone density and strength
- Buffers acid in stomach and acts as antacid
- Helps regulate heartbeat, blood clotting, muscle contraction
- Treats neonatal hypocalcemia
- Promotes storage and release of some body hormones
- Lowers phosphate concentrations in people with chronic kidney disease
- Helps reduce blood pressure in certain people

Possible Additional Benefits

- May help decrease risk of kidney stones
- May reduce leg cramps

MINERALS

→

- Potential treatment for toxemia in pregnant women
- May reduce the risk of colon cancer

Who May Benefit from Additional Amounts?

- Anyone with inadequate caloric or dietary intake or increased nutritional requirements or those who do not like or consume milk products
- People allergic to milk and milk products
- People with untreated lactase deficiency who avoid milk and dairy products
- People over 55 years old, particularly women
- Women throughout adult life, especially during pregnancy and lactation, but not limited to these times
- Those who abuse alcohol or other drugs
- People with a chronic wasting illness
- Those under excess stress for long periods
- Anyone who has recently undergone surgery
- People with bone fractures
- Adolescents with low dietary calcium intake

Deficiency Symptoms

Osteoporosis (late symptoms):

- Frequent fractures in spine and other bones
- Deformed spinal column with humps
- Loss of height

Osteomalacia:

- Frequent fractures
- Muscle contractions
- Convulsive seizures
- Muscle cramps

Usage Information

What this mineral does:

- Participates in metabolic functions necessary for normal activity of nervous, muscular, skeletal systems
- Plays important role in normal heart function, kidney function, blood clotting, blood-vessel integrity
- Helps utilize vitamin B-12

Miscellaneous information:

- Bones serve as a storage site for calcium in the body. There is a constant interchange between calcium in bone and in the bloodstream.
- Foods rich in calcium (or supplements) help maintain the balance between bone needs and blood needs.
- Exercise, a balanced diet, calcium from natural sources or supplements and estrogens are important in treating and preventing osteoporosis.
- The aluminum found in some antacids may interfere with the absorption of calcium.
- Recent studies indicate that bone mineral content is increased when calcium supplements are given during adolescence.
- Those who live in geographic areas with low sun exposure and home-bound or institutionalized persons should take vitamin D with calcium to improve absorption.

Available as:

- Tablets: Swallow whole with a full glass of liquid. Don't chew or crush. Take with or 1 to 1-1/2 hours after meals unless otherwise directed by your doctor.
- Chewable tablets: Chew well before swallowing.
- Calcium is available as carbonate, citrate, and gluconate, with varying levels of bioavailability (see Glossary).

Warnings and Precautions

Don't take if you:
- Are allergic to calcium or antacids
- Have a high blood-calcium level
- Have sarcoidosis

Consult your doctor if you have:
- Kidney disease
- Chronic constipation, colitis, diarrhea
- Stomach or intestinal bleeding
- Irregular heartbeat
- Heart problems or high blood pressure for which you are taking a calcium channel blocker

Over 55:
- Adverse reactions and side effects are more likely.
- Diarrhea or constipation are particularly likely.

Pregnancy:
- Pregnant women may need extra calcium. Consult your doctor about supplements.
- Don't take megadoses (see Optimal Daily Intake Information, page 476).

Breastfeeding:
- The drug passes into milk. Consult your doctor about supplements.
- Don't take megadoses (see Optimal Daily Intake Information, page 476).

Effect on lab tests:
- Serum-amylase and serum-11 hydroxycorticosteroid concentrations can be increased.
- Excessive, prolonged use decreases serum-phosphate concentration.

Storage:
- Store in cool, dry area away from direct light, but don't freeze.
- Store safely out of reach of children.
- Don't store in bathroom medicine cabinet. Heat and moisture may change the action of the mineral.

Others:
- Dolomite and bone meal are probably unsafe sources of calcium because they contain lead.
- Avoid taking calcium within 1 or 2 hours of meals or ingestion of other medicines, if possible.
- Some calcium carbonate is derived from oyster shells. Calcium carbonate derived from this source is not recommended!

 Overdose/Toxicity

Signs and symptoms:
Confusion, slow or irregular heartbeat, bone or muscle pain, nausea, vomiting (signs and symptoms of toxicity have not been seen, even at doses of 2 to 3 grams/day).

What to do:
For symptoms of overdose:
Discontinue mineral and consult doctor immediately. Also see *Adverse Reactions or Side Effects* section below.

For accidental overdose (such as child taking entire bottle): Dial 911 (emergency), 0 for operator or call your nearest Poison Control Center.

 Adverse Reactions or Side Effects

Reaction or effect	What to do
Early signs of too much calcium in blood:	
Constipation	Increase fluid intake. Discontinue. Call doctor when convenient.
Headache	Discontinue. Call doctor when convenient.
Late signs of too much calcium in blood:	
Confusion	Discontinue. Call doctor immediately.

MINERALS

➔

Muscle or bone pain	Discontinue. Call doctor immediately.
Nausea or vomiting	Discontinue. Call doctor immediately.
Slow or irregular heartbeat	Seek emergency treatment.

Interaction with Medicine, Vitamins or Minerals

Interacts with	Combined effect
Cellulose sodium phosphate	Decreases effect of cellulose sodium phosphate.
Digitalis preparations	Causes heartbeat irregularities.
Etidronate	Decreases effects of etidronate. Don't take within 2 hours of calcium supplements.
Gallium nitrate	Inhibits function of gallium nitrate.
Iron supplements	Decreases absorption of iron unless vitamin C is taken at the same time.
Magnesium-containing medications or supplements	Increases absorption of magnesium and calcium.
Oral contraceptives and estrogens	May increase calcium absorption.
Phenytoin	Decreases effect of both calcium and phenytoin. Do not take calcium within 1 to 3 hours of phenytoin.
Tetracyclines (oral)	Decreases absorption of tetracycline.
Vitamin D	Increases absorption of calcium supplements.

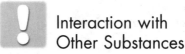

Interaction with Other Substances

Alcohol decreases absorption.

Beverages:
Caffeine (coffee, tea, cola, chocolate) can decrease absorption but has not been shown to decrease bone density.

Lab Tests to Detect Deficiency

- 24-hour urine collection to measure calcium levels (Sulkowitch)
- Imaging procedures to scan for bone density (more reliable than above test)

Chloride

 Basic Information

- Available from natural sources? Yes
- Available from synthetic sources? Yes
- Prescription required? No

 Natural Sources

Salt substitutes (potassium chloride)
Sea salt
Table salt (sodium chloride)
Note: Chloride is found in combination with other molecules.

 Benefits

- Regulates body's electrolyte (see Glossary) balance
- Regulates body's acid-base balance
- Promotes nerve and muscle function

 Possible Additional Benefits

None are known.

 Who May Benefit from Additional Amounts?

- People with Bartter's syndrome
- Individuals with renal tubular disorders or cystic fibrosis

 Deficiency Symptoms

Note: Chloride deficiency is basically unheard of in the United States except in people with acute acid-base disorders.

Causes:

- Continuous vomiting can lead to a deficiency.
- When chloride is intentionally neglected in infant-formula preparations, the infant develops metabolic alkalosis, hypovolemia and significant urinary loss. Psychomotor defects, memory loss and growth retardation also occur. This is not a problem with commercially available formulas.

Symptoms:

- Upsets balance of acids and bases in body fluids (rare)
- Nausea
- Vomiting
- Confusion
- Weakness
- Coma

 Usage Information

What this mineral does:

- Chloride is a constituent of acid in the stomach (hydrochloric acid).
- It interacts with sodium, potassium and carbon dioxide to maintain acid-base balance in body cells and fluids. It is crucial to normal health.
- Concentrations of sodium, potassium, carbon dioxide and chlorine are controlled by mechanisms inside each body cell.

Miscellaneous information:

- Healthy people do not have to make any special efforts to maintain sufficient chloride.
- Eating a balanced diet supplies all daily needs.

MINERALS

- Extremely ill patients, with acid-base imbalance, require hospitalization, frequent lab studies and skillful professional care.

Available as:
- Sodium-chloride (salt) tablets: These may cause stomach distress and overload on kidneys.
- Chloride is a constituent of many multivitamin/mineral preparations.

 ## Warnings and Precautions

Chloride supplement is not warranted except with significant alterations in acid-base balance, which would require medical care.

 ## Overdose/Toxicity

Signs and symptoms:

Upset in balance of acids and bases in body fluids can occur with too much chloride or with too little chloride. Symptoms of either include weakness, confusion and coma.

Consumption of reasonable amounts of chloride in the form of table salt or potassium replacement is not problematic.

What to do:

For symptoms of overdose: Discontinue mineral and consult doctor.

For accidental overdose (such as child taking a large amount): Dial 911 (emergency), 0 for operator or call your nearest Poison Control Center.

 ## Adverse Reactions or Side Effects

None are expected.

 ## Interaction with Medicine, Vitamins or Minerals

Interacts with	Combined effect
Chlorine	Maintains normal acid-base balance in body.
Potassium	Maintains normal acid-base balance in body.
Sodium	Maintains normal acid-base balance in body.

 ## Interaction with Other Substances

None are known.

 ## Lab Tests to Detect Deficiency

Serum chloride

Chromium

Basic Information

- Available from natural sources? Yes
- Available from synthetic sources? No
- Prescription required? No
- *Optimal Intake,* see page 476

Natural Sources

Apples	Eggs
Beef	Molasses
Brewer's yeast	Sweet potatoes
Calf liver	Tomatoes
Cheese	Whole-grain
Chicken	products
Corn on the cob	

Benefits

- Promotes glucose metabolism
- Helps insulin regulate blood sugar
- Decreases insulin requirements and improves glucose tolerance of some people with type II diabetes
- Aids in protein synthesis

Possible Additional Benefits

- May promote a decrease in total cholesterol and LDL (see Glossary)
- Possible weight loss and increase in muscle tissue

Who May Benefit from Additional Amounts?

- Those who abuse alcohol or other drugs
- People with a chronic wasting illness
- Anyone who has recently undergone surgery
- Possibly diabetics

Deficiency Symptoms

- Reduced tissue sensitivity to glucose, similar to diabetes
- Disturbances of glucose, fat and protein metabolism
- Numbness in extremities

Usage Information

What this mineral does:

- Aids transport of glucose into cells
- Enhances effect of insulin in glucose utilization

Miscellaneous information:

- Chromium toxicity can result from industrial overexposure, such as tanning, electroplating, steel making, abrasives manufacturing, cement manufacturing, diesel-locomotive repairs, furniture polishing, fur processing, glass making, jewelry making, metal cleaning, oil drilling, photography, textile dyeing and wood preservative manufacturing.
- Nutritional science has yet to determine the exact amounts of chromium in most foods. Less than 1 percent of dietary chromium is absorbed.

Available as:

- A constituent of many multivitamin/mineral preparations
- An individualized supplement

MINERALS

Warnings and Precautions

Don't take if you:
Work in an environment that has high concentrations of chromium.

Consult your doctor if you have:
• Diabetes
• Lung disease
• Liver disease
• Kidney disease

Over 55:
No special needs if you eat a balanced diet.

Pregnancy:
Avoid chromium during pregnancy until further information is available.

Breastfeeding:
Avoid chromium during breastfeeding until further information is available.

Effect on lab tests:
Diagnostic tests, such as red-blood-cell-survival studies performed after radioactive-hexavalent chromium is used for 3 months, may cause falsely elevated levels in blood.

Storage:
• Store in cool, dry place away from direct light, but don't freeze.
• Store safely out of reach of children.
• Don't store in bathroom medicine cabinet. Heat and moisture may change the action of the mineral.

 Overdose/Toxicity

Signs and symptoms:
The dietary form has very low toxicity. Long-term exposure to environmental chromium may lead to skin problems, liver impairment or kidney impairment.

What to do:
For symptoms of overdose:
Discontinue mineral and consult doctor.

For accidental overdose (such as child taking entire bottle): Dial 911 (emergency), 0 for operator or call your nearest Poison Control Center.

 Adverse Reactions or Side Effects

None are expected.

 Interaction with Medicine, Vitamins or Minerals

Interacts with	Combined effect
Insulin	May decrease amount of insulin needed to treat diabetes if taken at high levels.

 Lab Tests to Detect Deficiency

• Serum chromium
• Hair analysis not reliable test for deficiency or toxicity

Cobalt

 Basic Information

- Available from natural sources? Yes
- Available from synthetic sources? Yes
- Prescription required? No, but supplements are hard to find, so adequate food intake is important.

 Natural Sources

Clams	Liver
Dairy products	Meats
Kidney	Oysters

Note: Small amounts in diet satisfy requirements, except under unusual circumstances. Small amounts exist in some plant foods but are best utilized as part of B-12-rich foods.

 Benefits

- Promotes normal red-blood-cell formation
- Constituent of B-12
- Involved in enzyme reactions
- Aids in forming myelin nerve coverings

 Possible Additional Benefits

- May play a role in treating anemia that does not respond to other treatment
- May treat fatigue, digestive disorders and neuromuscular problems
- May treat certain cancers (radioactive cobalt-60)

 Who May Benefit from Additional Amounts?

- People with recent severe burns or injuries
- Those with anorexia nervosa or bulimia
- Vegan vegetarians with inadequate B-12 intake

 Deficiency Symptoms

Pernicious anemia, with the following symptoms:

- Weakness, especially in arms and legs
- Sore tongue
- Nausea, appetite loss, weight loss
- Bleeding gums
- Numbness and tingling in hands and feet
- Difficulty maintaining balance
- Pale lips, tongue, gums
- Confusion and dementia
- Headache
- Poor memory

 Usage Information

What this mineral does:

Cobalt acts as a catalyst in complex reactions to form vitamin B-12.

Miscellaneous information:

- Cobalt is a trace element stored mainly in the liver.
- Deficiency is extremely rare.
- It is a necessary ingredient to manufacture vitamin B-12 in the body. A deficiency of cobalt may lead to a deficiency of vitamin B-12 and therefore to pernicious anemia.

Available as:

Capsules: Swallow whole with a full glass of liquid. Don't chew or crush. Take with or 1 to 1-1/2 hours after meals unless otherwise directed by your doctor.

MINERALS

➜

Warnings and Precautions

Consult your doctor if you:
No problems are expected.

Over 55:
Eat a balanced diet to prevent deficiency.

Pregnancy:
Take as B-12 if your doctor advises.

Breastfeeding:
Take as B-12 if your doctor advises.

Effect on lab tests:
None are expected.

Storage:
- Store in cool, dry place away from direct light, but don't freeze.
- Store safely out of reach of children.
- Don't store in bathroom medicine cabinet. Heat and moisture may change the action of the mineral.

 ## Overdose/Toxicity

Signs and symptoms:
- In large doses (20–30mg/day), cobalt can produce polycythemia, enlargement of thyroid gland and enlargement of the heart leading to congestive heart failure (See Glossary).
- Cobalt toxicity can cause thyroid overgrowth in infants.

What to do:
For symptoms of overdose:
Discontinue mineral and consult doctor. Also see *Adverse Reactions or Side Effects* section below.

For accidental overdose (such as child taking large amounts): Dial 911 (emergency), 0 for operator or call your nearest Poison Control Center.

 ## Adverse Reactions or Side Effects

Reaction or effect	What to do
With megadoses:	
Enlargement of heart	Discontinue. Call doctor immediately.
Enlargement of thyroid gland	Discontinue. Call doctor immediately.
Polycythemia	Discontinue. Call doctor immediately.

 ## Interaction with Medicine, Vitamins or Minerals

Interacts with	Combined effect
Colchicine	May cause inaccurate lab studies of cobalt or vitamin B-12.
Neomycin	May cause inaccurate lab studies of cobalt or vitamin B-12.
Para-aminosalicylic acid	May cause inaccurate lab studies of cobalt or vitamin B-12.
Phenytoin	May cause inaccurate lab studies of cobalt or vitamin B-12.

 ## Interaction with Other Substances

Some beer contains cobalt as a stabilizer. People who consume large quantities of cobalt-stabilized beer over long periods may develop cobalt toxicity leading to cardiomyopathy (see Glossary) and congestive heart failure (see Glossary).

 ## Lab Tests to Detect Deficiency

- Concentration in human plasma
- Measured in bioassay as part of vitamin B-12

Copper

Basic Information

- Available from natural sources? Yes
- Available from synthetic sources? No
- Prescription required? No
- *DV and Optimal Intake,* see page 476

Natural Sources

Avocados	Oysters
Fish	Peanuts
Legumes	Raisins
Lentils	Salmon
Liver	Shell fish
Lobster	Soybeans
Nuts	Spinach
Oats	

Note: Copper-bottom pans and pipes can also raise the copper content of water and food supply.

Benefits

- Promotes normal red-blood-cell formation
- Acts as a catalyst in storage and release of iron to form hemoglobin for red blood cells
- Assists in production of several enzymes involved in respiration
- Promotes connective-tissue formation and central-nervous-system function
- Assists in production of several enzymes involved in forming melanin
- Promotes normal insulin function
- Helps maintain myelin
- Part of superoxide dismutase and its antioxidant (see Glossary) capacity

Possible Additional Benefits

- May be used to treat nutritional anemias along with iron, B-12 and/or folate
- May protect against cardiovascular disease; however, balance is critical because high levels of copper have been seen in patients with cardiovascular disease
- Possibly reduces inflammation associated with arthritis
- May enhance immune function

Who May Benefit from Additional Amounts?

- Anyone with inadequate caloric or dietary intake or increased nutritional requirements
- People over 55 years old
- Those who abuse alcohol or other drugs
- People with a chronic wasting illness, particularly those with chronic diarrhea, malabsorption disorders (see Glossary), kidney disease
- Anyone on long-term zinc supplementation
- People with recent severe burns or injuries

Deficiency Symptoms

- Anemia
- Low white-blood-cell count associated with reduced resistance to infection
- Faulty collagen formation
- Bone demineralization (see Glossary)
- Loss of hair, skin pigmentation

➔

MINERALS

Usage Information

What this mineral does:
Copper is an essential component of a number of proteins and enzymes, including lysyl, hydroxylase and dopamine beta-hydroxylase.

Miscellaneous information:
- Plasma-copper levels may increase in people with rheumatoid arthritis, pregnancy, cirrhosis of the liver, myocardial infarction (heart attack), schizophrenia, tumors or severe infections.
- Copper supplementation of 2mg/day is recommended for people on long-term zinc therapy supplementation.
- Menkes syndrome is a genetic defect in copper metabolism, which requires medical intervention.
- Processed foods may reduce normal copper absorption.
- Plasma-copper levels decrease with hypothyroidism, neutropenia, leukopenia, kwashiorkor, sprue, and nephrosis.
- Most nutritionists recommend a balanced diet rather than extra supplementation that could upset the body's delicate mineral balance.

Available as:
- Tablets: Swallow whole with a full glass of liquid. Don't chew or crush. Take with or 1 to 1-1/2 hours after meals unless otherwise directed by your doctor.
- Copper is a constituent of many multivitamin/mineral preparations.

Warnings and Precautions

Don't take if you:
Have Wilson's disease.

Consult your doctor if you are:
Considering taking a copper supplement.

Over 55:
No problems are expected.

Pregnancy:
Consult your doctor.

Breastfeeding:
Consult your doctor.

Effect on lab tests:
Cobalt, iron, nickel and oral contraceptives with estrogens can cause false-positive or elevated copper values.

Storage:
- Store in cool, dry place away from direct light, but don't freeze.
- Store safely out of reach of children.
- Don't store in bathroom medicine cabinet. Heat and moisture may change the action of the mineral.

Overdose/Toxicity

Signs and symptoms:
Nausea, vomiting, muscle aches, abdominal pain, anemia.

What to do:
For symptoms of overdose:
Discontinue mineral and consult doctor.

For accidental overdose (such as child taking entire bottle): Dial 911 (emergency), 0 for operator or call your nearest Poison Control Center.

Adverse Reactions or Side Effects

None are expected.

Interaction with Medicine, Vitamins or Minerals

Interacts with	Combined effect
Cadmium	May interfere with copper absorption and utilization.
Fiber	May interfere with copper absorption and utilization. Not clinically significant.
Molybdenum	Maintains appropriate ratio of copper to molybdenum in body. If you have excessive amounts of copper, your molybdenum level drops. If you have excessive amounts of molybdenum, your copper level drops.
Oral contraceptives	Increases copper level. Significance unknown at present.
Phytates (cereals, vegetables)	May interfere with copper absorption and utilization. Not clinically significant.
Vitamin C	Decreases absorption of copper. Large doses of vitamin C must be taken to produce this effect.
Zinc	May interfere with copper absorption and utilization. Copper supplement advised.

Interaction with Other Substances

None are known.

Lab Tests to Detect Deficiency

- Plasma-copper levels
- Urine-copper levels in 24-hour collection

MINERALS

Fluoride

Basic Information

Fluoride is available commercially as *sodium fluoride.*

- Available from natural sources? Yes
- Available from synthetic sources? Yes
- Prescription required? Yes, for some forms
- *DRI and Optimal Intake,* see page 476

Natural Sources

Apples	Salmon, canned
Calf liver	Sardines, canned
Cod	Tea
Eggs	Water
Kidney	

Note: The fluoride content of foods varies tremendously. It is relatively high where soils are rich and water is fluoridated and low otherwise.

Benefits

- Prevents dental caries (cavities) in children when level of fluoride in water is inadequate
- Treats osteoporosis with calcium and vitamin D, but use must be carefully monitored by a physician

Possible Additional Benefits

May play a role in preventing osteoporosis

→

Who May Benefit from Additional Amounts?

People living in an area with low-fluoride water content (check with your doctor, dentist or local health department)

 ## Deficiency Symptoms

Significant increase in dental cavities

 ## Usage Information

What this mineral does:

- Contributes to solid bone and tooth formation by helping body retain calcium
- Interferes with growth and development of bacteria that cause dental plaque

Miscellaneous information:

- Taking fluoride does not remove the need for good dental habits, including a good diet, brushing and flossing teeth and regular dental visits.
- If fluoride supplementation is needed in your area, continue until your child is 16. Subsequent topical applications every year or two may be continued to prevent cavities.

Available as:

- Tablets: Swallow whole with a full glass of liquid. Don't chew or crush. Take with or 1 to 1-1/2 hours after meals unless otherwise directed by your doctor.
- Drops: Dilute in at least 1/2 glass of water or other liquid. Take with or 1 to 1-1/2 hours after meals unless otherwise directed by your doctor. Do not take with milk or dairy products.

- Rinses: Follow directions and use just before bedtime, after proper brushing and flossing.
- Gels: Follow directions and use just before bedtime, after proper brushing and flossing.
- Paste: Follow directions and use just before bedtime, after proper brushing and flossing.

 ## Warnings and Precautions

Don't take if:

Fluoride intake from drinking water exceeds 0.7 parts fluoride/million. Too much fluoride stains teeth permanently (fluorosis).

Consult your doctor if you have:

- Osteoporosis
- Underactive thyroid function

Over 55:

No problems are expected.

Pregnancy:

Reports do not agree on benefit and risk to unborn child. Follow your doctor's instructions.

Breastfeeding:

Consult your doctor. Infant supplementation may be advised.

Effect on lab tests:

- Serum acid phosphatase, serum calcium and protein-bound iodine may be falsely decreased.
- Serum aspartate aminotransferase—SGOT (see Glossary)—may be falsely increased.

Storage:

- Store in cool, dry place away from direct light, but don't freeze.
- Keep in original plastic container. Fluoride decomposes glass.
- Store safely out of reach of children.

- Don't store in bathroom medicine cabinet. Heat and moisture may change the action of the mineral.

Overdose/Toxicity

Signs and symptoms:
- Stomach cramps or pain, faintness, vomiting (possibly bloody), diarrhea, black stools, shallow breathing, tremors, increased saliva, unusual excitement.
- Whitish streaks or patches or brown streaking (dental fluorosis) may occur in children whose tooth enamel is not completely formed.

What to do:

For symptoms of overdose:
Discontinue mineral and consult doctor. Also see *Adverse Reactions or Side Effects* section below.

For accidental overdose (such as child taking entire bottle): Dial 911 (emergency), 0 for operator or call your nearest Poison Control Center.

Adverse Reactions or Side Effects

Reaction or effect	What to do
With excessive amounts of fluoride:	
Appetite loss	Discontinue. Call doctor when convenient.
Constipation	Discontinue. Call doctor when convenient.
Mottling of teeth with brown, black or white discoloration	Discontinue. Call doctor when convenient.
Nausea	Discontinue. Call doctor when convenient.
Skin rash	Discontinue. Call doctor immediately.

Interaction with Medicine, Vitamins or Minerals

Interacts with	Combined effect
Aluminum hydroxide	Decreases absorption of fluoride.
Calcium supplements	Decreases absorption of fluoride.

Interaction with Other Substances

Beverages: Milk decreases absorption of fluoride. Take dose 2 hours before or after drinking milk.

Lab Tests to Detect Deficiency

None are available. Examinations of mouth for dental cavities once or twice a year yield all necessary evidence.

MINERALS

Germanium

 Basic Information

The oil form is used in aromatherapy.

- Available from natural sources? Yes
- Available from synthetic sources? Yes
- Prescription required? No

 Natural Sources

Aloe vera	Ginseng
Comfrey	Onions
Chlorella	Shiitake mushrooms
Garlic	Suma

 Benefits

Boosts oxygenation (see Glossary) of tissue

 Possible Additional Benefits

- May aid immune system
- May help rid the body of toxins and poisons
- Possible treatment for rheumatoid arthritis
- May treat food allergies
- Potential treatment for candidiasis
- May promote wound healing
- Oil form may be useful in treating wounds and burns, stress, menopausal and menstrual difficulties, athlete's foot, eczema, shingles, sore throat, mouth ulcers, insect stings, headaches, hemorrhoids

 Who May Benefit from Additional Amounts?

Those with immune suppression

 Deficiency 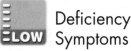 Symptoms

No proven symptoms exist.

 Usage Information

What this mineral does:
Germanium is involved in cellular oxygenation (see Glossary).

Miscellaneous information:
- Used to make computer chips
- Best taken by eating foods rich in germanium

Available as:
- Tablets– take as directed by manufacturer or your doctor.
- Powder– take as directed by manufacturer or your doctor.
- Capsules– take as directed by manufacturer or your doctor.
- Oil– take as directed by manufacturer or your doctor.
- "Organic" form: 25 mg/day (GE-132)—other forms may cause kidney damage.

STOP Warnings and Precautions

Pregnancy: **Breastfeeding:**
Do not use.   Do not use.

Storage:
- Store in a cool, dry place away from direct light, but don't freeze.
- Store safely out of reach of children.
- Don't store in bathroom medicine cabinet. Heat and moisture may change the action of the mineral.

Others:
Do not use oils around eyes.

Overdose/Toxicity

Signs and symptoms:
Large doses may harm kidneys, liver, muscles, nerves and brain.

What to do:
For symptoms of overdose:
Discontinue mineral and consult doctor immediately.

For accidental overdose (such as child taking entire bottle): Dial 911 (emergency), 0 for operator or call your nearest Poison Control Center.

Adverse Reactions or Side Effects

None are expected.

Interaction with Medicine, Vitamins or Minerals

None are known.

Interaction with Other Substances

None are known.

Lab Tests to Detect Deficiency

None are available.

MINERALS

Iodine

Basic Information

- Available from natural sources? Yes
- Available from synthetic sources? No
- Prescription required? Yes, for strengths over 130mg
- *DV/RDA and Optimal Intake,* see page 476

Natural Sources

Lobster	Saltwater fish
Milk	(cod, haddock,
Nutritional yeast	herring)
Oysters	Sea salt
Salmon, canned	Seaweed
Salted nuts, seeds,	Shrimp
snack foods	Table salt (iodized)

Benefits

- Promotes normal function of thyroid gland
- Promotes normal cell function
- Shrinks thyroid prior to thyroid surgery
- Tests thyroid function before and after administration of a radioactive form of iodine
- Keeps skin, hair, nails healthy
- Prevents goiter

Possible Additional Benefits

None are known.

➜

Who May Benefit from Additional Amounts?

Anyone who lives in a region where the soil is deficient in iodine (deficiency is usually treated by using iodized table salt)

Deficiency Symptoms

Children:
• Depressed growth
• Delayed sexual development
• Mental retardation
• Deafness

Adults:
Goiter

Symptoms of low thyroid-hormone level (children and adults):
• Listlessness
• Sluggish behavior

Usage Information

What this mineral does:
Iodine is an integral part of the thyroid hormones tetraiodothyronine (thyroxin) and triiodothyronine.

Miscellaneous information:
Iodized salt and the use of iodophors as antiseptics by the dairy industry are the main source of iodine in most diets.

Available as:
• Tablets: Swallow whole with a full glass of liquid. Don't chew or crush. Take with or 1 to 1-1/2 hours after meals unless otherwise directed by your doctor.
• Oral solution: Dilute in at least 1/2 glass of water or other liquid.

Take with or 1 to 1-1/2 hours after meals unless otherwise directed by your doctor.
• Enteric-coated tablets are not recommended. They may cause obstruction, bleeding and perforation of the small bowel.

Warnings and Precautions

Don't take if you have:
• Elevated serum potassium (determined by lab study)
• Myotonia congenita

Consult your doctor if you have:
• Hyperthyroidism
• Kidney disease
• Taken or are taking amiloride, antithyroid medications, lithium, spironolactone, triamterene

Over 55:
No problems are expected.

Pregnancy:
If you consume too much iodine during pregnancy, the infant may have thyroid enlargement, hypothyroidism or cretinism (dwarfism and mental deficiency).

Breastfeeding:
• Avoid supplements while nursing.
• Iodine in milk can cause skin rash and suppression of normal thyroid function in infant.

Effect on lab tests:
• May cause false elevation in all thyroid-function studies
• Interferes with test for naturally occurring steroids in urine

Storage:
• Store in cool, dry place away from direct light, but don't freeze.
• Store safely out of reach of children.

- Don't store in bathroom medicine cabinet. Heat and moisture may change the action of the mineral.

Overdose/Toxicity

Signs and symptoms:
Irregular heartbeat; confusion; difficulty breathing; swollen neck or throat; bloody or black, tarry stools.

What to do:
For symptoms of overdose:
Discontinue mineral and consult doctor. Also see *Adverse Reactions or Side Effects* section below.

For accidental overdose (such as child taking entire bottle): Dial 911 (emergency), 0 for operator or call your nearest Poison Control Center.

Adverse Reactions or Side Effects

Reaction or effect	What to do
Note: These reactions are all rare.	
Abdominal pain	Discontinue. Call doctor immediately.
Burning in mouth or throat	Discontinue. Call doctor immediately.
Diarrhea	Discontinue. Call doctor immediately.
Fever	Discontinue. Call doctor immediately.
Headache	Discontinue. Call doctor immediately.
Heavy legs	Discontinue. Call doctor when convenient.
Increased salivation	Discontinue. Call doctor immediately.
Metallic taste	Discontinue. Call doctor when convenient.
Nausea	Continue. Tell doctor at next visit.
Numbness, tingling or pain in hands or feet	Discontinue. Call doctor immediately.
Skin rash	Discontinue. Call doctor immediately.
Sore teeth or gums	Discontinue. Call doctor immediately.
Swelling of salivary gland	Seek emergency treatment.
Tiredness or weakness	Discontinue. Call doctor immediately.

Interaction with Medicine, Vitamins or Minerals

Interacts with	Combined effect
Lithium carbonate for manic-depressive illness	Produces abnormally low thyroid activity. People taking lithium carbonate should avoid iodine, which suppresses the thyroid gland.

Interaction with Other Substances

None are known.

Lab Tests to Detect Deficiency

Tests may indicate lower than normal thyroid function, implying a deficiency of iodine in some cases.

MINERALS

Iron

Basic Information

Ferrous sulfate is the most common form of iron.

- Available from natural sources? Yes
- Available from synthetic sources? Yes
- Prescription required? Yes, for some forms
- *DV/RDA and Optimal Intake,* see page 476

Natural Sources

Bread, enriched
Egg yolk
Fish
Garbanzo beans (chickpeas)
Lentils
Liver
Molasses, blackstrap

Mussels
Oysters
Red meats
Seaweed, greens
Whole-grain products, enriched

Note: Only about 10 percent of food iron is absorbed from food consumed by an individual with normal iron stores; however, an iron-deficient person may absorb 20 to 30 percent.

Benefits

- Prevents and treats iron-deficiency anemia due to dietary iron deficiency or other causes
- Stimulates bone-marrow production of hemoglobin, the red-blood-cell pigment that carries oxygen to body cells
- Forms part of several enzymes and proteins in the body

Possible Additional Benefits

- May help alleviate menstrual discomfort
- May stimulate immunity in iron-deficient people
- May promote learning in children with iron deficiency

Who May Benefit from Additional Amounts?

- Many women, of child-bearing age, with heavy menstrual flow and women with long menstrual periods or short menstrual cycles (common in teenage girls)
- Anyone with inadequate caloric or dietary intake or increased nutritional requirements
- People over 55 years old
- Pregnant or breastfeeding women
- Those who abuse alcohol or other drugs
- People with a chronic wasting illness
- Those under excess stress for long periods
- Anyone who has recently undergone surgery
- Athletes and workers who participate in vigorous physical activities
- Anyone who has lost blood recently, such as from heavy menstrual periods, an accident or long-term, undetected gastrointestinal bleeding
- Vegetarians with inadequate dietary intake
- Infants from 2 to 24 months

Deficiency Symptoms

- Listlessness
- Heart palpitations upon exertion
- Fatigue
- Irritability
- Pale appearance to skin, mucous membranes, nails
- Decreased mental capacity, learning deficit
- Pica

Usage Information

What this mineral does:

- Iron is an essential component of hemoglobin, myoglobin and a cofactor (see Glossary) of several essential enzymes. Of the total iron in the body, 60 to 70 percent is stored in hemoglobin (the red part of red blood cells).
- Hemoglobin is also a component of myoglobin, an iron-protein complex in muscles. This complex helps muscles get extra energy when they work hard.

Miscellaneous information:

- Iron-deficiency anemia in older men is usually due to a slow loss of blood.
- Iron content of foods, especially acidic foods, can be dramatically increased when prepared in iron cookware.
- You may require 3 weeks of treatment before you receive the maximum benefit.
- Vitamin C (ascorbic acid) enhances iron absorption.
- Elevated iron levels have been associated with a high risk of heart disease.

Available as:

- Tablets and capsules: Swallow whole with a full glass of liquid. Don't chew

or crush. Take with food or immediately after eating to decrease stomach irritation.
- Oral solution: Dilute in at least 1/2 glass of water or other liquid. Take with or 1 to 1-1/2 hours after meals unless otherwise directed by your doctor.
- Chewable tablets: Chew well before swallowing.
- Enteric-coated tablets: Swallow whole with a full glass of liquid. Take with meals or 1 to 1-1/2 hours after meals unless otherwise directed by your doctor.

Warnings and Precautions

Don't take if you have:

- An allergy to any iron supplement
- Acute hepatitis
- Hemosiderosis or hemochromatosis (conditions involving excess iron in body)
- Hemolytic anemia
- Had repeated blood transfusions

Consult your doctor if you have:

- Plans to become pregnant while taking medication
- Had peptic-ulcer disease, enteritis, colitis
- Had pancreatitis or hepatitis
- Alcoholism
- Kidney disease
- Intestinal disease
- Excess vitamin C—problematic in people with iron-storage disorder

Over 55:

- Deficiency is not uncommon. Check frequently with your doctor for anemia symptoms or slow blood loss in stool.
- If there is a history of heart disease in your family, consult your doctor before supplementing your diet with iron.

MINERALS

→

Pregnancy:

Pregnancy increases need. Check with doctor. During first 3 months of pregnancy, take only if your doctor prescribes it.

Breastfeeding:

- Supplements probably aren't necessary if you are healthy and eat a balanced diet. Consult your doctor.
- Your baby may need supplementation, especially premature infants. Consult your doctor.

Effect on lab tests:

Iron may cause abnormal results in serum bilirubin, serum calcium, serum iron, special radioactive studies of bones using technetium (Tc-99m-labeled agents) and stool studies for blood.

Storage:

- Store in cool, dry place away from direct light, but don't freeze.
- Store safely out of reach of children, with childproof cap. Iron tablets look like candy, and children have been known to overdose.
- Don't store in bathroom medicine cabinet. Heat and moisture may change the action of the mineral.

Others:

- Iron can accumulate to harmful levels (hemosiderosis) in patients with chronic kidney failure, Hodgkins disease or rheumatoid arthritis.
- Prolonged use in high doses can cause hemochromatosis (iron-storage disease), leading to bronze skin, diabetes, liver damage, impotence and heart problems.

 Overdose/Toxicity

Signs and symptoms:

- Early signs: Diarrhea with blood, severe nausea, abdominal pain, vomiting with blood.
- Late signs: Weakness; collapse; pallor; blue lips, hands, fingernails; shallow breathing; convulsions; coma; weak, rapid heartbeat.
- Too much iron may result in an increased risk of cancer and coronary disease.

What to do:

For symptoms of overdose:
Discontinue mineral and consult doctor. Also see *Adverse Reactions or Side Effects* section below.

For accidental overdose (such as child taking entire bottle): Dial 911 (emergency), 0 for operator or call your nearest Poison Control Center.

 Adverse Reactions or Side Effects

Reaction or effect	What to do
Abdominal pain	Discontinue. Call doctor immediately.
Black or gray stools (always)	Nothing.
Blood in stools	Seek emergency treatment.
Chest pain	Seek emergency treatment.
Drowsiness	Discontinue. Call doctor when convenient.
Stained tooth (with liquid forms)	Mix with water or juice to lessen effect. Brush teeth with baking soda or hydrogen peroxide to help remove stain.
Throat pain	Discontinue. Call doctor immediately.

Interaction with Medicine, Vitamins or Minerals

Interacts with	Combined effect
Allopurinol	May cause excess iron storage in liver.
Antacids	Causes poor iron absorption.
Calcium	Combination necessary for efficient calcium absorption.
Cholestyramine	Decreases iron effect.
Copper	Assists in copper absorption.
Iron supplements (other)	May cause excess iron storage in liver.
Pancreatin	Decreases iron absorption.
Penicillamine	Decreases penicillamine effect.
Sulfasalazine	Decreases iron effect.
Tetracyclines	Decreases tetracycline effect. Take iron 3 hours before or 2 hours after taking tetracycline.
Vitamin C	Increases iron effect. Necessary for red-blood-cell and hemoglobin formation.
Vitamin E	Decreases iron absorption.
Zinc (large doses)	Decreases iron absorption.

Interaction with Other Substances

Alcohol increases iron utilization and may cause organ damage. Avoid or use in moderation.

Food and beverages:
- Milk, cheese, yogurt and eggs decrease iron absorption.
- Tea decreases iron absorption.
- Coffee decreases iron absorption.
- Spinach decreases iron absorption.
- Bran, whole-grain breads and cereals decrease iron absorption.

Lab Tests to Detect Deficiency

- Red-blood-cell count
- Microscopic exam of red blood cells
- Serum iron, total iron-binding capacity
- Hemoglobin, low hematocrit determinations
- Serum ferritin

MINERALS

Magnesium

Basic Information

- Available from natural sources? Yes
- Available from synthetic sources? No
- Prescription required? Yes, for some forms
- *DV/DRI and Optimal Intake,* see page 477

Natural Sources

Almonds	Herring
Avocados	Leafy, green vegetables
Bananas	Mackerel
Bluefish	Molasses
Carp	Nuts
Cod	Ocean perch
Collards, beet greens	Shrimp
Dairy products	Swordfish
Flounder	Wheat germ
Halibut	Whole wheat bread

Benefits

- Aids bone growth
- Aids function of nerves and muscles, including regulation of normal heart rhythm
- Conducts nerve impulses
- Works as laxative in large doses
- Acts as antacid in small doses
- Strengthens tooth enamel

Possible Additional Benefits

- May help reduce the effects of lead poisoning
- May reduce kidney stones
- May be used to treat heart disease

Who May Benefit from Additional Amounts?

- Anyone with inadequate caloric or dietary intake or increased nutritional requirements
- Those who abuse alcohol or other drugs
- People with a chronic wasting illness
- Anyone who has recently undergone surgery
- Vomiting and diarrhea may increase need
- With medical supervision, may supplement treatment of acute myocardial infarction, cardiac surgery, digitalis toxicity and congestive heart failure

Deficiency Symptoms

Following symptoms occur rarely:

- Muscle contractions
- Convulsions
- Confusion, delirium, memory and concentration difficulties
- Irritability
- Nervousness
- Skin problems
- Hardening of soft tissues
- Hypertension
- Arrhythmia

Usage Information

What this mineral does:

- Activates essential enzymes
- Affects metabolism of proteins and nucleic acids
- Helps transport sodium and potassium across cell membranes
- Influences calcium levels inside cells
- Aids muscle contractions

Available as:

- Tablets, capsules, extended-release: Swallow whole with a full glass of liquid. Don't chew or crush. Take with or 1 to 1-1/2 hours after meals unless otherwise directed by your doctor.
- Liquid or powder: Follow manufacturer's instructions. Swallow with *at least* one full glass of liquid. Drink plenty of fluids throughout the day.
- Magnesium is a constituent of many multivitamin/mineral preparations.
- Injectable forms are administered by doctor or nurse.

Warnings and Precautions

Don't take if you have:

- Kidney failure
- Heart block (unless you have a pacemaker)
- Had an ileostomy

Consult your doctor if you have:

- Chronic constipation, colitis, diarrhea
- Symptoms of appendicitis
- Stomach or intestinal bleeding

Over 55:

Adverse reactions and side effects are more likely.

Pregnancy:

Risk to fetus. Don't use.

Breastfeeding:

Avoid magnesium except under advice of your physician.

Effect on lab tests:

- Inaccurate test for stomach-acid secretion
- May increase or decrease serum-phosphate concentrations
- May decrease serum and urine pH

Storage:

- Store in cool, dry place away from direct light, but don't freeze.
- Store safely out of reach of children.
- Don't store in bathroom medicine cabinet. Heat and moisture may change the action of the mineral.

Others:

- Chronic kidney disease causes body to retain excess magnesium.
- Adverse reactions, side effects and interactions with medicines, vitamins or minerals occur only rarely when you take too much magnesium for too long or if you have kidney disease.

 Overdose/Toxicity

Signs and symptoms:

Severe nausea and vomiting, extremely low blood pressure, extreme muscle weakness, difficulty breathing, heartbeat irregularity.

What to do:

For symptoms of overdose:
Discontinue mineral and consult doctor immediately. Also see *Adverse Reactions or Side Effects* section below.

For accidental overdose (such as child taking entire bottle): Dial 911 (emergency), 0 for operator or call your nearest Poison Control Center.

 Adverse Reactions or Side Effects

Reaction or effect	What to do
Abdominal pain	Discontinue. Call doctor immediately.
Appetite loss	Discontinue. Call doctor when convenient.
Diarrhea	Discontinue. Call doctor when convenient.
Irregular heartbeat	Seek emergency treatment.
Mood changes or mental changes	Discontinue. Call doctor when convenient.
Nausea	Discontinue. Call doctor when convenient.
Tiredness or weakness	Discontinue. Call doctor when convenient.
Urination discomfort	Discontinue. Call doctor when convenient.
Vomiting	Discontinue. Call doctor immediately.

 Interaction with Medicine, Vitamins or Minerals

Interacts with	Combined effect
Antibiotics (some)	Decreases magnesium levels.
Cellulose sodium phosphate	Decreases magnesium effect. Take 1 or more hours apart.
Diuretics (some)	Decreases magnesium level.
Ketoconazole	Reduces absorption of ketoconazole. Take 2 hours apart.
Mecamylamine	May slow urinary excretion of mecamylamine. Avoid combination
Tetracycline	Decreases absorption of tetracycline.
Vitamin D	May raise magnesium level too high.

MINERALS

→

Interaction with Other Substances

None are known.

Lab Tests to Detect Deficiency

Serum magnesium

Manganese

Basic Information

- Available from natural sources? Yes
- Available from synthetic sources? Yes
- Prescription required? Yes, for some forms
- *Optimal Intake,* see page 477

Natural Sources

Beans, dried
Blue- and
   blackberries
Bran
Buckwheat
Carrots
Chestnuts
Hazelnuts
   (filberts)

Oatmeal
Peanuts
Peas
Pecans
Seaweed
Spinach
Tea
Whole grains

Benefits

- Promotes normal growth and development
- Helps many enzymes generate energy
- Aids in carbohydrate metabolism
- Promotes nerve function
- Aids in formation of connective tissue
- Involved in antioxidation process

Possible Additional Benefits

- May reduce asthmatic symptoms
- May enhance fertility
- May promote glucose transport

Who May Benefit from Additional Amounts?

Anyone with inadequate caloric or nutritional dietary intake or increased nutritional requirements

Deficiency Symptoms

Note: Deficiencies are extremely rare because manganese is widely available in the food supply and requirements are very small.

- Abnormal growth and development of children
- No proven symptoms caused by manganese deficiency in adults

Usage Information

What this mineral does:

- Manganese is concentrated in the cells of the pituitary gland, liver, pancreas, kidney and bone. It stimulates production of cholesterol by the liver and is a cofactor (see Glossary) in many enzymes.

- Manganese works with vitamin K to promote blood clotting.

Miscellaneous information:

- Manganese is abundant in many foods.
- Manganese and magnesium are *not* related!

Available as:

- Capsules: Swallow whole with a full glass of liquid. Don't chew or crush. Take with food or immediately after eating to decrease stomach irritation.
- Manganese is a constituent of many multivitamin/mineral preparations.
- Injection

Warnings and Precautions

Don't take if you:
Are healthy and eat well.

Consult your doctor if you have:
- Liver disease
- Iron deficiency

Over 55:
No problems are expected.

Pregnancy:
Don't take supplements that contain manganese unless prescribed by your doctor.

Breastfeeding:
Don't take supplements that contain manganese unless prescribed by your doctor.

Effect on lab tests:
Excess manganese can reduce serum iron.

Storage:

- Store in cool, dry place away from direct light, but don't freeze.
- Store safely out of reach of children.
- Don't store in bathroom medicine cabinet. Heat and moisture may change the action of the mineral.

Others:
Check with your industrial health office if you are a miner or industrial worker to make sure your work environment does not contain toxic amounts of manganese.

Overdose/Toxicity

Signs and symptoms:
Delusions, hallucinations, insomnia, depression, impotence.

What to do:

For symptoms of overdose:
Discontinue mineral and consult doctor. Also see *Adverse Reactions or Side Effects* section below.

For accidental overdose (such as child taking entire bottle): Dial 911 (emergency), 0 for operator or call your nearest Poison Control Center.

Adverse Reactions or Side Effects

Reaction or effect	What to do
Appetite loss	Discontinue. Call doctor when convenient
Breathing problems	Seek emergency treatment.
Headaches	Discontinue. Call doctor when convenient.
Unusual tiredness	Discontinue. Call doctor when convenient.

M I N E R A L S

Interaction with Medicine, Vitamins or Minerals

Interacts with	Combined effect
Calcium (from food or supplements)	May decrease manganese absorption when taken in large doses.
Iron (from food or supplements)	Excess manganese interferes with iron absorption and can lead to iron-deficiency anemia.
Magnesium (from food or supplements)	May decrease manganese absorption when taken in large doses.
Oral contraceptives	Decreases manganese in blood.
Phosphate (from food or supplements)	When taken in large doses, may decrease manganese absorption.

Interaction with Other Substances

None are known.

Lab Tests to Detect Deficiency

Serum manganese

Molybdenum

Basic Information

- Available from natural sources? Yes
- Available from synthetic sources? No
- Prescription required? Yes, for some forms
- *Optimal Intake,* see page 477

Natural Sources

Beans
Cereal grains, whole grains
Dark green, leafy vegetables
Lean meats
Organ meats (liver, kidney, sweetbreads)
Peas and other legumes
Note: The dietary concentration of molybdenum may vary according to the status of the soil in which grains and vegetables are raised. Deficiencies are extremely rare.

Benefits

- Promotes normal growth and development
- Is a component of xanthine oxidase, an enzyme involved in converting nucleic acid to uric acid, a waste product eliminated in the urine

Possible Additional Benefits

- May protect teeth
- May enhance iron absorption

Who May Benefit from Additional Amounts?

- Anyone with inadequate caloric or nutritional dietary intake or increased nutritional requirements
- People with recent severe burns or injuries

- Extremely ill people who must be fed intravenously or by nasogastric tube

Deficiency Symptoms

No symptoms in humans. Deficiency is rare and only in conjunction with other disorders.

Usage Information

What this mineral does:
- Becomes a part of bones, liver, kidney
- Forms part of the enzyme system of xanthine oxidase

Miscellaneous information:
A balanced diet provides all the molybdenum that is necessary in a healthy child or adult.

Available as:
- Capsules: Swallow whole with a full glass of liquid. Don't chew or crush. Take with or 1 to 1-1/2 hours after meals unless otherwise directed by your doctor.
- Injectable forms are administered by a doctor or nurse.
- Molybdenum is a constituent of many multivitamin/mineral preparations.

Warnings and Precautions

Don't take if you:
No problems are expected at 0.15 to 0.5mg/day. Don't take higher doses without a doctor's prescription.

Consult your doctor if you have:
- High levels of uric acid
- Gout
- Copper deficiency
- Kidney or liver disease

Over 55:
No problems are expected.

Pregnancy:
Don't take.

Breastfeeding:
Don't take.

Effect on lab tests:
Excess molybdenum causes serum-copper level to drop.

Storage:
- Store in cool, dry place away from direct light, but don't freeze.
- Store safely out of reach of children.
- Don't store in bathroom medicine cabinet. Heat and moisture may change the action of the mineral.

Overdose/Toxicity

Signs and symptoms:
Gout and a gout-like syndrome can be produced by massive intake (10 to 15mg/day). Moderate excess (up to 0.54mg/day) can cause excess loss of copper in urine.

What to do:
For symptoms of overdose:
Discontinue mineral and consult doctor.

For accidental overdose (such as child taking entire bottle): Dial 911 (emergency), 0 for operator or call your nearest Poison Control Center.

MINERALS

→

Adverse Reactions or Side Effects

None are expected.

 Interaction with Other Substances

None are known.

 Interaction with Medicine, Vitamins or Minerals

Interacts with	Combined effect
Copper	Maintains appropriate ratio of molybdenum and copper in body. With excess molybdenum, copper level drops. With excess copper, molybdenum level drops.
Sulfur	Increased sulfur intake causes decline in molybdenum concentration.

 Lab Tests to Detect Deficiency

None are available, except for experimental purposes.

Phosphorus

 Basic Information

- Available from natural sources? Yes
- Available from synthetic sources? No
- Prescription required? Yes, for medical purposes
- *RDA/DRI and Optimal Intake,* see page 477

 Natural Sources

Almonds
Beans, dried
Calf liver
Cheese, cheddar
Cheese, pasteurized
Eggs
Fish
Milk
Milk products
Peanuts
Peas
Poultry
Pumpkin seeds
Red meat
Sardines, canned
Scallops
Soda
Soybeans
Sunflower seeds
Tuna
Whole-grain products

Benefits

- Builds strong bones and teeth (with calcium)
- Promotes energy metabolism
- Promotes growth, maintenance and repair of all body tissues
- Buffers body fluids for acid-base balance
- Acidifies urine and reduces possibility of kidney stones

 Possible Additional Benefits

None are known.

 Who May Benefit from Additional Amounts?

- Anyone suffering prolonged vomiting
- Those with inadequate caloric or dietary intake or increased nutritional requirements
- Those who take excessive amounts of antacid
- People with a chronic wasting illness
- Those under excess stress for long periods
- Anyone who has recently undergone surgery
- Those with liver disease
- People with hyperparathyroidism
- Alcoholics

 Deficiency Symptoms

- Bone pain
- Loss of appetite
- Weakness
- Easily broken bones

 Usage Information

What this mineral does:
- Necessary for utilization of many B-complex vitamins
- An important constituent of all fats, proteins, carbohydrates and many enzymes

Available as:
- Tablets: Swallow whole with a full glass of liquid. Don't chew or crush. Take with or 1 to 1-1/2 hours after meals unless otherwise directed by your doctor.
- Capsules for oral solution: Empty contents into at least 1/2 glass of water or other liquid. Don't swallow filled capsule. Take with or 1 to 1-1/2 hours after meals unless otherwise directed by your doctor.
- Oral solution: Dilute in at least 1/2 glass of water or other liquid. Take with or 1 to 1-1/2 hours after meals unless otherwise directed by your doctor.
- Phosphorus is a constituent of many multivitamin/mineral preparations.

 Warnings and Precautions

Don't take if you have:
- Kidney disease
- Kidney stones, and analysis has shown their composition to be magnesium ammonium phosphate

Consult your doctor if you have:
- Hypoparathyroidism
- Osteomalacia
- Acute pancreatitis
- Chronic kidney disease
- Rickets
- Adrenal insufficiency (Addison's disease)
- Dehydration
- Severe burns
- Heart disease
- Edema
- High blood pressure
- Toxemia of pregnancy

Over 55:
No problems are expected.

Pregnancy:
Take under doctor's supervision only. Don't take megadoses.

Breastfeeding:
Take under doctor's supervision only. Don't take megadoses.   →

MINERALS

Effect on lab tests:

May show false decrease in bone uptake in technetium-labeled diagnostic-imaging tests

Storage:

• Store in cool, dry place away from direct light, but don't freeze.
• Store safely out of reach of children.
• Don't store in bathroom medicine cabinet. Heat and moisture may change the action of the mineral.

Overdose/Toxicity

Signs and symptoms:

• Seizures, heartbeat irregularities, shortness of breath.
• Overconsumption may increase calcium excretion and lead to osteoporosis.

What to do:

For symptoms of overdose: Discontinue mineral and seek emergency treatment. Also see *Adverse Reactions or Side Effects* section below.

For accidental overdose (such as child taking entire bottle): Dial 911 (emergency), 0 for operator or call your nearest Poison Control Center.

Adverse Reactions or Side Effects

Reaction or effect	What to do
Abdominal pain	Discontinue. Call doctor immediately.
Bone or joint pain	Discontinue. Call doctor immediately.
Breathing problems	Discontinue. Call doctor immediately.
Confusion	Discontinue. Call doctor immediately.
Convulsions	Discontinue. Call doctor immediately.
Decreased volume of urine in one day	Seek emergency treatment.
Fast, slow or irregular heartbeat	Discontinue. Call doctor immediately.
Headaches	Discontinue. Call doctor immediately.
Muscle cramps	Discontinue. Call doctor when convenient.
Numbness or tingling in hands or feet	Discontinue. Call doctor when convenient.
Tremor	Discontinue. Call doctor immediately.
Unusual thirst	Discontinue. Call doctor when convenient.

Interaction with Medicine, Vitamins or Minerals

Interacts with	Combined effect
Anabolic steroids	Increases risk of edema.
Antacids with aluminum or magnesium	May prevent absorption of phosphates.
Calcium-containing supplements and antacids	May decrease phosphate absorption.
Captopril	Increases risk of too much potassium (hyperkalemia).
Corticosteroids	Decreases phosphate absorption.
Cortisone drugs or ACTH	Increases serum sodium.
Digitalis preparations	Increases risk of too much potassium (hyperkalemia).
Dilantin	May decrease phosphate absorption.
Enalapril	Increases risk of too much potassium (hyperkalemia).
Iron supplements	Do not take within 1 to 2 hours of taking potassium phosphate as it may interfere with iron supplement.
Salicylates	May increase plasma concentration of salicylates.

Testosterone	Increases risk of edema.
Vitamin D	Enhances phosphate absorption but may increase chance of too much phosphorus in blood and body cells.

Lab Tests to Detect Deficiency

Serum phosphorus

Interaction with Other Substances

Alcohol decreases available phosphorus for vital body functions.

Potassium

Basic Information

Potassium chloride is the most common form. This combination is also called *trikates.*

- Available from natural sources? Yes
- Available from synthetic sources? Yes
- Prescription required? Yes, for some forms
- *DV and Optimal Intake,* see page 477

Natural Sources

Asparagus	Molasses
Avocados	Nuts
Bananas	Parsnips
Beans	Peas (fresh)
Cantaloupe	Potatoes
Carrots	Raisins
Chard	Salt substitute
Citrus fruit	Sardines, canned
Juices (grapefruit,	Spinach, fresh
tomato, orange)	Whole-grain cereal
Milk	

Benefits

- Promotes regular heartbeat
- Promotes normal muscle contraction
- Regulates transfer of nutrients to cells
- Maintains water balance in body tissues and cells
- Preserves or restores normal function of nerve cells, heart cells, skeletal-muscle cells, kidneys, stomach-juice secretion
- Treats potassium deficiency from illness or taking diuretics (water pills), cortisone drugs or digitalis preparations

Possible Additional Benefits

- May cure alcoholism
- May cure acne
- Possible allergy cure
- Possible heart disease cure
- May help heal burns
- May prevent high blood pressure

MINERALS

→

Who May Benefit from Additional Amounts?

- People who take diuretics, cortisone drugs or digitalis preparations
- Anyone with inadequate caloric or nutritional dietary intake or increased nutritional requirements
- People over 55 years old
- Pregnant or breastfeeding women
- Women taking oral contraceptives
- People who abuse alcohol, tobacco or other drugs
- People with a chronic wasting illness
- Those under excess stress for long periods
- Anyone who has recently undergone surgery
- Athletes and workers who participate in vigorous physical activities, especially when endurance is an important aspect of the activity
- Those with part of the gastrointestinal tract surgically removed
- People with malabsorption disorders (See Glossary)
- Those with recent severe burns or injuries
- Vegetarians

 ## Deficiency Symptoms

- Hypokalemia
- Weakness, paralysis
- Low blood pressure
- Irregular or rapid heartbeat that can lead to cardiac arrest and death

 ## Usage Information

What this mineral does:

Potassium is the predominant positive electrolyte (see Glossary) in body cells. An enzyme (adenosine triphosphatase) controls the flow of potassium and sodium into and out of cells to maintain normal function of the heart, brain, skeletal muscles and kidney, and to maintain acid-base balance.

Miscellaneous information:

Avoid cooking food in large amounts of water.

Available as:

- Oral solution: Dilute in at least 1/2 glass of water or other liquid. Take with or 1 to 1-1/2 hours after meals unless otherwise directed by your doctor.
- Potassium is not recommended for children.
- Some forms are available by generic name.

 ## Warnings and Precautions

Don't take if you:

- Take potassium-sparing diuretics, such as spironolactone, triamterene or amiloride
- Are allergic to any potassium supplement
- Have kidney disease

Consult your doctor if you:

- Have Addison's disease
- Have diabetes
- Have heart disease
- Have intestinal blockage
- Have a stomach ulcer
- Take diuretics
- Take heart medicine
- Take laxatives or if you have chronic diarrhea
- Use salt substitutes or low-salt milk

Over 55:

- Observe dose schedule strictly; potassium balance is critical. Deviation above or below normal levels can have serious results.
- There is a greater risk of hyperkalemia.

Pregnancy:
No problems are expected. Consult your doctor.

Breastfeeding:
Studies are inconclusive on risk to infants. Consult your doctor about supplements.

Effect on lab tests:
• ECG and kidney function studies can be affected by too much or too little potassium.
• No effect is expected on blood studies, except serum-potassium levels.

Storage:
• Store in cool, dry area away from direct light, but don't freeze.
• Store safely out of reach of children.
• Don't store in bathroom medicine cabinet. Heat and moisture may change the action of the mineral

Others:
Take with food.

 Overdose/Toxicity

Signs and symptoms:
Irregular or fast heartbeat, paralysis of arms and legs, blood-pressure drop, convulsions, coma, cardiac arrest.

What to do:
For symptoms of overdose:
Discontinue mineral and consult doctor immediately. Also see *Adverse Reactions or Side Effects* section below.

For accidental overdose (such as child taking entire bottle): Dial 911 (emergency), 0 for operator or call your nearest Poison Control Center. If person's heart has stopped beating, render CPR until trained help arrives.

 Adverse Reactions or Side Effects

Reaction or effect	What to do
Black, tarry stool	Seek emergency treatment.
Bloody stool	Seek emergency treatment.
Breathing difficulty	Seek emergency treatment.
Confusion	Discontinue. Call doctor immediately.
Diarrhea	Discontinue. Call doctor immediately.
Extreme fatigue	Discontinue. Call doctor when convenient.
Heaviness in legs	Discontinue. Call doctor when convenient.
Irregular heartbeat	Seek emergency treatment.
Nausea	Discontinue. Call doctor when convenient.
Numbness in hands or feet	Discontinue. Call doctor when convenient.
Stomach discomfort	Discontinue. Call doctor when convenient.
Tingling in hands or feet	Discontinue. Call doctor when convenient.
Vomiting	Discontinue. Call doctor immediately.
Weakness	Discontinue. Call doctor immediately.

 Interaction with Medicine, Vitamins or Minerals

Interacts with	Combined effect
Amiloride	Causes dangerous rise in blood potassium.
Atropine	Increases possibility of intestinal ulcers, which may occur with oral potassium.
Belladonna	Increases possibility of intestinal ulcers, which may occur with oral potassium.

MINERALS

Calcium	Increases possibility of heartbeat irregularities.
Captopril	Increases chance of excessive amounts of potassium.
Cortisone	Decreases effect of potassium.
Digitalis preparations	May cause irregular heartbeat.
Enalapril	Increases chance of excessive amounts of potassium.
Laxatives	May decrease potassium effect.
Spironolactone	Increases blood potassium.
Triamterene	Increases blood potassium.
Vitamin B-12	Extended-release tablets may decrease vitamin B-12 absorption and increase vitamin B-12 requirements.

Alcohol intensifies gastrointestinal symptoms.

Cocaine may cause irregular heartbeat.

Marijuana may cause irregular heartbeat.

Beverages:
• Salty drinks, such as tomato juice and commercial thirst quenchers, cause increased fluid retention.
• Coffee decreases potassium absorption and intensifies gastrointestinal symptoms.
• Low-salt milk increases fluid retention.

Foods:
• Salty foods increase fluid retention.
• Sugar decreases potassium absorption.

Interaction with Other Substances

Tobacco decreases absorption. Smokers may require supplemental potassium.

Lab Tests to Detect Deficiency

• Serum-potassium determinations
• Serum creatinine
• Electrocardiograms
• Serum-pH determinations

Selenium

Basic Information

• Available from natural sources? Yes
• Available from synthetic sources? No
• Prescription required? No
• *RDA and Optimal Intake,* see page 477

Natural Sources

Bran
Broccoli
Brown rice
Cabbage
Chicken
Garlic (grown in selenium-rich soil)
Kidney
Liver
Milk
Mushrooms
Nutritional yeast
Oatmeal
Onions
Seafood
Tuna
Whole-grain products

Note: The selenium content of food varies greatly because of the wide variability of this element in the soil. Foods grown in the southeastern United States are known to have lower selenium content.

Benefits

- Complements vitamin E as an efficient antioxidant (see Glossary)
- Promotes normal growth and development
- Functions as antioxidant itself
- Stimulates immune system
- Protects against prostate cancer

Possible Additional Benefits

- May protect against increased oxidation (see Glossary) associated with aging
- May protect against cardiovascular disease, strokes and heart attacks
- Potentially decreases platelet clumping in bloodstream and prevents clots at site of blood-vessel damage in heart and brain
- May protect against damage caused by tobacco smoking
- May be extremely strong antioxidant (see Glossary)
- May reduce cataract formation through antioxidation

Who May Benefit from Additional Intake?

- Anyone with inadequate caloric or nutritional dietary intake or increased nutritional requirements
- People who live in areas where soil is selenium-deficient, such as China, New Zealand and central and southeastern United States (check with your local county agricultural agent)
- Anyone with celiac disease
- HIV/AIDS patients

Deficiency Symptoms

Selenium deficiency has resulted in cardiomyopathy and myocardial deaths in humans

Usage Information

What this mineral does:
Selenium helps defend against damage from oxidation.

Miscellaneous information:
- Selenium should be part of a well-balanced vitamin and mineral regimen.
- Protection from human degenerative disorders has yet to be proved.
- Experimental studies are trying to prove that selenium plays a big part as an antioxidant (see Glossary) nutrient to help protect against damaging free radicals.
- Organic forms (from foods or brewer's yeast) are less toxic than inorganic sodium selenide.
- No one can be sure of the correct amount to be ingested each day. People who eat a balanced diet of food grown in the western United States probably get enough from food.

Available as:
- Tablets or capsules: Swallow whole with a full glass of liquid. Don't chew or crush. Take with or 1 to 1-1/2 hours after meals unless otherwise directed by your doctor.
- Selenium is a constituent of many multivitamin/mineral preparations.

MINERALS

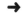

Warnings and Precautions

Don't take if you:
Plan to use it on the scalp or skin for seborrheic dermatitis or dandruff if you have any inflammation or oozing.

Consult your doctor if you:
Plan to take more than the dose recommended by the manufacturer.

Over 55:
No problems are expected with usual doses.

Pregnancy:
No problems are expected with usual doses.

Breastfeeding:
No problems are expected with usual doses.

Storage:
• Store in cool, dry place away from direct light, but don't freeze.
• Store safely out of reach of children.
• Don't store in bathroom medicine cabinet. Heat and moisture may change the action of the mineral.

Others:
Workers at industrial sites that manufacture glass, pesticides, rubber, semiconductors, copper and film are at increased risk of developing toxic symptoms from inhalation, absorption through the skin and ingestion. These symptoms may include bronchial pneumonia, asthma, precipitous drop in blood pressure, red eyes, garlic odor on breath and in urine, headaches, metallic taste, nose and throat irrita-tion, difficulty breathing, vomiting and weakness.

 ## Overdose/Toxicity

Signs and symptoms:
• Toxicity is unlikely to develop with organic selenium if you don't consume more than the regular dose recommended by the manufacturer.
• Individuals in industrial settings have been reported to suffer toxic symptoms of selenium overdoses, including liver disease and cardiomyopathy.
• Children reared in selenium-rich areas show a higher incidence of decayed, missing and filled teeth.
• Selenium is toxic in megadoses and may cause alopecia (hair loss), loss of nails, fatigue, nausea, vomiting, lesions and sour-milk breath.

What to do:
For symptoms of overdose:
Discontinue mineral and consult doctor. Also see *Adverse Reactions or Side Effects* section below.

For accidental overdose (such as child taking entire bottle): Dial 911 (emergency), 0 for operator or call your nearest Poison Control Center.

 ## Adverse Reactions or Side Effects

Reaction or effect	What to do
Dizziness and nausea, without other apparent cause	Discontinue. Call doctor immediately.
Fragile or black fingernails	Discontinue. Call doctor when convenient.
Persistent garlic odor on breath and skin	Discontinue. Call doctor when convenient.
Unusual dryness when used on scalp or skin	Discontinue. Call doctor when convenient.
Unusual hair loss or discoloration of hair	Discontinue. Call doctor when convenient.

Interaction with Medicine, Vitamins or Minerals

Interacts with	Combined effect
Vitamin C	May decrease selenium absorption if taken with an inorganic form of selenium.
Vitamin E	Prevents oxidation that might cause breakdown of body chemicals.

Interaction with Other Substances

None are known.

Lab Tests to Detect Deficiency

24-hour urine collection

Silicon

Basic Information

- Available from natural sources? Yes
- Available from synthetic sources? Yes
- Prescription required? No

Natural Sources

Apples	Legumes
Beets	Root vegetables
Brown rice	Soybeans
Horsetail	Whole grains

Benefits

Essential for collagen formation

Possible Additional Benefits

- May aid early stages of calcium absorption
- May boost immune system
- May prevent osteoporosis
- May improve nails, skin and hair
- May reduce risk of cardiovascular disease
- May help reduce blood pressure

Who May Benefit from Additional Amounts?

Unknown

Deficiency Symptoms

Deficiency is not known because silicon is available in so many foods.

Usage Information

What this mineral does:

- Plays a role in bone growth
- Strengthens blood vessels, cartilage and tendons

Miscellaneous information:

- Most of the silicon present in the body is found in connective tissue.
- Studies on chicks showed that silicon deficiency causes skull, bone and joint abnormalities.

Available as:

- Liquid- take as directed by manufacturer or your doctor.
- Tablet- take as directed by manufacturer or your doctor.

MINERALS

→

Warnings and Precautions

Pregnancy:
Do not take.

Breastfeeding:
Do not take.

Storage:
- Store in cool, dry place away from direct light, but don't freeze.
- Store safely out of reach of children.
- Don't store in bathroom medicine cabinet. Heat and moisture may change the action of the mineral.

 ## Overdose/Toxicity

What to do:

For symptoms of overdose:
Discontinue mineral and consult doctor immediately.

For accidental overdose (such as child taking entire bottle): Dial 911 (emergency), 0 for operator or call your nearest Poison Control Center.

 ## Adverse Reactions or Side Effects

None are known.

 ## Interaction with Medicine, Vitamins or Minerals

Interacts with	Combined effect
Aluminum	Counteracts effect of aluminum.
Boron	Helps body utilize silicon.
Calcium	Helps body utilize silicon.
Magnesium	Helps body utilize silicon.
Manganese	Helps body utilize silicon.
Potassium	Helps body utilize silicon.

 ## Interaction with Other Substances

None are known.

 ## Lab Tests to Detect Deficiency

No existing tests because deficiency doesn't occur.

Sodium

 ## Basic Information

- Available from natural sources? Yes
- Available from synthetic sources? No
- Prescription required? No
- *DV and Optimal Intake,* see page 477

 ## Natural Sources

Bacon
Beef, dried and fresh
Bread
Butter
Clams
Green beans
Ham
Margarine
Milk
Olives
Pickles
Processed meat
Salted nuts, snack foods
Sardines, canned
Table salt (chief source of sodium)
Tomatoes, canned

Note: In most commercially canned vegetables and processed foods, salt is added to improve taste. "Highly processed" foods (also high in sodium) include soups, bouillon, pickles, potato chips, snack foods and ham.

 Benefits

- Helps regulate water balance in body
- Plays a crucial role in maintaining normal blood pressure
- Aids muscle contraction and nerve transmission
- Regulates body's acid-base balance

 Possible Additional Benefits

Low-sodium diets appear to reduce high blood pressure in some individuals.

 Who May Benefit from Additional Amounts?

- Anyone who suffers prolonged loss of body fluids from vomiting or diarrhea
- Those with Addison's disease
- Those who drink water excessively for prolonged periods (usually a psychiatric condition)
- People who suffer some types of cancers of the adrenal glands
- Those who sweat excessively due to heavy exercise or workload
- People who use diuretics (generally low-sodium diet is also prescribed to prevent fluid retention)
- Those with chronic kidney disease

 Deficiency Symptoms

- Muscle and stomach cramps
- Nausea
- Fatigue
- Mental apathy
- Muscle twitching and cramping (usually in legs)
- Appetite loss

In severe cases:
- Shock resulting from a decrease in blood pressure

 Usage Information

What this mineral does:
As an electrolyte (see Glossary), sodium is present in all body cells. Its most important function is to regulate the balance of water inside and outside cells.

Miscellaneous information:
- We consume most of our sodium as sodium chloride—ordinary table salt.
- The most common problem with sodium in a healthy person is too much, rather than too little. A typical diet contains 3,000 to 12,000mg of sodium a day. Recommended intake is 2,400mg/day.
- Excessive amounts of sodium can be a major factor in the development of high blood pressure. Decreasing sodium intake helps control high blood pressure.
- There is speculation that the relationship between sodium intake and high blood pressure is actually more closely related to the sodium-potassium ratio. Certain people are "sodium sensitive" and will have lower blood pressure in response to a low-sodium diet.

Available as:
Sodium-chloride tablets, but these may cause stomach distress and an overload on the kidneys.

MINERALS

→

Warnings and
Precautions

Don't take if you have:
- Congestive heart failure
- Hepatic cirrhosis
- Hypertension
- Edema from any cause
- A family history of high
  blood pressure

Consult your doctor if you have:
- Any heart or blood-vessel disease
- Bleeding problems
- Epilepsy
- Kidney disease

Over 55:
No problems are expected in healthy
individuals.

Pregnancy:
Dietary restriction of sodium in
healthy women during pregnancy is
not recommended.

Breastfeeding:
Dietary restriction of sodium in
healthy women during lactation is
not recommended.

Effect on lab tests:
None are expected.

Storage:
- Store in cool, dry place away from
  direct light, but don't freeze.
- Store safely out of reach of children.
- Don't store in bathroom medicine
  cabinet. Heat and moisture may
  change the action of the mineral.

Others:
- Too little sodium occurs almost
  entirely in people desperately ill with
  dehydration, recovering from recent
  surgery or after excessive sweating
  from heavy physical activity in a hot
  environment.

- Proper replacement of sodium
  deficiencies requires care by your
  doctor and frequent lab studies.

 Overdose/Toxicity

Signs and symptoms:
Tissue swelling (edema), stupor, coma.

What to do:
For symptoms of overdose:
Discontinue mineral and consult
doctor. Also see *Adverse Reactions or
Side Effects* section below.

For accidental overdose (such as
child taking entire bottle): Dial 911
(emergency), 0 for operator or call
your nearest Poison Control Center.

 Adverse Reactions
or Side Effects

Reaction or effect   What to do

With excessive amounts of sodium:

Reaction or effect	What to do
Anxiety	Discontinue. Call doctor immediately.
Confusion	Discontinue. Call doctor immediately.
Edema	Discontinue. Call doctor immediately.
Nausea	Discontinue. Call doctor immediately.
Restlessness	Discontinue. Call doctor immediately.
Vomiting	Seek emergency treatment.
Weakness	Discontinue. Call doctor immediately.

 Interaction with
Medicine, Vitamins
or Minerals

None are expected.

Interaction with Other Substances

None are known.

 Lab Tests to Detect Deficiency

Serum sodium

 # Sulfur

 Basic Information

- Available from natural sources? Yes
- Available from synthetic sources? No
- Prescription required? No

 Natural Sources

Beans, dried	Lean beef, meats
Eggs	Milk
Fish	Poultry
Garlic	Wheat germ

 Benefits

- Plays a role in oxidation-reduction reactions (see Glossary)
- Aids bile secretion in liver
- Aids in metabolism

 Possible Additional Benefits

- May extend life span
- May protect against toxic substances
- May reduce arthritis symptoms
- Methyl sulfonyl methane has been used to treat allergies

 Who May Benefit from Additional Amounts?

Supplements are probably not needed—no recorded deficiency states.

 Deficiency Symptoms

No proven symptoms exist.

 Usage Information

What this mineral does:

- Sulfur is part of the chemical structure of cysteine, methionine, taurine and glutathione.
- Sulfur aids treatment of aluminum, cadmium, mercury and lead poisoning.
- It is a component of biotin and B-1.

Available as:

A constituent of many multivitamin/mineral preparations.

STOP Warnings and Precautions

Don't take if you:
No problems are expected.

Consult your doctor if you have:
No problems are expected.

Over 55:
No problems are expected.

Pregnancy:
No problems are expected.

Breastfeeding:
No problems are expected.

MINERALS

Effect on lab tests:
None are expected.

Storage:
• Store in cool, dry place away from direct light, but don't freeze.
• Store safely out of reach of children.
• Don't store in bathroom medicine cabinet. Heat and moisture may change the action of the mineral.

 Overdose/Toxicity

Signs and symptoms:
Unlikely to threaten life or cause significant symptoms.

What to do:
For symptoms of overdose:
Discontinue mineral and consult doctor.

For accidental overdose (such as child taking entire bottle): Dial 911 (emergency), 0 for operator or call your nearest Poison Control Center.

 Adverse Reactions or Side Effects

None are known.

 Interaction with Medicine, Vitamins or Minerals

None are known.

 Interaction with Other Substances

Tobacco decreases absorption. Smokers may require supplemental sulfur.

 Lab Tests to Detect Deficiency

None are available, except for experimental purposes.

Vanadium

 Basic Information

• Available from natural sources? Yes
• Available from synthetic sources? No
• Prescription required? No

 Natural Sources

Cereals	Mushrooms
Dill	Parsley
Fish/seafood	Soy
Liver	

 Benefits

Plays role in metabolism of bones and teeth

 Possible Additional Benefits

May help prevent heart attacks

Who May Benefit from Additional Amounts?

Supplements are probably not needed—no recorded deficiency states.

Deficiency Symptoms

A vanadium-deficient diet fed to laboratory animals resulted in impaired reproductive ability and increased infant mortality.

Usage Information

What this mineral does:

- Unknown in humans, but believed to be essential
- May be a part of cholesterol metabolism as well as hormone production

Miscellaneous information:

- Even the most nutritionally inadequate diet contains sufficient quantities to prevent a deficiency.
- Research is being conducted regarding the role of vanadium intake and thyroid.

Available as:

- Capsules: Swallow whole with a full glass of liquid. Don't chew or crush. Take with or 1 to 1-1/2 hours after meals unless otherwise directed by your doctor.
- Vanadium is a constituent of many multivitamin/mineral preparations.

Warnings and Precautions

Don't take if you:
No problems are expected.

Consult your doctor if you have:
No problems are expected.

Over 55:
No problems are expected.

Pregnancy:
No problems are expected.

Breastfeeding:
No problems are expected.

Effect on lab tests:
None are expected.

Storage:
- Store in cool, dry place away from direct light, but don't freeze.
- Store safely out of reach of children.
- Don't store in bathroom medicine cabinet. Heat and moisture may change the action of the mineral.

Overdose/Toxicity

Signs and symptoms:
Toxicity would likely affect kidney, liver or spleen function, and bone marrow.

What to do:

For symptoms of overdose:
Discontinue mineral and consult doctor.

For accidental overdose (such as child taking entire bottle): Dial 911 (emergency), 0 for operator or call your nearest Poison Control Center.

Adverse Reactions or Side Effects

None are expected.

MINERALS

Interaction with Medicine, Vitamins or Minerals

Interacts with	Combined effect
Chromium	Chromium and vanadium may interfere with each other.

Interaction with Other Substances

None are known.

Lab Tests to Detect Deficiency

None are available, except for experimental purposes.

Zinc

Basic Information

- Available from natural sources? Yes
- Available from synthetic sources? No
- Prescription required? No
- *DV/RDA and Optimal Intake,* see page 477

Natural Sources

Beef, lean	Pork
Chicken heart	Sesame seeds
Egg yolk	Soybeans
Fish	Sunflower seeds
Herring	Turkey
Lamb	Wheat bran
Maple syrup	Wheat germ
Milk	Whole-grain
Molasses,	products
blackstrap	Yeast
Oysters	

Benefits

- Functions in antioxidant reactions (see Glossary)
- Maintains normal taste and sense of smell
- Promotes normal growth and development
- Aids wound healing
- Promotes normal fetal growth
- Helps synthesize DNA and RNA
- Promotes cell division, repair and growth
- Maintains normal level of vitamin A in blood
- Boosts immunity in zinc-deficient people
- Treats Wilson's disease

Possible Additional Benefits

- May promote normal fertility
- May increase attention span and improve short-term memory

Who May Benefit from Additional Amounts?

- Anyone with inadequate caloric or nutritional dietary intake or increased nutritional requirements, such as vegetarians
- Preschool children with inadequate diet

- People over 55 years old
- Those who abuse alcohol or other drugs
- People with a chronic wasting illness
- Those under excess stress for long periods
- Anyone who has recently undergone surgery
- People with recent severe burns or injuries
- Anyone taking diuretics (water pills) for any reason, such as high blood pressure, congestive heart failure, liver disease
- Those who live in areas where soil is deficient in zinc
- Babies born with acrodermatitis enteropathica
- Anyone with Crohn's or celiac disease
- People with chronic diarrhea

Deficiency Symptoms

Moderate deficiency:
- Loss of taste and smell
- Slow growth in children
- Alopecia
- Rashes
- Multiple skin lesions
- Glossitis (See Glossary)
- Stomatitis (See Glossary)
- Blepharitis (See Glossary)
- Paronychia (See Glossary)
- Sterility
- Low sperm count
- Delayed wound healing

Serious deficiency:
- Delayed bone maturation
- Enlarged spleen or liver
- Decreased size of testicles
- Testicular function less than normal
- Decreased growth or dwarfism
- Problems relating to the eye such as optic neuritis, poor color discrimination, cataract formation

Usage Information

What this mineral does:

Zinc is a part of the molecular structure of 80 or more known enzymes. These particular enzymes work with red blood cells to move carbon dioxide from tissues to lungs.

Miscellaneous information:
- Zinc toxicity from inhalation is rare but can occur in the following industries and occupations: alloy manufacturing, brass foundry, bronze foundry, electric-fuse manufacturing, gas welding, electroplating, galvanizing, paint manufacturing, metal cutting, metal spraying, rubber manufacturing, roof manufacturing and zinc manufacturing.
- If you take zinc supplements, take with food to decrease gastric irritation.
- If taking zinc long term, copper at 2 to 3mg/day should also be prescribed.
- Large doses of zinc may decrease HDL (see Glossary) cholesterol levels.

Available as:
- Tablets: Swallow whole with a full glass of liquid. Don't chew or crush. Take with or 1 to 1-1/2 hours after meals unless otherwise directed by your doctor.
- Zinc is a constituent of many multivitamin/mineral preparations.

Warnings and Precautions

Don't take if you have:

Stomach or duodenal ulcers.

Consult your doctor if you:
- Plan to take more than the manufacturer's recommended dose

→

MINERALS

- Plan to take any calcium supplement or tetracycline drugs (zinc may interfere with absorption of these medicines)

Over 55:
Deficiency is more likely.

Pregnancy:
- Many diets are marginally low in zinc and may not supply the zinc required during pregnancy. Ask your doctor about supplementation.
- Overconsumption is dangerous and can lead to premature labor or stillbirth.
- Deficiency may be a factor in toxemia and could also be a factor in low-birthweight babies. Ask your doctor for advice.
- Zinc treats nausea in pregnancy.

Breastfeeding:
Some diets are marginally low in zinc and may not supply the zinc required while breastfeeding. Ask your doctor about supplementation.

Effect on lab tests:
- Zinc decreases high-density lipoprotein levels in young males. High-density lipoproteins decrease risk of coronary-artery disease.
- High doses decrease copper in blood.

Storage:
- Store in cool, dry place away from direct light, but don't freeze.
- Store safely out of reach of children.
- Don't store in bathroom medicine cabinet. Heat and moisture may change the action of the mineral.

Overdose/Toxicity

Signs and symptoms:
- Toxicity at RDA doses is highly unlikely. Toxic symptoms are extremes of the *Adverse Reactions or Side Effects* listed below.

- Overdose produces drowsiness, lethargy, lightheadedness, difficulty writing, staggering gait, restlessness and excessive vomiting leading to dehydration.

What to do:
For symptoms of overdose:
Discontinue mineral and consult doctor. Also see *Adverse Reactions or Side Effects* section below.

For accidental overdose (such as child taking entire bottle): Dial 911 (emergency), 0 for operator or call your nearest Poison Control Center.

Adverse Reactions or Side Effects

Reaction or effect	What to do
Abdominal pain	Seek emergency treatment.
Abnormal bleeding	Seek emergency treatment.
Diarrhea (mild)	Discontinue. Call doctor when convenient.
Gastric ulceration (burning pain in upper chest relieved by food or antacid)	Discontinue. Call doctor immediately.
Nausea or vomiting	Discontinue. Call doctor immediately.

Interaction with Medicine, Vitamins or Minerals

Interacts with	Combined effect
Calcium	Interferes with calcium absorption.
Copper	Decreases absorption of copper. Large or long-term doses of zinc must be taken to produce this effect.
Cortisone drugs	May interfere with lab tests measuring zinc.
Diuretics	Increases zinc excretion. Greater amounts of zinc required.

Iron	Decreases absorption of iron. Large doses of zinc must be taken to produce this effect.
Oral contraceptives	Lowers zinc blood levels.
Tetracycline	Decreases amount of tetracycline absorbed into bloodstream. Zinc and tetracycline should not be mixed. Take at least 2 hours apart.
Vitamin A	Assists in absorption of vitamin A.

Interaction with Other Substances

Alcohol, even in moderate amounts, can increase the excretion of zinc in urine and can impair the body's ability to combine zinc into its proper enzyme combinations in the liver.

Beverages: Coffee should not be consumed at the same time as zinc because it may decrease absorption of zinc.

Lab Tests to Detect Deficiency

Serum zinc (by atomic absorption spectroscopy)

MINERALS

Amino Acids and Nucleic Acids

Amino Acids

Amino acids are a chemical group containing nitrogen, carbon, oxygen and hydrogen. The amino acids form the chief structure of proteins, several of which are essential for human growth, development and nutrition.

Supplementation with commercially available forms should not be necessary.

Nucleic Acids

These chemicals contain sugars, phosphoric acid, purines and pyrimidine bases (see Glossary). The two most studied nucleic acids are chemicals found in the genes: ribonucleic acid (RNA) and deoxyribonucleic acid (DNA) (see Glossary). Nucleic acids taken as supplements have little or no value. Nucleic acids taken as injections can be dangerous.

AMINO ACIDS

Arginine

 Basic Information

Arginine is an amino acid.

- Available from natural sources? Yes
- Available from synthetic sources? Yes
- Prescription required? No

 Natural Sources

Brown rice	Popcorn
Carob	Raisins
Chocolate	Raw cereals
Nuts	Sesame seeds
Oatmeal	Sunflower seeds
Peanuts/peanut	Whole-wheat
butter	products

 Benefits

- Functions as building block of all proteins
- Stimulates human-growth hormone
- Stimulates immune system
- Helps treat HIV infection by boosting activity of immune-system fighting cells
- Used to treat liver disorders
- Increases metabolism in fat cells to decrease obesity
- Builds muscle
- Speeds wound healing

 Possible Additional Benefits

May inhibit cancer and growth of tumors

 Who May Benefit from Additional Amounts?

- Those with inadequate protein dietary intake
- Children and pregnant or lactating women who are vegan vegetarians
- People with recent severe burns or injuries
- Premature infants
- People with diseases that suppress the immune system, such as AIDS

 Deficiency Symptoms

Single amino-acid deficiencies are unknown except in people on crash diets consisting of only a few foods. Amino-acid deficiencies appear more commonly as a result of total protein deficiency, which is rare in the United States and Canada.

- Impaired insulin production
- Impaired liver-lipid metabolism

 Usage Information

What this amino acid does:

- Provides part of all proteins
- Stimulates activity and size of thymus gland, causing it to increase production of cells that are crucial to the immune system

Miscellaneous information:

- Arginine has been reported to increase the activity of some herpes viruses and inhibit others.
- If you take arginine as a supplement, take it on an empty stomach before retiring at night.

Available as:

- Tablets or capsules: Swallow whole with a full glass of liquid. Don't chew or crush. Take with or 1 to 1-1/2 hours after meals unless otherwise directed by your doctor.
- Powder for oral solution: Dissolve powder in cold water or juice. Take with or 1 to 1-1/2 hours after meals unless otherwise directed by your doctor.

 ## Warnings and Precautions

Don't take if you are:

- A child or adolescent not fully grown
- Allergic to any food protein, such as eggs, milk, wheat
- At risk of poor nutrition for any reason

Consult your doctor if you have:
Any bone disease.

Over 55:
Don't take amino-acid supplements if you are healthy.

Pregnancy:
Don't take amino-acid supplements.

Breastfeeding:
Don't take amino-acid supplements.

Effect on lab tests:
None are known.

Storage:

- Store in cool, dry place away from direct light, but don't freeze.
- Store safely out of reach of children.
- Don't store in bathroom medicine cabinet. Heat and moisture may change the action of the amino acid.

Others:
Children and adolescents should not take any arginine supplement. It may cause bone deformities.

 ## Overdose/Toxicity

Signs and symptoms:
Unlikely to threaten life or cause significant symptoms.

What to do:
For symptoms of overdose:
Discontinue amino acid and consult doctor. Also see *Adverse Reactions or Side Effects* section below.

For accidental overdose (such as child taking entire bottle): Dial 911 (emergency), 0 for operator or call your nearest Poison Control Center.

 ## Adverse Reactions or Side Effects

Note: Impurities in amino-acid supplements have resulted in diverse health problems.

Reaction or effect	What to do
Diarrhea (from large doses)	Decrease dose or discontinue.
Nausea (from large doses)	Decrease dose or discontinue.

 ## Interaction with Medicine, Vitamins or Minerals

None are known.

 ## Interaction with Other Substances

None are known.

 ## Lab Tests to Detect Deficiency

None are available, except for experimental purposes.

AMINO ACIDS

Glutamine

Basic Information

Glutamine converts to the amino acid called *glutamic acid.*

- Available from natural sources? Yes
- Available from synthetic sources? Yes
- Prescription required? No

Natural Sources

Raw parsley
Spinach

Benefits

- Functions as building block of all proteins
- Aids digestive tract
- Important for muscle growth and maintenance
- Decreases muscle wasting
- Enhances digestive-system function in trauma patients and cancer patients on chemotherapy

Possible Additional Benefits

- May treat intestinal disorders and peptic ulcers
- Possible treatment for connective-tissue diseases and damage to tissue from radiation treatment
- May enhance brain function and mental activity by boosting GABA (gamma-aminobutyric acid) levels (see Glossary)

Who May Benefit from Additional Amounts?

- Those with inadequate protein dietary intake
- People who experience muscle wasting due to disease (such as cancer or AIDS) or lengthy bed rest
- Trauma patients or patients on high-dose chemotherapy such as bone marrow-transplant patients

Deficiency Symptoms

Single amino-acid deficiencies are unknown except in people on crash diets consisting of only a few foods. Amino-acid deficiencies appear more commonly as a result of total protein deficiency, which is rare in the United States and Canada.

Usage Information

What this amino acid does:

- Converts into glutamic acid when it passes through the blood-brain barrier (Glutamic acid is critical for cerebral function.)
- Participates in regulating the proper acid/alkaline balance
- Participates in the synthesis of RNA and DNA (see Glossary)

Miscellaneous information:

- Poorly nourished people have a greater chance of adverse side effects from taking amino-acid supplements, including an amino-acid imbalance.
- Muscles contain large amounts of glutamine.

• Glutamine is considered a non-essential amino acid; however, recent findings indicate that in high-stress situations, such as trauma, it may be essential.

Available as:
Powder: Follow manufacturer's instructions.

 ## Warnings and Precautions

Don't take if you have:
• Kidney problems
• Cirrhosis of the liver
• Reye's syndrome

Consult your doctor if you are:
Undergoing chemotherapy.

Over 55:
Don't take amino-acid supplements if you are healthy.

Pregnancy:
Don't take amino-acid supplements.

Breastfeeding:
Don't take amino-acid supplements.

Effect on lab tests:
None are known.

Storage:
• Store safely out of reach of children.
• Don't store in bathroom medicine cabinet. Heat and moisture may change the action of the amino acid.
• Keep completely dry or the quality of the supplement will deteriorate.

Others:
• It is best to consume complete proteins rather than individual amino acids.

 ## Overdose/Toxicity

Signs and symptoms:
• May decrease production of growth hormone
• Decreases bicarbonate buffer (which may upset the acid-base balance of the stomach)

What to do:
For symptoms of overdose:
Discontinue amino acid and consult doctor.

For accidental overdose (such as child taking entire bottle): Dial 911 (emergency), 0 for operator or call your nearest Poison Control Center.

 ## Adverse Reactions or Side Effects
None are expected.

 ## Interaction with Medicine, Vitamins or Minerals
None are expected.

 ## Interaction with Other Substances
None are known.

 ## Lab Tests to Detect Deficiency
None are available, except for experimental purposes.

AMINO ACIDS

L-Cysteine

 ## Basic Information

L-cysteine is an amino acid.

- Available from natural sources? Yes
- Available from synthetic sources? Yes
- Prescription required? No

 ## Natural Sources

Cereals (some)
Dairy products
Eggs
Meat
Whole grains

 ## Benefits

- Functions as building block of all proteins
- Eliminates certain toxic chemicals, rendering them harmless (antioxidant—see Glossary)

 ## Possible Additional Benefits

- One of the amino acids containing sulfur in a form believed to inactivate free radicals—if so, it protects and preserves cells
- May help build muscle
- May burn fat
- May protect against toxins and pollutants, including some found in cigarette smoke and alcohol
- May combat arthritis
- May participate in some forms of DNA (see Glossary) repair and theoretically extend life span
- Potential aid in treatment of respiratory disorders

- May slow viral replication in HIV
- May help treat asthma when inhaled in mist form

 ## Who May Benefit from Additional Amounts?

- Those with inadequate protein dietary intake
- Children and pregnant or breast-feeding women who are vegan vegetarians
- People with recent severe burns or injuries
- Premature infants

 ## Deficiency Symptoms

Single amino-acid deficiencies are unknown except in people on crash diets consisting of only a few foods. Amino-acid deficiencies appear more commonly as a result of total protein deficiency, which is rare in the United States and Canada.

Moderate deficiency:

- Slowed growth in children
- Low levels of essential proteins in blood

Severe deficiency:

- Apathy
- Depigmentation of hair
- Edema (excess fluid in connective tissue)
- Lethargy
- Liver damage
- Loss of muscle and fat
- Skin lesions
- Weakness

Usage Information

What this amino acid does:
- Provides part of all proteins
- Functions in synthesis of glutathione, a substance that may neutralize environmental pollutants, including tobacco

Miscellaneous information:
- Poorly nourished people have a greater chance of adverse side effects from taking amino-acid supplements, including an amino-acid imbalance.
- Take l-cysteine supplements with vitamin C. Take 2 to 3 times as much vitamin C as cysteine, milligram to milligram, as a precaution against kidney- or bladder-stone formation.
- L-cysteine is used under medical supervision in emergency rooms to protect against liver damage caused by overdoses of acetaminophen.

Available as:
Capsules: Swallow whole with a full glass of liquid. Don't chew or crush. Take with or 1 to 1-1/2 hours after meals unless otherwise directed by your doctor.

Warnings and Precautions

Don't take if you are:
- Allergic to any food protein, such as eggs, milk, wheat
- Diabetic
- Self-prescribing without medical supervision

Consult your doctor if you have:
- Diabetes mellitus
- Cystinuria

Over 55:
Don't take amino-acid supplements if you are healthy.

Pregnancy:
Don't take amino-acid supplements.

Breastfeeding:
Don't take amino-acid supplements.

Effect on lab tests:
None are known.

Storage:
- Store in cool, dry place away from direct light, but don't freeze.
- Store safely out of reach of children.
- Don't store in bathroom medicine cabinet. Heat and moisture may change the action of the amino acid.

Overdose/Toxicity

Signs and symptoms:
Unlikely to threaten life or cause significant symptoms.

What to do:
For symptoms of overdose:
Discontinue amino acid and consult doctor.

For accidental overdose (such as child taking entire bottle): Dial 911 (emergency), 0 for operator or call your nearest Poison Control Center.

Adverse Reactions or Side Effects
None are expected.

Interaction with Medicine, Vitamins or Minerals

Interacts with	Combined effect
Insulin	May inactivate insulin effect.

AMINO ACIDS

→

Monosodium-glutamate (MSG)	L-cysteine may increase toxicity of monosodium glutamate in individuals who suffer from the "Chinese-restaurant syndrome." Causes headache, dizziness, disorientation and burning sensations.
Vitamin C	Taken with l-cysteine, vitamin C helps prevent l-cysteine from converting to cystine, which may cause bladder or kidney stones.

Interaction with Other Substances

None are known.

Lab Tests to Detect Deficiency

None are available, except for experimental purposes.

L-Lysine

Basic Information

L-lysine is an amino acid.

- Available from natural sources? Yes
- Available from synthetic sources? Yes
- Prescription required? No

Natural Sources

Cheese	Potatoes
Eggs	Red meat
Fish	Soy products
Lima beans	Yeast
Milk	

Benefits

- Functions as essential building block of all proteins
- Promotes growth, tissue repair and production of antibodies, hormones, enzymes

Possible Additional Benefits

- May protect against herpes viruses
- May prevent recurrence of cold sores and lessen severity of outbreaks

Who May Benefit from Additional Amounts?

- Those with inadequate protein dietary intake
- Children and pregnant or breastfeeding women who are vegan vegetarians

Deficiency Symptoms

Single amino-acid deficiencies are unknown except in people on crash diets consisting of only a few foods. Amino-acid deficiencies appear more commonly as a result of total protein deficiency, which is rare in the United States and Canada.

Moderate deficiency:
- Slowed growth in children
- Low levels of essential proteins in blood

Severe deficiency:
- Apathy
- Depigmentation of hair
- Edema (excess fluid in connective tissue)
- Lethargy
- Liver damage
- Loss of muscle and fat
- Skin lesions
- Weakness

Usage Information

What this amino acid does:
- L-lysine is one of eight essential amino acids that the body does not manufacture.
- All biological amino acids participate in the synthesis of proteins in animal bodies.

Miscellaneous information:
- There is no scientific evidence to show that supplements are needed or helpful.
- Poorly nourished people have a greater chance of adverse side effects from taking amino-acid supplements, including an amino-acid imbalance.

Available as:
- Capsules: Swallow whole with a full glass of liquid. Don't chew or crush. Take with or 1 to 1-1/2 hours after meals unless otherwise directed by your doctor.
- Lysine is a constituent of many multivitamin/mineral preparations.

Warnings and Precautions

Don't take if you are:
- Allergic to any food protein, such as eggs, milk, wheat

- At risk of poor nutrition for any reason
- Self-prescribing without medical supervision

Consult your doctor if you have:
Diabetes mellitus.

Over 55:
Don't take amino-acid supplements if you are healthy.

Pregnancy:
Don't take amino-acid supplements.

Breastfeeding:
Don't take amino-acid supplements.

Effect on lab tests:
None are known.

Storage:
- Store in cool, dry place away from direct light, but don't freeze.
- Store safely out of reach of children.
- Don't store in bathroom medicine cabinet. Heat and moisture may change the action of the amino acid.

Overdose/Toxicity

Signs and symptoms:
Unlikely to threaten life or cause significant symptoms.

What to do:
For symptoms of overdose:
Discontinue amino acid and consult doctor.

For accidental overdose (such as child taking entire bottle): Dial 911 (emergency), 0 for operator or call your nearest Poison Control Center.

Adverse Reactions or Side Effects
None are expected.

➜

AMINO ACIDS

Interaction with Medicine, Vitamins or Minerals

None are expected.

 Interaction with Other Substances

Foods high in arginine (nuts, chocolate, seeds, carob and raisins) decrease the ability of l-lysine to prevent or reduce cold sore outbreaks.

 Lab Tests to Detect Deficiency

None are available, except for experimental purposes.

Methionine

 Basic Information

Methionine is an amino acid. S-adenosyl-methionine (SAM), a by-product of methionine, is more widely used in Europe.

- Available from natural sources? Yes
- Available from synthetic sources? Yes
- Prescription required? No

 Natural Sources

Beans	Lentils
Eggs	Meat
Fish	Milk
Garlic	Onions

 Benefits

Functions as building block of all proteins

 Possible Additional Benefits

- May be effective adjuvant treatment for depression—consult doctor

- Cysteine and taurine may rely on methionine for synthesis in the human body

 Who May Benefit from Additional Amounts?

- Those with inadequate protein dietary intake
- Vegan vegetarians
- People with recent severe burns or injuries
- Premature infants

 Deficiency Symptoms

Single amino-acid deficiencies are unknown except in people on crash diets consisting of only a few foods. Amino-acid deficiencies appear more commonly as a result of total protein deficiency, which is rare in the United States and Canada.

Moderate deficiency:
- Slowed growth in children
- Low levels of essential proteins in blood

Severe deficiency:
- Apathy
- Depigmentation of hair
- Edema (excess fluid in connective tissue)
- Lethargy
- Liver damage
- Loss of muscle and fat
- Skin lesions
- Weakness

Usage Information

What this amino acid does:
Methionine provides part of all proteins.

Miscellaneous information:
- This sulfur-containing amino acid (like choline and taurine) may help eliminate fatty substances that could cause occlusion (see Glossary) of vital arteries.
- Poorly nourished people have a greater chance of adverse side effects from taking amino-acid supplements, including an amino-acid imbalance.
- Few people need methionine supplements.

Available as:
- Tablets: Swallow whole with a full glass of liquid. Don't chew or crush. Take with or 1 to 1-1/2 hours after meals unless otherwise directed by your doctor.
- Capsules: Swallow whole with a full glass of liquid. Don't chew or crush. Take with food or immediately after eating to decrease stomach irritation.

Warnings and Precautions

Don't take if you are:
- Allergic to any food protein, such as eggs, milk, wheat
- At risk of poor nutrition for any reason

Consult your doctor if you have:
Self-prescribed methionine without medical supervision.

Over 55:
Don't take amino-acid supplements if you are healthy.

Pregnancy:
Don't take amino-acid supplements.

Breastfeeding:
Don't take amino-acid supplements.

Effect on lab tests:
None are known.

Storage:
- Store in cool, dry place away from direct light, but don't freeze.
- Store safely out of reach of children.
- Don't store in bathroom medicine cabinet. Heat and moisture may change the action of the amino acid.

Overdose/Toxicity

Signs and symptoms:
Unlikely to threaten life or cause significant symptoms.

What to do:
For symptoms of overdose:
Discontinue amino acid and consult doctor.

For accidental overdose (such as child taking entire bottle): Dial 911 (emergency), 0 for operator or call your nearest Poison Control Center.

➡

AMINO ACIDS

Adverse Reactions or Side Effects

None are expected.

 Interaction with Other Substances

None are known.

 Interaction with Medicine, Vitamins or Minerals

None are known.

 Lab Tests to Detect Deficiency

None are available, except for experimental purposes.

Phenylalanine

 Basic Information

Phenylalanine is an amino acid.

- Available from natural sources? Yes
- Available from synthetic sources? Yes
- Prescription required? No

 Natural Sources

Almonds	Peanuts
Avocados	Pickled herring
Bananas	Pumpkin seeds
Cheese	Sesame seeds
Cottage cheese	Sugar products with
Lima beans	aspartame
Nonfat dried milk	

 Benefits

- Functions as building block of all proteins
- Can induce significant short-term increases of blood levels of norepinephrine, dopamine and epinephrine, which may be harmful at times and helpful at others (Don't take without medical supervision!)

 Possible Additional Benefits

No proven additional benefits exist.

Who May Benefit from Additional Amounts?

- Those with inadequate protein dietary intake
- Children and pregnant or breastfeeding women who are vegan vegetarians
- People with recent severe burns or injuries
- Premature infants

 Deficiency Symptoms

Single amino-acid deficiencies are unknown except in people on crash diets consisting of only a few foods. Amino-acid deficiencies appear more commonly as a result of total protein deficiency, which is rare in the United States and Canada.

Moderate deficiency:

- Slowed growth in children
- Low levels of essential proteins in blood

Severe deficiency:

- Apathy
- Depigmentation of hair

- Edema (excess fluid in connective tissue)
- Lethargy
- Liver damage
- Loss of muscle and fat
- Skin lesions
- Weakness

 ## Usage Information

What this amino acid does:

It is involved in the production of dopamine and epinephrine, which affect transmission of impulses in the human brain and other parts of the nervous system.

Miscellaneous information:

- Supplements taken by healthy people will not make them healthier.
- Poorly nourished people have a greater chance of adverse side effects from taking amino-acid supplements, including an amino-acid imbalance.

Available as:

- Tablets: Swallow whole with a full glass of liquid. Don't chew or crush. Take with or 1 to 1-1/2 hours after meals unless otherwise directed by your doctor.
- There are three different forms of phenylalanine: L, D and D L. The most common type is L. Consult your doctor about the proper type for you.

 ## Warnings and Precautions

Don't take if you:

- Are allergic to any food protein, such as eggs, milk, wheat
- Are at risk of poor nutrition for any reason
- Suffer from migraine headaches

- Have phenylketonuria (PKU)
- Have pigmented malignant melanoma, a deadly form of skin cancer
- Take any monoamine oxidase inhibitor as an antidepressant, including pargyline, isocarboxazid, phenelzine, procarbazine, tranylcypromine
- Have diabetes
- Are pregnant
- Suffer from anxiety attacks

Consult your doctor if you have:

- High blood pressure
- Self-medicated with phenylalanine for any reason without medical supervision

Over 55:

Don't take amino-acid supplements if you are healthy.

Pregnancy:

- Don't take amino-acid supplements.
- Pregnant women and children with PKU must follow a phenylalanine-free or -low diet to maintain health. Consult your doctor.

Breastfeeding:

Don't take amino-acid supplements.

Effect on lab tests:

None are known.

Storage:

- Store in cool, dry place away from direct light, but don't freeze.
- Store safely out of reach of children.
- Don't store in bathroom medicine cabinet. Heat and moisture may change the action of the amino acid.

Others:

- Phenylalanine may cause high blood pressure to rise even higher.
- It can cause mental retardation in children with PKU.

AMINO ACIDS

→

Overdose/Toxicity

Signs and symptoms:
Unlikely to threaten life or cause significant symptoms.

What to do:

For symptoms of overdose:
Discontinue amino acid and consult doctor. Also see *Adverse Reactions or Side Effects* section below.

For accidental overdose (such as child taking entire bottle): Dial 911 (emergency), 0 for operator or call your nearest Poison Control Center.

Adverse Reactions or Side Effects

Reaction or effect	What to do
Lowers blood pressure	Discontinue. Call doctor immediately.
Migraine headaches	Discontinue. Call doctor immediately.
Raises blood pressure	Discontinue. Call doctor immediately.

Interaction with Medicine, Vitamins or Minerals

Interacts with	Combined effect
Antidepressant drugs (containing monoamine oxidase inhibitors)	Dangerous or life-threatening blood-pressure elevation.
Tyrosine	Additive effect with phenylalanine greatly increases chance of undesirable side effects.

Interaction with Other Substances

None are known.

Lab Tests to Detect Deficiency

None are available, except for experimental purposes.

Serine

Basic Information

Serine is an amino acid.

• Available from natural sources? Yes
• Available from synthetic sources? Yes
• Prescription required? No

Natural Sources

Dairy products
Meat
Peanuts
Soy
Wheat gluten

Benefits

- Functions as building block of all proteins
- Aids metabolism of fats
- Important for muscle growth and maintenance
- Used in skin care products as a natural moisturizer

Possible Additional Benefits

None are known.

Who May Benefit from Additional Intake?

Anyone with inadequate caloric or nutritional dietary intake or increased nutritional requirements

Deficiency Symptoms

Single amino-acid deficiencies are unknown except in people on crash diets consisting of only a few foods. Amino-acid deficiencies appear more commonly as a result of total protein deficiency, which is rare in the United States and Canada.

Usage Information

What this amino acid does:
Serine helps produce antibodies.

Miscellaneous information:
- Poorly nourished people have a greater chance of adverse side effects from taking amino-acid supplements, including an amino-acid imbalance.
- Serine is considered a nonessential amino acid.

Available as:
A constituent of some amino-acid supplements.

Warnings and Precautions

Don't take if you are:
- Allergic to any food protein, such as eggs, milk, wheat
- Self-prescribing without medical supervision

Consult your doctor if you are:
Considering taking serine.

Over 55:
Don't take amino-acid supplements if you are healthy.

Pregnancy:
Don't take amino-acid supplements.

Breastfeeding:
Don't take amino-acid supplements.

Effect on lab tests:
None are known.

Storage:
- Store in cool, dry area away from direct light, but don't freeze.
- Store safely out of reach of children.
- Don't store in bathroom medicine cabinet. Heat and moisture may change the action of the amino acid.

Overdose/Toxicity

Signs and symptoms:
Unknown.

AMINO ACIDS

→

What to do:

For symptoms of overdose:
Discontinue amino acid and consult doctor.

For accidental overdose (such as child taking entire bottle): Dial 911 (emergency), 0 for operator or call your nearest Poison Control Center.

Adverse Reactions or Side Effects

None are expected.

Interaction with Medicine, Vitamins or Minerals

None are known.

Interaction with Other Substances

None are known.

Lab Tests to Detect Deficiency

None are available, except for experimental purposes.

Taurine

Basic Information

Taurine is an amino acid that is nonessential—it can be made by the body.

• Available from natural sources? Yes
• Available from synthetic sources? Yes
• Prescription required? No

Natural Sources

Breast milk
Eggs
Fish (especially clams and oysters)
Meat
Milk
Note: Not available from plant sources.

Benefits

• Helps regulate fluid balance

Possible Additional Benefits

• May stabilize heart rhythm
• May contribute to antioxidant (see Glossary) defense
• May be essential for growth of infants, children, adolescents
• May strengthen heart muscle
• May reduce Adriamycin toxicity
• May aid in controlling high blood pressure
• May reduce platelet clumping

Who May Benefit from Additional Amounts?

- Those with inadequate protein dietary intake
- Children and pregnant or breast-feeding women who are vegan vegetarians
- People with recent severe burns or injuries
- Premature infants

Deficiency Symptoms

Single amino-acid deficiencies are unknown except in people on crash diets consisting of only a few foods. Amino-acid deficiencies appear more commonly as a result of total protein deficiency, which is rare in the United States and Canada.

Moderate deficiency:
- Slowed growth in children
- Low levels of essential proteins in blood

Severe deficiency:
- Apathy
- Depigmentation of hair
- Edema (excess fluid in connective tissue)
- Lethargy
- Liver damage
- Loss of muscle and fat
- Skin lesions
- Weakness

Usage Information

Miscellaneous information:
- Taurine is synthesized from methionine and cystine. Vitamin B-6 is needed for this synthesis.
- Healthy people who eat well-balanced diets don't need supplements.

- Poorly nourished people have a greater chance of adverse side effects from taking amino-acid supplements, including an amino-acid imbalance.
- Breast milk is rich in taurine.

Available as:
- Tablets: Swallow whole with a full glass of liquid. Don't chew or crush. Take with or 1 to 1-1/2 hours after meals unless otherwise directed by your doctor.
- Capsules: Swallow whole with a full glass of liquid. Don't chew or crush. Take with or 1 to 1-1/2 hours after meals unless otherwise directed by your doctor.

Warnings and Precautions

Don't take if you:
- Are allergic to any food protein such as eggs, milk, wheat
- Are at risk of poor nutrition for any reason
- Have stomach ulcers

Consult your doctor if you have:
- Epilepsy
- Eye problems
- Self-prescribed taurine without medical supervision

Over 55:
Don't take amino-acid supplements if you are healthy.

Pregnancy:
Don't take amino-acid supplements.

Breastfeeding:
Don't take amino-acid supplements.

Effect on lab tests:
None are known.

Storage:
- Store in cool, dry place away from direct light, but don't freeze.

AMINO ACIDS

- Store safely out of reach of children.
- Don't store in bathroom medicine cabinet. Heat and moisture may change the action of the amino acid.

Overdose/Toxicity

Signs and symptoms:
Unlikely to threaten life or cause significant symptoms.

What to do:
For symptoms of overdose:
Discontinue amino acid and consult doctor. Also see *Adverse Reactions or Side Effects* section below.

For accidental overdose (such as child taking entire bottle): Dial 911 (emergency), 0 for operator or call your nearest Poison Control Center.

Adverse Reactions or Side Effects

Reaction or effect	What to do
Depression of central nervous system	Discontinue. Call doctor immediately.
Memory deficits	Discontinue. Call doctor when convenient.

Interaction with Medicine, Vitamins or Minerals

Interacts with	Combined effect
Anticonvulsants	May decrease frequency of seizures.

Interaction with Other Substances

Alcohol: Excessive alcohol intake causes large urinary loss of taurine and impaired utilization of taurine.

Food and beverages: Intake of monosodium glutamate (MSG) and aspartame may reduce taurine levels.

Lab Tests to Detect Deficiency

None are available, except for experimental purposes.

Tryptophan Declared unsafe: DO NOT TAKE!

Basic Information

Tryptophan is an amino acid.

- Available from natural sources? Yes
- Available from synthetic sources? Yes
- Prescription required? No

Natural Sources

Barley
Brown Rice
Cottage cheese
Fish (tuna, crab, shellfish)

Meats (beef, chicken, duck, turkey)
Milk
Peanuts
Soybean

Note: You cannot get enough tryptophan from natural sources to cause adverse reactions.

Benefits

Functions as building block of all proteins

 Possible Additional Benefits

- May reduce alcohol cravings
- May be an effective sleep aid
- Potential antidepressant
- May help treat cocaine addiction
- May decrease sensitivity to moderate pain

 Who May Benefit from Additional Amounts?

- Those with inadequate protein dietary intake
- Children and pregnant or breastfeeding women who are vegan vegetarians
- People with recent severe burns or injuries
- Premature infants

 Deficiency Symptoms

Single amino-acid deficiencies are unknown except in people on crash diets consisting of only a few foods. Amino-acid deficiencies appear more commonly as a result of total protein deficiency, which is rare in the United States and Canada.

Moderate deficiency:
- Slowed growth in children
- Low levels of essential proteins in blood

Severe deficiency:
- Apathy
- Depigmentation of hair
- Edema (excess fluid in connective tissue)
- Lethargy
- Liver damage
- Loss of muscle and fat
- Skin lesions
- Weakness

 Usage Information

What this amino acid does:
- Provides part of all proteins
- Participates in biosynthesis of a neurotransmitter (see Glossary) called serotonin, which may induce certain stages of sleep

Miscellaneous information:
Contaminated supplements have been related to several deaths in the United States.

Available as:
- Tryptophan has been withdrawn from the United States market by the U.S. Food and Drug Administration.
- 5-hydroxytryptophan (5-HTP), a supplement that contains a form of tryptophan, is now available.

 Warnings and Precautions

Don't take:
May cause eosinophilia-myalgia, a potentially fatal adverse reaction. Declared unsafe by the United States Food and Drug Administration and withdrawn from the U.S. market.

Consult your doctor if you:
- Take medicines to induce sleep
- Have asthma—tryptophan may increase breathing problems
- Have taken or are taking antidepressants

AMINO ACIDS

Over 55:
Don't take tryptophan.

Pregnancy:
Don't take tryptophan.

Breastfeeding:
Don't take tryptophan.

Effect on lab tests:
None are known.

Others:
• Tryptophan has caused eosinophilia-myalgia, a potentially fatal adverse reaction. (The adverse reaction of eosinophiliamyalgia was caused by a contaminant found in supplements, not tryptophan itself.)
• In experimental animal studies of animals with vitamin B-6 deficiency, large doses of tryptophan caused bladder cancer.
• If you have any tryptophan in your medicine cabinet, throw it out.

 Overdose/Toxicity

Signs and symptoms:
May cause eosinophilia-myalgia, a potentially fatal adverse reaction.

What to do:
For symptoms of overdose:
Discontinue amino acid and consult doctor. Also see *Adverse Reactions or Side Effects* section below.

For accidental overdose (such as child taking entire bottle): Dial 911 (emergency), 0 for operator or call your nearest Poison Control Center.

 Adverse Reactions or Side Effects

Tryptophan has caused eosinophilia-myalgia, a potentially fatal adverse reaction.

 Interaction with Medicine, Vitamins or Minerals

None are known.

 Interaction with Other Substances

None are known.

 Lab Tests to Detect Deficiency

None are available, except for experimental purposes.

Tyrosine

Basic Information

- Available from natural sources? Yes
- Available from synthetic sources? Yes
- Prescription required? No

Natural Sources

Canned beans with pork	Lima beans
	Meat
Cheese, especially cheddar	Miso
	Peanuts
Cottage cheese	Pumpkin seeds
Eggs	Shellfish
Fish	Soybeans
Ice cream	

Benefits

- Functions as building block of all proteins
- Can induce significant short-term increases of blood levels of norepinephrine, dopamine and epinephrine, which may be harmful at times and helpful at others (Don't take without medical supervision!)

Possible Additional Benefits

- May regulate and elevate moods
- May help to reduce mental depression
- May improve memory
- May diminish pain
- May increase mental alertness
- May reduce Parkinson's disease symptoms (under medical care)
- May treat chronic fatigue and narcolepsy
- May reduce stress
- May reduce body fat
- May help with withdrawal from cocaine addiction (under medical supervision)

Who May Benefit from Additional Amounts?

- Those with inadequate protein dietary intake
- Children and pregnant or breastfeeding women who are vegan vegetarians
- People with recent severe burns or injuries
- Premature infants

Deficiency Symptoms

Single amino-acid deficiencies are unknown except in people on crash diets consisting of only a few foods. Amino-acid deficiencies appear more commonly as a result of total protein deficiency, which is rare in the United States and Canada.

Moderate deficiency:
- Slowed growth in children
- Low levels of essential proteins in blood

Severe deficiency:
- Apathy
- Depigmentation of hair
- Edema (excess fluid in connective tissue)
- Lethargy
- Liver damage
- Loss of muscle and fat
- Skin lesions
- Weakness

AMINO ACIDS

→

Unproved speculated symptoms:
• Lack of sexual interest
• Impotence
• Poor memory
• Obesity

 Usage Information

What this amino acid does:
It is involved in the production of dopamine and epinephrine, which affect transmission of impulses in the human brain and other parts of the nervous system.

Miscellaneous information:
• Supplements taken by healthy people will not make them healthier.
• Poorly nourished people have a greater chance of adverse side effects from taking amino-acid supplements, including an amino-acid imbalance.
• Take with a high carbohydrate meal or at bedtime.

Available as:
Tablets: Swallow whole with a full glass of liquid. Don't chew or crush. Take with or 1 to 1-1/2 hours after meals unless otherwise directed by your doctor.

 Warnings and Precautions

Don't take if you:
• Are allergic to any food protein, such as eggs, milk, wheat
• Are at risk of poor nutrition for any reason
• Suffer from migraine headaches
• Have phenylketonuria (PKU)
• Have pigmented malignant melanoma, a deadly form of skin cancer
• Take any monamine oxidase inhibitor as an antidepressant, including pargyline, isocarboxazid, phenelzine, procarbazine, tranylcypromine

Consult your doctor if you have:
• High blood pressure
• Self-medicated with tyrosine for any reason without medical supervision

Over 55:
Don't take amino-acid supplements if you are healthy.

Pregnancy:
Don't take amino-acid supplements.

Breastfeeding:
Don't take amino-acid supplements.

Effect on lab tests:
None are known.

Storage:
• Store in cool, dry place away from direct light, but don't freeze.
• Store safely out of reach of children.
• Don't store in bathroom medicine cabinet. Heat and moisture may change the action of the amino acid.

Others:
Tyrosine may cause high blood pressure to rise even higher at times.

 Overdose/Toxicity

Signs and symptoms:
Unlikely to threaten life or cause significant symptoms.

What to do:
For symptoms of overdose:
Discontinue amino acid and consult doctor. Also see *Adverse Reactions or Side Effects* section below.

For accidental overdose (such as child taking entire bottle): Dial 911 (emergency), 0 for operator or call your nearest Poison Control Center.

Adverse Reactions
or Side Effects

Reaction or effect	What to do
Lowers blood pressure	Discontinue. Call doctor immediately.
Migraine headaches	Discontinue. Call doctor immediately.
Raises blood pressure	Discontinue. Call doctor immediately.

 Interaction with
Medicine, Vitamins
or Minerals

Interacts with	Combined effect
Antidepressant drugs (containing mono-amine oxidase inhibitors)	Dangerous or life-threatening blood-pressure elevation.
Phenylalanine	Additive effect with tyrosine greatly increases chance of undesirable side effects.

 Interaction with
Other Substances

None are known.

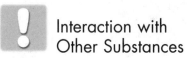 Lab Tests to Detect
Deficiency

None are available, except for experimental purposes.

Food Supplements

The substances discussed in this section are not vitamins, minerals or herbs. There are many more supplements available than those listed. Many people continue to debate their value in human nutrition and health.

Acidophilus (Lactobacillus)

 ## Basic Information

Acidophilus is a bacterium found in yogurt, kefir and other products.

Chemical this supplement contains: Enzymes to aid digestion.

 ## Known Effects

- Helps maintain normal bacteria balance in lower intestines
- Kills monilia, yeast and fungus on contact

Miscellaneous information:

Acidophilus is made by fermenting milk using *lactobacillus acidophilus* and other bacteria.

 ## Possible Additional Effects

- May lower cholesterol
- May clear up skin problems
- May help prevent vaginal yeast infections in women who take antibiotics or who have diabetes
- May extend life span
- Potential aid for digestion of milk and milk products in people with lactase deficiency
- May enhance immunity
- May reduce symptoms from spastic colon
- May reduce diarrhea related to long-term antibiotic use

STOP Warnings and Precautions

Don't take if you:
- Have intestinal problems, except under medical supervision
- Plan to use in vaginal area for yeast infections

Consult your doctor if you:

Take any medicinal drugs or herbs including aspirin, laxatives, cold and cough remedies, antacids, vitamins, minerals, amino acids, supplements, other prescription or nonprescription drugs.

Pregnancy:

Problems in pregnant women taking small or usual amounts have not been proved, but the chance of problems does exist. Don't use unless prescribed by your doctor.

Breastfeeding:

Problems in breast-fed infants of lactating mothers taking small or usual amounts have not been proved, but the chance of problems does exist. Don't use unless prescribed by your doctor.

Infants and children:

Treating infants and children under 2 with any supplement is hazardous.

Storage:
- Refrigerate but don't freeze.
- Store safely out of reach of children.

Safe dosage:
- At present no "safe" dosage has been established.
- It is available as a liquid, in capsules or tablets, as a powder or in milk products, such as yogurt or kefir.

Toxicity

Comparative-toxicity rating is not available from standard references.

Adverse Reactions, Side Effects or Overdose Symptoms

None are expected.

Bee Pollen

Basic Information

Bee pollen is the microscopic male seed in flowering plants. It is expensive and provides inadequate, uncertain quantities of nutrients.

Chemicals this supplement contains:
- Amino acids
- Minerals
- Vitamins (some)

Known Effects

None are proven.

Miscellaneous information:
Bee pollen from a local source is preferable as it is more likely to decrease allergy symptoms.

Possible Additional Effects

- May produce antimicrobial (see Glossary) effect
- May renew skin
- May boost immunity
- May decrease allergy symptoms

Warnings and Precautions

Don't take if you are:
Pregnant, think you may be pregnant or plan pregnancy in the near future.

Consult your doctor if you:
Take this herb for any medical problem that doesn't improve in 2 weeks (There may be safer, more effective treatments.)

Pregnancy:
Problems in pregnant women taking small or usual amounts have not been proved, but the chance of problems does exist. Don't use unless prescribed by your doctor.

Breastfeeding:
Problems in breast-fed infants of lactating mothers taking small or usual amounts have not been proved, but the chance of problems does exist. Don't use unless prescribed by your doctor.

Infants and children:
Treating infants and children under 2 with any supplement is hazardous.

FOOD SUPPLEMENTS

→

Storage:

- Keep cool and dry, but don't freeze.
- Store safely away from children.
- Store in tightly sealed container.

Safe dosage:

- At present no "safe" dosage has been established.
- Bee pollen is available in injectable form and capsules.

Toxicity

Comparative-toxicity rating is not available from standard references.

For symptoms of toxicity: See *Adverse Reactions, Side Effects or Overdose Symptoms* section below.

Adverse Reactions, Side Effects or Overdose Symptoms

Signs and symptoms	What to do
May cause allergic reactions in those sensitive to pollens: Mild allergic response is characterized by itching, pain at injection site and swelling occurring within 24 to 48 hours.	Discontinue. Call doctor immediately.
Life-threatening anaphylaxis may follow injection: Symptoms include immediate severe itching, paleness, low blood pressure, loss of consciousness, coma	Yell for help. Don't leave victim. Begin CPR (cardio-pulmonary resuscitation), mouth-to-mouth breathing and external cardiac massage. Have someone dial "0" (operator) or 911 (emergency). Don't stop CPR until help arrives.

Bioflavonoids, Phytochemicals (Vitamin P)

Basic Information

Bioflavonoids are a brightly colored, chemical constituent of the pulp and rind of citrus fruits, green pepper, apricots, cherries, grapes, papaya, tomatoes and broccoli.

There are at least 4,000 compounds found in fruits, vegetables, wine and tea.

For information about specific phytochemicals, their food sources and disease prevention, see the *Phytochemicals and Health* chart, page 478.

Chemicals this supplement contains:

- Eriodictyol
- Hesperetin
- Hesperidin
- Nobiletin
- Quercetin
- Rutin
- Sinensetin
- Tangeretin

Known Effects

Treats rare bioflavonoid deficiency characterized by fragile capillaries and unusual bleeding

Miscellaneous information:

- Enough bioflavonoids are present in food to make supplements unnecessary in healthy humans.
- Commercial products such as tablets or capsules often contain vitamin C.

Possible Additional Effects

- Quercetin may help regulate blood-sugar levels in diabetics
- May act as an antioxidant (see Glossary), preventing vitamin C and adrenaline from being oxidized by copper-containing enzymes (see Glossary)
- May increase effectiveness of vitamin C
- May prevent hemorrhoids
- May prevent miscarriages
- May prevent retinal bleeding in people with diabetes and hypertension
- May prevent capillary fragility
- May prevent nosebleed
- May prevent post-partum hemorrhage
- May prevent menstrual disorders
- May prevent blood clotting and platelet clumping
- May prevent easy bruising
- May prevent or treat cataracts
- May lessen symptoms of oral herpes when taken with vitamin C
- May decrease cholesterol levels
- Quercetin may lessen or prevent asthma symptoms

Warnings and Precautions

Don't take if you:

Have a bleeding problem, until studies are done to diagnose the underlying disease.

Consult your doctor if you:

- Self-medicate
- Take any medicinal drugs or herbs including aspirin, laxatives, cold and cough remedies, antacids, vitamins, minerals, amino acids, supplements, other prescription or nonprescription drugs

Pregnancy:

Notify your doctor if you take supplements.

Breastfeeding:

Notify your doctor if you take supplements.

Infants and children:

Treating infants and children under 2 with any supplement is hazardous.

Others:

None are expected if you are beyond childhood and under 45, basically healthy and take supplements for only a short time.

Storage:

- Store in cool, dry place away from direct light, but don't freeze.
- Store safely out of reach of children.
- Don't store in bathroom medicine cabinet. Heat and moisture may change the action of the supplement.

Safe dosage:

- At present no "safe" dosage has been established.
- Bioflavonoids are sold under the brand names Rutin and Hesperiden and are included in numerous vitamin/mineral supplements.

Toxicity

Comparative-toxicity rating is not available from standard references.

Adverse Reactions, Side Effects or Overdose Symptoms

None are expected.

FOOD SUPPLEMENTS

Brewer's Yeast

 Basic Information

Brewer's yeast is nonleavening with a slightly bitter taste. It is an excellent source of B vitamins, protein and minerals.

Chemicals this supplement contains:
- B vitamins
- DNA and RNA (see Glossary)
- Trace mineral, chromium

 Known Effects

- Supplies B vitamins, protein and minerals
- Provides bulk to prevent constipation
- Good source of enzyme-producing vitamins
- Chromium in brewer's yeast helps regulate sugar metabolism

Miscellaneous information:
- Out of the can, the bitter taste of brewer's yeast may be unpleasant. Adding it to foods with a strong taste makes it tolerable.
- Brewer's yeast is a good, inexpensive food supplement for aging adults and growing, developing children.

 Possible Additional Effects

- May reduce risk of high cholesterol in blood
- Possible treatment for contact dermatitis
- May increase energy
- May reduce risk of prostate cancer

 Warnings and Precautions

Don't take if you have:
Intestinal disease.

Consult your doctor if you:
- Have an acute intestinal upset
- Take any medicinal drugs or herbs including aspirin, laxatives, cold and cough remedies, antacids, vitamins, minerals, amino acids, supplements, other prescription or nonprescription drugs
- Have osteoporosis

Pregnancy:
Safe to use in doses of 1 to 2 tablespoons per day.

Breastfeeding:
Safe to use in doses of 1 to 2 tablespoons per day.

Infants and children:
Treating infants and children under 2 with any supplement is hazardous.

Others:
- The quality and quantity of nutrients vary greatly among commercially available products.
- Brewer's yeast is usually nontoxic if you consume 1 tablespoon or less of the powder or equivalent amounts of tablets or flakes.

Storage:
- Store in cool, dry place away from direct light, but don't freeze.
- Store safely out of reach of children.
- Don't store in bathroom medicine cabinet. Heat and moisture may change the action of the supplement.

Safe dosage:
- Brewer's yeast is available in powder, flakes and tablets.
- It can be used in baking, soups, chili and casseroles to increase nutritional content.

 Toxicity

Comparative-toxicity rating is not available from standard references.

For symptoms of toxicity: See *Adverse Reactions, Side Effects or Overdose Symptoms* section below.

 Adverse Reactions, Side Effects or Overdose Symptoms

Signs and symptoms	What to do
Diarrhea	Discontinue. Call doctor immediately.
Nausea	Discontinue. Call doctor immediately.

Chondroitin Sulfate

 Basic Information

This substance is found in the cartilage of most mammals.

Chemicals this supplement contains: Complex protein molecules.

 Known Effects

None are proven.

Miscellaneous information:

Chondroitin sulfate is found in bone, cartilage and connective tissue.

 Possible Additional Effects

- May lower cholesterol levels
- May prolong clotting time
- May reduce urine acid levels associated with gout
- Anti-inflammatory effects may reduce osteoarthritis symptoms (generally taken with glucosamine)

 Warnings and Precautions

Don't take if you:
- Have bleeding problems
- Are pregnant, think you may be pregnant or plan pregnancy in the near future

Consult your doctor if you take:
- Anticoagulants
- Any medicinal drugs or herbs including aspirin, laxatives, cold and cough remedies, antacids, vitamins, minerals, amino acids, supplements, other prescription or nonprescription drugs

Pregnancy:
Don't use unless prescribed by your doctor.

FOOD SUPPLEMENTS

➜

Breastfeeding:
Don't use unless prescribed by
your doctor.

Infants and children:
Treating infants and children under
2 with any supplement is hazardous.

Others:
No precautions if you are beyond
childhood and under 45, basically
healthy and take for only a short time.

Storage:
• Store in cool, dry place away from
  direct light, but don't freeze.
• Store safely out of reach of children.
• Don't store in bathroom medicine
  cabinet. Heat and moisture may
  change the action of the supplement.

Safe dosage:
• At present no "safe" dosage has been
  established.
• Chondroitin sulfate is available in
  capsule form.

Toxicity

Comparative-toxicity rating is not available from standard references.

Adverse Reactions, Side Effects or Overdose Symptoms

None are expected.

Coenzyme Q (CoQ) (Ubiquinone)

Basic Information

Coenzyme Q is part of the mitochondria (see Glossary) of cells and is
necessary for energy production.

Chemical this supplement contains:
Coenzyme Q10 (a nutrient) found in
• Beef   • Salmon
• Mackerel   • Sardines
• Peanuts   • Spinach

Known Effects

• Controls flow of oxygen within
  individual cells
• Increases circulation
• Boosts the immune system

Possible Additional Effects

• May improve heart-muscle
  metabolism
• Potential treatment for chest pain
  caused by narrowed coronary
  arteries (coronary insufficiency)
• May lower blood pressure
• May treat congestive (see Glossary)
  heart failure by enhancing pumping
  action of heart
• May be effective in congestive heart
  failure, ischemic (see Glossary)
  heart disease

Warnings and Precautions

Don't take if you have:
Heart disease, without consulting
your doctor.

Consult your doctor if you:

Take any medicinal drugs or herbs including aspirin, laxatives, cold and cough remedies, antacids, vitamins, minerals, amino acids, supplements, other prescription or nonprescription drugs.

Pregnancy:

Dangers outweigh any benefits. Don't use.

Breastfeeding:

Dangers outweigh any benefits. Don't use.

Infants and children:

Treating infants and children under 2 with any supplement is hazardous.

Others:

No problems are expected if you are not pregnant and do not take amounts larger than the manufacturer's recommended dosage.

Storage:

- Keep cool and dry, but don't freeze.
- Store safely away from children.
- Store away from heat and light.

Safe dosage:

- 200–300mg, 2 to 3 times per day.
- Oral products are available: Lozenges, chewable tablets and oil-based gelcaps.
- The best forms to use are liquid or oil that contain a small portion of vitamin E to preserve ubiquinone.

 Toxicity

Comparative-toxicity rating is not available from standard references.

 Adverse Reactions, Side Effects or Overdose Symptoms

None are expected.

Conjugated Linoleic Acid (CLA)

 Basic Information

Conjugated linoleic acid is a fatty acid found in corn oil, safflower oil, sunflower oil, canola oil, nuts, seeds, beef and dairy products.

 Known Effects

The following effects have been found in studies conducted on animals, not in humans:

- Reduces body fat
- Inhibits tumor growth
- Boosts immune system

Miscellaneous information:

- CLA is not damaged by cooking or storage.
- CLA is an omega-6 fatty acid.
- The balance between omega-6 and omega-3 fatty acids is important to overall health and disease prevention.
- Linoleic acid is an essential fatty acid which should be included in all diets to prevent a deficiency.
- CLA prevents essential-fatty-acid deficiency due to lack of linoleic acid.

FOOD SUPPLEMENTS

→

Possible
Additional Effects

- May reduce risk of arteriosclerosis
- May reduce cholesterol levels
- May reduce symptoms of psoriasis

 Warnings and
Precautions

Don't take if you are:
Healthy and eat a well-balanced diet.

Consult your doctor if you are:
On anticoagulant therapy.

Pregnancy:
Decide with your doctor if any benefits of CLA justify the risk to your unborn child. Risk is unknown because CLA is not regulated by the FDA.

Breastfeeding:
Breast milk is considered balanced in fatty acids to best meet the infant's needs. Supplements should not be necessary. Consult doctor before taking.

Infants and children:
Treating infants and children under 2 with any supplement is hazardous.

Safe dosage:
CLA, as a product, is marketed as a dietary supplement and is not reviewed by the U.S. Food and Drug Administration (FDA) for effectiveness and safety. The best dosage amounts are unknown. Use with caution.

 Toxicity

Comparative-toxicity rating is not available from standard references.

 Adverse Reactions,
Side Effects or
Overdose Symptoms

None are known.

Creatine

 Basic Information

Creatine is manufactured in the liver and also found in meats.

Chemicals this supplement contains: proteins.

 Known Effects

Promotes weight gain

Miscellaneous information:
- Competitive athletes may benefit from additional amounts of creatine.
- Creatine aids the release of energy in muscles by increasing the production and circulation of adenosine triphosphate (ATP).
- Creatine is not researched carefully as yet for use in humans.

 Possible
Additional Effects

- May improve strength and power

- May enhance performance in activities that require intense short-term effort such as weight-lifting or swimming
- May decrease fatigue

Warnings and Precautions

Don't take if you are:
Allergic to creatine.

Consult your doctor if you:
- Have any chronic health problem
- Are allergic to any medication, food or other substance
- Are considering taking creatine (safety of creatine supplements is currently being investigated by the U.S. Food and Drug Administration)

Pregnancy:
Risk is unknown. Do not use.

Breastfeeding:
Risk is unknown. Do not use.

Infants and children:
Treating infants and children under 2 with any supplement is hazardous.

Others:
- Don't take with any prescription or nonprescription medicine without consulting your doctor or pharmacist.
- Not much is known about the effects of long-term use.

Safe dosage:
- Creatine, as a product, is marketed as a dietary supplement. The U.S. Food and Drug Administration (FDA) recently labeled creatine supplements as unsafe due to deaths in three athletes. It is unknown if creatine or some impurity in the supplement led to the deaths. The best dosage amounts are unknown. Use with caution.
- Creatine is available as chewable tablets, capsules or powder: Follow instructions on the label or consult your doctor or pharmacist. Different brands supply different doses.
- At present no "safe" dosage has been established.

Toxicity

Comparative-toxicity rating is not available from standard references.

For symptoms of toxicity: See *Adverse Reactions, Side Effects or Overdose Symptoms* section below.

Adverse Reactions, Side Effects or Overdose Symptoms

Signs and symptoms	What to do
Gastrointestinal problems	Discontinue. Call doctor when convenient.
Increased blood pressure	Discontinue. Call doctor when convenient.
Muscle cramping	Discontinue. Call doctor when convenient.
Nausea	Discontinue. Call doctor when convenient.

FOOD SUPPLEMENTS

Dehydroepiandrosterone (DHEA)

 Basic Information

DHEA is a steroid produced in the human body by the adrenal glands (which sit on top of the kidney).

 Known Effects

Improves overall feeling of well-being in some individuals

Miscellaneous information:

- DHEA concentration peaks at about age 20 and then decreases progressively with advancing age. Supplements are sold as an anti-aging remedy.
- Although it is not known whether DHEA itself causes hormonal effects, the body breaks DHEA down into two hormones: estrogen and testosterone. Some people's bodies make large amounts of estrogen and testosterone from DHEA, while others make smaller amounts.

 Possible Additional Effects

- May improve energy
- May increase strength
- May boost immunity
- May increase muscle
- May decrease fat
- May improve sense of well-being in those with AIDS or multiple sclerosis

 Warnings and Precautions

Don't take if you are:
Allergic to DHEA.

Consult your doctor if you have:
- Any chronic health problem
- A family history of cancer
- Allergies to any medication, food or other substance

Pregnancy:
Decide with your doctor if any benefits of DHEA justify risk to the unborn child. Risk is unknown because DHEA is not regulated by the FDA.

Breastfeeding:
It is unknown if DHEA passes into milk. Avoid it or discontinue nursing until you finish medicine. Consult doctor for advice on maintaining milk supply.

Infants and children:
Treating infants and children under 2 with any supplement is hazardous.

Others:
- Hormone supplements may not have the same effects on the body as naturally produced hormones have, because the body processes them differently. Higher doses of supplements may result in higher amounts of hormones in the blood than are healthy.
- DHEA is not researched carefully as yet for use in humans. Most research has been performed on animals. Studies are ongoing to find more definite answers about its effect on aging, muscles and the immune system. Studies in men and women

have shown an improvement in the feeling of well-being. AIDS patients and those with multiple sclerosis also reportedly experienced improvement in well-being, but without an outcome change.

- Researchers are concerned that DHEA supplements may cause high levels of estrogen or testosterone in some people. The body's own testosterone plays a role in prostate cancer, and high levels of naturally produced estrogen are suspected of increasing breast cancer risk. The effect of DHEA is unknown.
- Don't take with any prescription or nonprescription medicine without consulting your doctor or pharmacist.

Safe dosage:

- DHEA is available in tablet or capsule form: Follow instructions on the label or consult your doctor or pharmacist. Different brands supply different doses. DHEA, as a product, is marketed as a dietary supplement and is not reviewed by the U.S. Food and Drug Administration (FDA) for effectiveness and safety. The best dosage amounts are unknown. Use with caution.

- A lower starting dosage may be recommended for persons over 55 years old until a response is determined.

Toxicity

Comparative-toxicity rating is not available from standard references.

For symptoms of toxicity: See *Adverse Reactions, Side Effects or Overdose Symptoms* section below.

Adverse Reactions, Side Effects or Overdose Symptoms

Signs and symptoms	What to do
Infrequent:	
In women—acne, hair loss, facial hair growth (hirsutism), deepening of voice (the last two may be irreversible)	Discontinue. Call doctor when convenient.

Dessicated Liver

Basic Information

Dessicated liver is a concentrated form of dried liver.

Chemicals this supplement contains:
Calcium
Cholesterol
Copper
Iron
Phosphorus
Vitamins A, B-complex, C, D

Known Effects

Source of vitamins A, B-complex, C, D and iron, calcium, phosphorus, copper

Miscellaneous information:

Do not use. There is a high risk of impurities, especially hepatitis. There is no indication that any organ parts have biological activity after digestion: If you

➔

have liver damage or liver problems, eating liver supplements will not fix your liver.

 ## Possible Additional Effects

- May act as an antistress agent
- May cure gum problems
- Possible anemia treatment
- May create red blood cells
- May increase energy

 ## Warnings and Precautions

Don't take if you are:
Pregnant, think you may be pregnant or plan pregnancy in the near future.

Consult your doctor if you:
Take any medicinal drugs or herbs including aspirin, laxatives, cold and cough remedies, antacids, vitamins, minerals, amino acids, supplements, other prescription or nonprescription drugs.

Pregnancy:
Problems in pregnant women taking small or usual amounts have not been proved, but the chance of problems does exist. Don't use unless prescribed by your doctor.

Breastfeeding:
Problems in breast-fed infants of lactating mothers taking small or usual amounts have not been proved, but the chance of problems does exist. Don't use unless prescribed by your doctor.

Infants and children:
Treating infants and children under 2 with any supplement is hazardous.

Storage:
- Keep cool and dry, but don't freeze.
- Store safely away from children.
- Don't store in bathroom medicine cabinet. Heat and moisture may change the action of the supplement.

Safe dosage:
- At present no "safe" dosage has been established.
- Dessicated liver is available in tablet or powder form.

 ## Toxicity

Comparative-toxicity rating is not available from standard references.

 ## Adverse Reactions, Side Effects or Overdose Symptoms

None are expected.

Dietary Fiber

 ## Basic Information

Cell walls of plants are made of fiber that give a plant structure and stability. Fiber cannot be broken down by enzymes in the digestive tract, so fiber passes through without being absorbed.

Chemicals this supplement contains: Structured and nonstructured substances in plant carbohydrate (starches).

Soluble Food Sources	Insoluble Food Sources
Apples	Brown rice
Barley	Legumes
Citrus fruits	Nuts
Cooked dried beans	Raw vegetables
Oats/oat bran/oatmeal	Root vegetables
Strawberries	Seeds
	Wheat bran
	Whole-grain breads and cereals

Known Effects

- Absorbs many times its weight in water, causing bulkier stools and lessening chance of constipation
- Helps control blood-sugar level in diabetics
- Helps reduce cholesterol and triglycerides in blood
- Soluble fiber found in oats is particularly beneficial for lowering cholesterol

Miscellaneous information:

- The best sources of dietary fiber include fresh fruits, vegetables, nuts, seeds, whole-grain products and potatoes.
- Increase in diet gradually over several weeks to avoid gastro-intestinal distress.

Possible Additional Effects

- May reduce risk of heart disease
- May reduce risk of colon and rectum cancer
- May reduce risk of diverticulitis
- May reduce risk of hemorrhoids
- May reduce risk of obesity
- Wheat, bran fiber may reduce risk of breast cancer

 ## Warnings and Precautions

Don't take if you have:
Crohn's disease.

Consult your doctor if you are:
Pregnant, think you may be pregnant or plan pregnancy in the near future.

Pregnancy:
Problems in pregnant women taking small or usual amounts have not been proved, but the chance of problems does exist. Don't use unless prescribed by your doctor.

Breastfeeding:
Problems in breast-fed infants of lactating mothers taking small or usual amounts have not been proved, but the chance of problems does exist. Don't use unless prescribed by your doctor.

Infants and children:
Treating infants and children under 2 with any supplement is hazardous.

Others:

- Intake of excessive amounts of fiber may decrease absorption of minerals, especially calcium, iron and zinc.
- Take fiber supplements separately from vitamin and mineral supplements.

Storage:

- Keep cool and dry, but don't freeze.
- Store safely away from children.
- Don't store in bathroom medicine cabinet. Heat and moisture may change the action of the supplement.

Safe dosage:

- Most experts feel that increasing fiber is healthful.
- Recommended intake to reduce risk of heart disease and cancer and promote blood-glucose control is 25–30 grams per day.

FOOD SUPPLEMENTS

- Fiber is available commercially in capsules, tablets, chewable tablets, oral suspension and flakes or wafers.

Toxicity

Comparative-toxicity rating is not available from standard references.

For symptoms of toxicity: See *Adverse Reactions, Side Effects or Overdose Symptoms* section below.

Adverse Reactions, Side Effects or Overdose Symptoms

Signs and symptoms	What to do
Bloating of abdomen	Discontinue. Call doctor when convenient.
Excess flatulence	Discontinue. Call doctor when convenient.
Obstruction of large intestine (rare, but more likely if there is pre-existing inflammatory disease): Symptoms of obstruction are tender, distended abdomen; abdominal pain; fever; no bowel movements.	Discontinue. Call doctor immediately.

Gamma-Linolenic Acid (GLA)

Basic Information

Gamma linolenic acid is found in a supplement called *evening primrose oil.*

Chemicals found in this supplement: Fatty acids found in

- Evening primrose (a plant)
- Fish
- Human mother's milk
- Spirulina (blue-green algae)

Known Effects

- Astringent
- Anti-inflammatory
- Reduces liver damage

- Anticoagulant properties, which make it useful in the prevention of heart attacks caused by thrombosis
- Helps people suffering from atopic eczema or eczema due to allergy
- Functions as one of the sources of essential fatty acids

Miscellaneous information:
- Deficiency can cause eczema.
- Those whose fat and oil intake is greatly restricted may require supplements.
- Evening primrose grows wild. A long spike of yellow flowers opens at night. Oil can be expressed from the tiny seeds of the flower.

Possible
Additional Effects

- Used in external preparations to treat skin eruptions, such as psoriasis
- May reduce inflammation associated with arthritis

 Warnings and Precautions

Don't take if you are:
- Healthy and eat a well-balanced diet
- On anticoagulant therapy—may increase bleeding time
- Taking other medicines such as phenothiazines

Consult your doctor if you have:
Any illness.

Pregnancy:
GLA appears to be safe. Consult your doctor before taking.

Breastfeeding:
GLA appears to be safe. Consult your doctor before taking.

Infants and children:
Treating infants and children under 2 with any supplement is hazardous.

Others:
- Gamma-linolenic acid, working with enzymes, becomes part of some prostaglandins. Prostaglandins sometimes limit inflammatory reactions in the body and sometimes cause inflammatory reactions. Taking evening primrose oil may cause unpredictable, harmful effects.
- Patients with schizophrenia should avoid taking gamma-linolenic acid.
- Discontinue at least 2 weeks prior to any surgery.
- Taking with vitamin E may prevent oxidation of the oil.

Storage:
- Store in cool, dry place away from direct light, but don't freeze.
- Store safely out of reach of children.
- Don't store in bathroom medicine cabinet. Heat and moisture may change the action of the supplement.

Safe dosage:
- GLA is available in capsule form: Swallow whole with a full glass of liquid. Don't chew or crush. Take with or 1 to 1-1/2 hours after meals unless otherwise directed by your doctor.
- At present, no "safe" dosage has been established.

 Toxicity

Unlikely to threaten life or cause significant symptoms.

For symptoms of toxicity: See *Adverse Reactions, Side Effects or Overdose Symptoms* section below.

 Adverse Reactions, Side Effects or Overdose Symptoms

Signs and symptoms	What to do
Headache, indigestion, nausea	Discontinue. Call doctor when convenient.

FOOD SUPPLEMENTS

Inositol

 Basic Information

Inositol is also called *myoinositol*. It is found naturally in breast milk, calf liver, cantaloupe, citrus fruit (except lemons), dried beans, garbanzo beans (chickpeas), lentils, milk, nuts, oats, pork, rice, veal, wheat germ and whole-grain products.

Chemicals this supplement contains: Sugars

 Known Effects

- Plays a role similar to choline in helping move fats out of liver
- Functions in nerve transmission
- Forms an important part of phospholipids, which are compounds manufactured in our bodies

Miscellaneous information:

- Individuals under medical supervision for sleep or anxiety disorders may benefit from supplements.
- Newborns benefit from inositol through breast milk.

 Possible Additional Effects

- May protect against peripheral neuropathy associated with diabetes (Some studies have shown promise for this use, but definitive, well-controlled studies have not been done.)
- May function as mild antianxiety agent
- May help control blood-cholesterol level

- Potential treatment for constipation with its stimulating effect on muscular action of alimentary canal
- May improve sleep
- Under study for anxiety disorders and Alzheimer's disease

 Warnings and Precautions

Don't take if you are:
Healthy.

Consult your doctor if you have:

- Diabetes with peripheral neuropathy: pain, numbness, tingling, alternating feelings of cold and hot in feet and hands—medical supervision is necessary
- A sleep or anxiety disorder

Pregnancy:
Don't take.

Breastfeeding:
Don't take.

Infants and children:
Treating infants and children under 2 with any supplement is hazardous

Others:
Excretion may increase with lithium treatment.

Storage:

- Store in cool, dry place away from direct light, but don't freeze.
- Store safely out of reach of children.
- Don't store in bathroom medicine cabinet. Heat and moisture may change the action of the supplement.

Safe dosage:

- At present, no "safe" dosage has been established.

- Inositol is available in capsule form: Swallow whole with a full glass of liquid. Don't chew or crush. Take with or 1 to 1-1/2 hours after meals unless otherwise directed by your doctor.

Adverse Reactions, Side Effects or Overdose Symptoms

None are expected.

Toxicity

Unlikely to threaten life or cause significant symptoms.

Jojoba (Goatnut)

Basic Information

Biological name: *Simmondsia chinensis.*

Chemical this supplement contains: Amino acids

Known Effects

Acts as soothing ingredient in many shampoos, toothpastes, pre-electric-shave conditioners, aftershave preparations, skin lotion, makeup remover

Miscellaneous information:

- Jojoba is unique among plants because its seeds contain a liquid wax oil.
- The plant grows in Arizona and is used as a medicinal herb among Southern Arizona Indians.
- Jojoba is used in perfume.

Possible Additional Effects

- May reduce joint pain associated with rheumatoid arthritis
- May relieve swelling
- May promote healing
- Potential dry skin treatment

Warnings and Precautions

Don't take if you:

No problems are expected if you are an adult and not pregnant or breastfeeding and do not take amounts larger than the manufacturer's recommended dosage.

Consult your doctor if you:

- Are pregnant, think you may be pregnant or plan pregnancy in the near future
- Take any medicinal drugs or herbs including aspirin, laxatives, cold and cough remedies, antacids, vitamins, minerals, amino acids, supplements, other prescription or nonprescription drugs

FOOD SUPPLEMENTS

→

Pregnancy:
Problems in pregnant women taking small or usual amounts have not been proved, but the chance of problems does exist. Don't use unless prescribed by your doctor.

Breastfeeding:
Problems in breast-fed infants of lactating mothers taking small or usual amounts have not been proved, but the chance of problems does exist. Don't use unless prescribed by your doctor.

Infants and children:
Treating infants and children under 2 with any supplement is hazardous.

Others:
No beneficial effects when taken by mouth have been proved.

Storage:
• Store in cool, dry place away from direct light, but don't freeze.

• Store safely out of reach of children.
• Don't store in bathroom medicine cabinet. Heat and moisture may change the action of the supplement.

Safe dosage:
At present no "safe" dosage has been established.

 Toxicity

Comparative-toxicity rating is not available from standard references.

 Adverse Reactions, Side Effects or Overdose Symptoms

None are expected.

L-Carnitine

 Basic Information

L-carnitine is synthesized in the body from the amino acids *lysine* and *methionine*. It is found naturally in avocados, breast milk, dairy products, red meats (especially lamb and beef) and tempeh (fermented soybean product).

 Known Effects

• Promotes normal growth and development

• Essential for infants, especially premature infants
• Transports long-chain fatty acids into mitochondria, which are the metabolic furnaces of cells (particularly heart and kidney cells), where they may be oxidized to yield energy
• Synthesized in human kidney and liver from the essential amino acids lysine and methionine, plus vitamin B-6, vitamin C and iron

Miscellaneous information:
• Because carnitine requires essential amino acids to be synthesized by the body, anyone with deficient protein or amino acids in their diet may require supplements.

• People with recent severe burns or injuries, hypothyroidism and vegan vegetarians may also require supplements. Consult your doctor.

 ## Possible Additional Effects

• Possible treatment for (and maybe prevention of) some forms of cardiovascular disease
• May protect against muscle disease
• May help build muscle
• May protect against liver disease
• May protect against diabetes
• May protect against kidney disease
• Potential diet aid
• May make low-calorie diets easier to tolerate by reducing feelings of hunger and weakness
• May increase energy and activity in people with congestive heart disease (see Glossary)

 ## Warnings and Precautions

Don't take if you are:
• Allergic to any food protein, such as eggs, milk, wheat
• At risk of poor nutrition for any reason
• Pregnant, think you may be pregnant or plan pregnancy in the near future

Consult your doctor if you have:
Any liver or kidney problems.

Pregnancy:
Problems in pregnant women taking small or usual amounts have not been proved, but the chance of problems does exist. Don't use unless prescribed by your doctor.

Breastfeeding:
Problems in breast-fed infants of lactating mothers taking small or usual amounts have not been proved, but the chance of problems does exist. Don't use unless prescribed by your doctor.

Infants and children:
Treating infants and children under 2 with any supplement is hazardous.

Others:
• Deficiency may cause muscle fatigue, cramps or low blood-sugar levels.
• AZT may reduce carnitine levels.

Storage:
• Store in cool, dry place away from direct light, but don't freeze.
• Store safely out of reach of children.
• Don't store in bathroom medicine cabinet. Heat and moisture may change the action of the supplement.

Safe dosage:
• At present no "safe" dosage has been established.
• Available as tablets: Swallow whole with a full glass of liquid. Don't chew or crush. Take with or 1 to 1-1/2 hours after meals unless otherwise directed by your doctor. Avoid dl-carnitine tablets; they may be toxic.
• Also available as acetyl l-carnitine.

 ## Toxicity

Comparative-toxicity rating is not available from standard references.

For symptoms of toxicity: See *Adverse Reactions, Side Effects or Overdose Symptoms* section below.

Adverse Reactions, Side Effects or Overdose Symptoms

Signs and symptoms	What to do
Muscle weakness	Discontinue. Consult doctor.
Symptoms of myasthenia (progressive weakness of certain muscle groups without evidence of atrophy or wasting) have been reported in kidney patients being maintained for prolonged periods on hemodialysis and supplemental dl-carnitine.	Don't take supplements without doctor's prescription and supervision.

Lecithin

Basic Information

Lecithin is also called *phosphatidyl-choline*.

Lecithin is found in all animal and plant products, including cabbage, cauliflower, caviar, eggs, garbanzo beans (chickpeas), green beans, lentils, organ meats, seeds/nuts, soy lecithin, soybeans and split peas.

Chemicals this supplement contains:

Choline
Fatty acids
Glycerin
Phosphorus

Known Effects

- Protects against damage to cells by oxidation
- Major source of the chemical nutrient choline—choline's benefits are also lecithin's benefits (see Choline)

Miscellaneous information:

- Lecithin must be present for choline synthesis in the human body.
- It is found in chemicals that aid passage of many nutrients from the bloodstream into cells.
- It is used as a thickener in several foods, including mayonnaise, margarine and ice cream.
- People taking niacin or nicotinic acid for treatment of high-serum cholesterol and triglycerides may need lecithin or choline supplements.

Possible
Additional Effects

- May protect against cardiovascular disease
- May treat liver damage caused by alcoholism
- May lower cholesterol level

 Warnings and Precautions

Don't take if you are:
Healthy and eat a well-balanced diet.

Consult your doctor if you have:
Plans to treat Alzheimer's disease with lecithin/choline.

Pregnancy:
Supplements are unnecessary.

Breastfeeding:
Supplements are unnecessary.

Infants and children:
Treating infants and children under 2 with any supplement is hazardous.

Others:
- Excess lecithin may increase phosphorus levels unless the diet is adequate in calcium.
- It may cause inaccurate results in a lecithin/sphingomyelin lab test as part of an examination of amniotic fluid.
- Nicotinic acid (nicotinamide, vitamin B-3) decreases lecithin effectiveness.

Storage:
- Store in cool, dry place away from direct light, but don't freeze.
- Store safely out of reach of children.
- Don't store in bathroom medicine cabinet. Heat and moisture may change the action of the supplement.

Safe dosage:
- Don't take more than 1 gram per day.
- Lecithin is available as tablets: Swallow whole with a full glass of liquid. Don't chew or crush. Take with or 1 to 1-1/2 hours after meals unless otherwise directed by your doctor.
- Lecithin is also available in liquid form: Dilute in at least 1/2 glass of water or other liquid. Take with or 1 to 1-1/2 hours after meals unless otherwise directed by your doctor.

 Toxicity

Comparative-toxicity rating is not available from standard references.

For symptoms of toxicity: See *Adverse Reactions, Side Effects or Overdose Symptoms* section below.

 Adverse Reactions, Side Effects or Overdose Symptoms

Signs and symptoms	What to do
Dizziness	Discontinue. Call doctor immediately.
Fishy body odor	Discontinue. Call doctor when convenient.
Nausea or vomiting	Discontinue. Call doctor immediately.

FOOD SUPPLEMENTS

Melatonin

 Basic Information

Melatonin is a hormone produced in the body by the pineal gland and secreted at night. In most people, melatonin levels are highest during the normal hours of sleep. The levels increase rapidly in the late evening, peaking after midnight and decreasing toward morning.

 Known Effects

- Fatigue
- Helps alleviate sleep disturbances
- Helps cure insomnia and restless leg syndrome

Miscellaneous information:
Melatonin is not researched carefully as yet for use in humans.

 Possible Additional Effects

- May slow aging
- May fight disease
- May enhance sex life
- May dimish the effects of jet lag

 Warnings and Precautions

Don't take if you are:
Allergic to melatonin.

Consult your doctor if you have:
- Any chronic health problem
- Allergies to any medication, food or other substance

- High blood pressure (hypertension) or cardiovascular disease (Some studies in animals suggest melatonin may constrict blood vessels, a condition that could be dangerous for people with these conditions.)

Pregnancy:
Decide with your doctor if the benefits of melatonin justify the risk to your unborn child. The risk is unknown because melatonin is not regulated by the FDA.

Breastfeeding:
It is unknown if melatonin passes into milk. Consult your doctor before taking.

Infants and children:
Treating infants and children under 2 with any supplement is hazardous.

Others:
- Don't take with any prescription or nonprescription medicine without consulting your doctor or pharmacist.
- Drivers, pilots or individuals involved in hazardous work should not work while using melatonin until it has been determined how it affects you.
- Alcohol and tobacco disrupt the nighttime melatonin effect. Avoid.

Storage:
- Store in cool, dry place away from direct light, but don't freeze.
- Store safely out of reach of children.
- Don't store in bathroom medicine cabinet. Heat and moisture may change the action of the supplement.

Safe dosage:
- Melatonin, as a product, is marketed as a dietary supplement and is not reviewed by the U.S. Food and Drug

Administration (FDA) for effectiveness and safety. The best dosage amounts are unknown. Use with caution.

- Hormone supplements may not have the same effects on the body as naturally produced hormones have, because the body processes them differently. Higher doses of supplements may result in higher amounts of hormones in the blood than are healthy.
- Melatonin is available in tablet or capsule form: Follow instructions on the label or consult your doctor or pharmacist. Different brands supply different doses.
- At present "safe" dosage information is unknown.
- A lower starting dosage is often recommended for people over 55 years old until a response is determined.

Toxicity

Comparative-toxicity rating is not available from standard references.

For symptoms of toxicity: See *Adverse Reactions, Side Effects or Overdose Symptoms* section below.

Adverse Reactions, Side Effects or Overdose Symptoms

Signs and symptoms	What to do
Drowsiness, confusion, headache or grogginess may occur the following morning.	Reduce dosage or discontinue. Call doctor when convenient.

Omega-3 Fatty Acids (Fish Oils)

Basic Information

Omega-3 fatty acids are a dietary supplement available in capsules or oil. These acids come from cold-water fish, particularly cod, tuna, salmon, halibut, shark and mackerel.

Chemicals this supplement contains:

Docosahexaenoic acid (DHA)
Eicosapentaenoic acid (EPA)

Known Effects

- Greenland Eskimos who eat foods high in omega-3 fatty acids have very low serum triglycerides and total cholesterol. They have high high-density-lipoprotein (HDL) cholesterol. This cholesterol is known to protect against deposits of plaque, which can occlude (see Glossary) critical blood vessels and cause heart attacks, strokes and other major health problems. Coastal Japanese people have similar diets and similar findings. Increasing omega-3 by supplementation may raise blood cholesterol.
- Omega-3 acids protect against coronary artery disease.
- They also protect against arteriosclerosis.

Miscellaneous information:

Increasing "oily" fish in the diet is preferable to taking omega-3 fatty-acid supplements.

→

Possible Additional Effects

- Potential anti-inflammatory for arthritis
- May protect against strokes
- May improve immune response
- May impede blood clotting
- May increase tendency toward anemia in menstruating women
- May reduce reclosure of arteries after angioplasty

Warnings and Precautions

Don't take if you:
- Are pregnant, think you may be pregnant or plan pregnancy in the near future
- Are diabetic, as supplements are high in fat
- Have a blood clotting problem (omega-3 acids may impede clotting)

Consult your doctor if you:
Take any medicinal drugs or herbs including aspirin, laxatives, cold and cough remedies, antacids, vitamins, minerals, amino acids, supplements, other prescription or nonprescription drugs.

Pregnancy:
Problems in pregnant women taking small or usual amounts have not been proved, but the chance of problems does exist. Don't use unless prescribed by your doctor.

Breastfeeding:
Problems in breast-fed infants of lactating mothers taking small or usual amounts have not been proved, but the chance of problems does exist. Don't use unless prescribed by your doctor.

Infants and children:
Treating infants and children under 2 with any supplement is hazardous.

Others:
- This fat becomes rancid easily and quickly.
- No one knows how much is beneficial and nontoxic.
- Omega-3 causes fishy breath odor, greasy stools, belching and abdominal distension.
- It reduces blood clotting capability and could cause excessive bleeding in an accident.
- People are generally advised to discontinue 3 to 4 weeks prior to elective surgery.
- Heat kills essential fatty acids, so they should not be processed or cooked.

Storage:
- Store in cool, dry place away from direct light, but don't freeze.
- Store safely out of reach of children.
- Don't store in bathroom medicine cabinet. Heat and moisture may change the action of the supplement.

Safe dosage:
At present no "safe" dosage has been established.

Toxicity

Comparative-toxicity rating is not available from standard references.

For symptoms of toxicity: See *Adverse Reactions, Side Effects or Overdose Symptoms* section below.

Adverse Reactions, Side Effects or Overdose Symptoms

Signs and symptoms	What to do
Large amounts may lead to bleeding problems, diminished immunity, predisposition to some malignancies	Discontinue. Call doctor immediately.

Para-Aminobenzoic Acid (PABA)

 ## Basic Information

Para-aminobenzoic acid is made by intestinal bacteria and can be found in the following foods: bran, brown rice, kidney, liver, molasses, sunflower seeds, wheat germ, whole-grain products and yogurt.

Chemicals this supplement contains: enzymes, to aid the breakdown and synthesis of protein.

 ## Known Effects

- Shields skin from ultraviolet radiation damage when used as a topical sunscreen
- Treats vitiligo, a condition characterized by discoloration or depigmentation of some areas of the skin
- Increases effectiveness of folic acid, vitamin-B complex and vitamin C

Miscellaneous information:

PABA stimulates intestinal bacteria, enabling them to produce folic acid, which aids in the production of pantothenic acid.

 ## Possible Additional Effects

- May rejuvenate skin
- May treat arthritis
- May treat constipation
- May treat gastrointestinal disorders
- May treat nervousness and irritability

 ## Warnings and Precautions

Don't take if you:

Take any sulfonamide or antibiotic internally because PABA prevents them from exerting their full effect.

Consult your doctor if you are:

Pregnant, think you may be pregnant or plan pregnancy in the near future.

Pregnancy:

- Don't take internally. Risks outweigh the benefits.
- No problems are expected if you use PABA topically.

Breastfeeding:

- Don't take internally. Risks outweigh the benefits.
- No problems are expected if you use PABA topically.

Infants and children:

Treating infants and children under 2 with any supplement is hazardous.

Others:

- Decreases effectiveness of antibiotics
- Decreases effectiveness of sulfonamides ("sulfa drugs")

Storage:

- Store in cool, dry place away from direct light, but don't freeze.
- Store safely out of reach of children.
- Don't store in bathroom medicine cabinet. Heat and moisture may change the action of the supplement.

Safe dosage:

- At present no "safe" dosage has been established.

FOOD SUPPLEMENTS

→

- PABA is a constituent of many multivitamin/mineral preparations: Don't take oral supplements without your doctor's supervision.
- PABA is a constituent of many topical sunscreen products.

Toxicity

PABA is stored in the tissues. In continued high doses, it may prove toxic to the liver. Symptoms of toxicity are nausea and vomiting.

For symptoms of toxicity:
Discontinue supplement and consult doctor. Also see *Adverse Reactions, Side Effects or Overdose Symptoms* section below.

Adverse Reactions, Side Effects or Overdose Symptoms

Signs and symptoms	What to do
Diarrhea	Discontinue. Call doctor immediately.
Fever	Discontinue. Call doctor immediately.
Liver disease, evidenced by abnormal liver-function tests, jaundice (yellow skin and eyes), vomiting	Discontinue. Call doctor immediately.
Nausea or vomiting	Discontinue. Call doctor immediately.
Skin rash	Discontinue. Call doctor immediately.

Pregnenolone

Basic Information

Pregnenolone is used by the body to make steroids. It increases estrogen and testosterone levels in the body.

Known Effects

None are proven.

Miscellaneous information:

- Pregnenolone is not researched carefully as yet for use in humans. Most research has been performed on animals. Studies are ongoing to find more definite answers about its effect on aging and memory.
- It is a precursor (see Glossary) of DHEA (see DHEA).

Possible Additional Effects

- May improve memory
- May slow the aging process
- May aid in treating spinal cord injury when used with anti-inflammatory agents
- May reduce inflammation associated with arthritis

Warnings and Precautions

Don't take if you:

- Are allergic to pregnenolone
- Have a hormone-dependent cancer or cancer history in your family

Consult your doctor if you have:
- Any chronic health problem
- Allergies to any medication, food or other substance

Pregnancy:
Decide with your doctor if the benefits of pregnenolone justify the risk to your unborn child. Risk is unknown because pregnenolone is not regulated by the FDA.

Breastfeeding:
It is unknown if pregnenolone passes into milk. Consult your doctor before taking.

Infants and children:
Treating infants and children under 2 with any supplement is hazardous.

Others:
Don't take with any prescription or nonprescription medicine without consulting your doctor or pharmacist.

Storage:
- Store in cool, dry area away from direct light, but don't freeze.
- Store safely out of reach of children.
- Don't store in bathroom medicine cabinet. Heat and moisture may change the action of the supplement.

Safe dosage:
- Pregnenonlone, as a product, is marketed as a dietary supplement and is not reviewed by the U.S. Food and Drug Administration (FDA) for effectiveness and safety. The best dosage amounts are unknown. Use with caution.

- Hormone supplements may not have the same effects on the body as naturally produced hormones have, because the body processes them differently. Higher doses of supplements may result in higher amounts of hormones in the blood than are healthy.
- A lower starting dosage may be recommended for persons over 55 years old until a response is determined.
- Pregnenolone is available in capsule form: Follow instructions on the label or consult your doctor or pharmacist. Different brands supply different doses.

Toxicity

Comparative-toxicity rating is not available from standard references.

For symptoms of toxicity: See *Adverse Reactions, Side Effects or Overdose Symptoms* section below.

Adverse Reactions, Side Effects or Overdose Symptoms

Signs and symptoms	What to do
Infrequent:	
In women— facial hair growth (hirsutism)	Discontinue. Call doctor when convenient.
In men— breast enlargement	

Royal Jelly

Basic Information

Royal jelly is a milky-white, gelatinous substance secreted by the salivary glands of worker bees to stimulate growth and development of queen bees.

Chemicals this supplement contains: Pantothenic acid (part of B-complex vitamins)

Known Effects

None are proven.

Miscellaneous information:
This substance must be given by injection.

Possible Additional Effects

• May extend life span
• May treat bone and joint disorders, such as rheumatoid arthritis
• May protect against leukemia
• May contain antibiotic properties
• May treat bronchial asthma
• May treat insomnia
• May treat liver and kidney disease

Warnings and Precautions

Don't take if you are:
Pregnant, think you may be pregnant or plan pregnancy in the near future.

Consult your doctor if you:
Take any medicinal drugs or herbs including aspirin, laxatives, cold and cough remedies, antacids, vitamins, minerals, amino acids, supplements, other prescription or nonprescription drugs.

Pregnancy:
Dangers outweigh any benefits. Don't use.

Breastfeeding:
Dangers outweigh any benefits. Don't use.

Infants and children:
Treating infants and children under 2 with any supplement is hazardous.

Others:
Dangers outweigh any benefits. Don't use.

Storage:
• Store safely away from children.
• Keep refrigerated in a tightly sealed container.

Safe dosage:
At present no "safe" dosage has been established.

Toxicity

Comparative-toxicity rating is not available from standard references.

For symptoms of toxicity: See *Adverse Reactions, Side Effects or Overdose Symptoms* section below.

Adverse Reactions, Side Effects or Overdose Symptoms

Signs and symptoms	What to do
Life-threatening anaphylaxis may follow injections: Symptoms include immediate severe itching, paleness, low blood pressure, loss of consciousness, coma.	Yell for help. Don't leave victim. Begin CPR (cardiopulmonary resuscitation), mouth-to-mouth breathing and external cardiac massage. Have someone dial "0" (operator) or 911 (emergency). Don't stop CPR until help arrives.

Shark Cartilage

Basic Information

Shark cartilage is made from the powderized cartilage of shark.

Chemicals this supplement contains:

Amino acids (some)
Calcium
Mucopolysaccharides
Phosphorus
Protein
Some amino acids

Known Effects

Mucopolysaccharides found in this cartilage inhibit the growth of new blood vessels (cellular angiogenesis).

Miscellaneous information:

Some doctors question the effectiveness of taking oral shark-cartilage supplements. They feel that the supplement's active ingredient may be destroyed during digestion, not allowing it to enter the blood stream.

Possible Additional Effects

- May boost immune system
- May decrease joint swelling and stiffness due to anti-inflammatory properties
- Because of angiogenesis-inhibition properties, it may be effective in the treatment of certain eye disorders that occur because of inappropriate growth of new blood vessels, as well as arthritis, psoriasis, bowel inflammation, scleroderma
- May protect against cancer

FOOD SUPPLEMENTS

→

Warnings and Precautions

Don't take if you:
- Have recently undergone surgery
- Have had a heart attack
- Are still growing

Consult your doctor if you:

Take any prescription or nonprescription medicine.

Pregnancy:

Decide with your doctor if any benefits of shark cartilage justify the risk to your unborn child. Risk is unknown because shark cartilage is not regulated by the FDA.

Breastfeeding:

It is unknown if shark cartilage passes into milk. Consult your doctor before taking.

Infants and children:

Treating infants and children under 2 with any supplement is hazardous.

Storage:
- Store in cool, dry area away from direct light, but don't freeze.
- Store safely out of reach of children.
- Don't store in bathroom medicine cabinet. Heat and moisture may change the action of the supplement.

Safe dosage:
- Shark cartilage, as a product, is marketed as a dietary supplement and is not reviewed by the U.S. Food and Drug Administration (FDA) for effectiveness and safety. The best dosage amounts are unknown. Use with caution.
- Shark cartilage is available in powder or capsule form: It is important to get a supplement that is 100-percent pure shark cartilage to get the maximum effect. The color should be white.

 ## Toxicity

Comparative-toxicity rating is not available from standard references.

 ## Adverse Reactions, Side Effects or Overdose Symptoms

Signs and symptoms	What to do
None are known.	

Spirulina (Blue-green Algae)

 ## Basic Information

Biological names: *Spirulina maxima, Spirulina platensis.*

Chemicals this supplement contains:

B-complex vitamins
Beta-carotene
Gamma-linolenic acid
Iron
Protein

 ## Known Effects

None are proven.

Miscellaneous information:
- Spirulina is expensive and tastes terrible.
- It is a blue-green microalgae that grows wild on the surface of brackish, alkaline lakes in the tropics.

- Spirulina is cultivated commercially in several places, including Mexico, Thailand, Japan and Southern California.

Possible Additional Effects

- Possible energy booster
- May protect immune system
- May lower cholesterol
- May decrease appetite
- May be beneficial for individuals with hypoglycemia

Warnings and Precautions

Don't take if you are:
Pregnant, think you may be pregnant or plan pregnancy in the near future.

Consult your doctor if you:
Take any medicinal drugs or herbs including aspirin, laxatives, cold and cough remedies, antacids, vitamins, minerals, amino acids, upplements, other prescription or nonprescription drugs.

Pregnancy:
Don't use unless prescribed by your doctor.

Breastfeeding:
Don't use unless prescribed by your doctor.

Infants and children:
Treating infants and children under 2 with any supplement is hazardous.

Others:
No problems are expected if you are not pregnant and do not take amounts larger than a reputable manufacturer recommends on the package.

Storage:
- Keep cool and dry, but don't freeze.
- Store safely away from children.
- Don't store in bathroom medicine cabinet. Heat and moisture may change the action of the supplement.

Safe dosage:
- At present no "safe" dosage has been established.
- Spirulina is available in powder and tablet form. Follow manufacturer's instructions or consult your doctor.

Toxicity

Comparative-toxicity rating is not available from standard references.

For symptoms of toxicity: See *Adverse Reactions, Side Effects or Overdose Symptoms* section below.

Adverse Reactions, Side Effects or Overdose Symptoms

Signs and symptoms	What to do
Diarrhea	Discontinue. Call doctor immediately.
Nausea	Discontinue. Call doctor immediately.
Vomiting	Discontinue. Call doctor immediately.

FOOD SUPPLEMENTS

Superoxide Dismutase

 Basic Information

Superoxide dismutase is an enzyme associated with copper, zinc and manganese.

Chemical this supplement contains: Enzyme that participates in utilization of copper, zinc and manganese by body cells.

 Known Effects

Neutralizes the free radical (see Glossary), superoxide

Miscellaneous information:
Superoxide dismutase protects against free radicals.

 Possible Additional Effects

• May reduce oxidative cell damage associated with cancer, cancer therapies
• May have antioxidant (see Glossary) properties (injectable forms only)

 Warnings and Precautions

Don't take if you have:
Any medical problems.

Consult your doctor if you:
Take any medicinal drugs or herbs including aspirin, laxatives, cold and cough remedies, antacids, vitamins, minerals, amino acids, supplements, other prescription or nonprescription drugs.

Pregnancy:
Don't use without medical supervision.

Breastfeeding:
Don't use without medical supervision.

Infants and children:
Treating infants and children under 2 with any supplement is hazardous.

Others:
• Available oral forms are worthless.
• Injectable forms may cause anaphylaxis.

Storage:
• Store in cool, dry place away from direct light, but don't freeze.
• Store safely out of reach of children.
• Don't store in bathroom medicine cabinet. Heat and moisture may change the action of the supplement.

Safe dosage:
• At present no "safe" dosage has been established.
• Oral superoxide dismutase is destroyed in the intestines before being absorbed, so oral forms are worthless unless pills are enteric-coated to allow absorption into the small intestines.
• It is available in injectable forms, but these should be used only under close medical supervision.

 Toxicity

Comparative-toxicity rating is not available from standard references.

For symptoms of toxicity: *See Adverse Reactions, Side Effects or Overdose Symptoms section below.*

Adverse Reactions, Side Effects or Overdose Symptoms

Signs and symptoms	What to do
Life-threatening anaphylaxis may follow injections: Symptoms include immediate severe itching, paleness, low blood pressure, loss of consciousness, coma.	Yell for help. Don't leave victim. Begin CPR (cardio-pulmonary resuscitation), mouth-to-mouth breathing and external cardiac massage. Have someone dial "0" (operator) or 911 (emergency). Don't stop CPR until help arrives.

Wheat Germ

Basic Information

Wheat germ is the embryo of the wheat grain located at the lower end. It is derived from both root and shoot.

Chemicals this supplement contains:

Calcium	Most B vitamins
Copper	Phosphorus
Magnesium	Vitamin E (one of
Manganese	the richest
	natural sources)

Known Effects

Excellent nutritional source of chemicals listed above

Possible Additional Effects

- May reduce symptoms of muscular dystrophy
- May improve physical stamina and performance

Warnings and Precautions

Don't take if you:

No problems are expected if you are not pregnant and do not take amounts larger than manufacturer's recommended dosage.

Consult your doctor if you:

- Are pregnant, think you may be pregnant or plan pregnancy in the near future
- Take any medicinal drugs or herbs including aspirin, laxatives, cold and cough remedies, antacids, vitamins, minerals, amino acids, supplements, other prescription or nonprescription drugs

Pregnancy:

Problems in pregnant women taking small or usual amounts have not been proved, but the chance of problems does exist. Don't use unless prescribed by your doctor.

FOOD SUPPLEMENTS

→

Breastfeeding:

Problems in breast-fed infants of lactating mothers taking small or usual amounts have not been proved, but the chance of problems does exist. Don't use unless prescribed by your doctor.

Infants and children:

Treating infants and children under 2 with any supplement is hazardous.

Others:

No problems are expected if you are beyond childhood and under 45, basically healthy and take for only a short time.

Storage:

• Keep cool and dry, but don't freeze.
• Store safely away from children.
• Wheat germ goes rancid quickly—keep refrigerated.

Safe dosage:

• At present no "safe" dosage has been established.
• Wheat germ is available in food and as flakes to mix with other foods. It is also available as oil, which should be kept tightly covered and refrigerated.

 Toxicity

Comparative-toxicity rating is not available from standard references.

 Adverse Reactions, Side Effects or Overdose Symptoms

None are expected.

Wheat Grass (Barley Grass, Plant Sprouts)

 Basic Information

These products are derived from roots and leaves.

Chemicals this supplement contains:

B vitamins
Chlorophyll
Select phytochemicals
Superoxide dismutase

 Known Effects

None are proven.

 Possible Additional Benefits

• May protect against cancer.
• May function as an antioxidant

 Warnings and Precautions

Don't take if you are:

Pregnant, think you may be pregnant or plan pregnancy in the near future.

Consult your doctor if you:

• Take this herb for any medical problem that doesn't improve in 2 weeks (There may be safer, more effective treatments.)

• Take any medicinal drugs or herbs including aspirin, laxatives, cold and cough remedies, antacids, vitamins, minerals, amino acids, supplements, other prescription or nonprescription drugs.

Pregnancy:

Problems in pregnant women taking small or usual amounts have not been proved, but the chance of problems does exist. Don't use unless prescribed by your doctor.

Breastfeeding:

Problems in breast-fed infants of lactating mothers taking small or usual amounts have not been proved, but the chance of problems does exist. Don't use unless prescribed by your doctor.

Infants and children:

Treating infants and children under 2 with any supplement is hazardous.

Others:

No problems are expected if you are not pregnant and do not take amounts larger than the manufacturer's recommended dosage.

Storage:

• Store in cool, dry place away from direct light, but don't freeze.
• Store safely out of reach of children.
• Don't store in bathroom medicine cabinet. Heat and moisture may change the action of the supplement.

Safe dosage:

At present no "safe" dosage has been established.

Toxicity

Comparative-toxicity rating is not available from standard references.

Adverse Reactions, Side Effects or Overdose Symptoms

None are expected.

FOOD SUPPLEMENTS

Medicinal Herbs

The following section attempts to provide you with enough knowledge to avoid toxicity if you choose to self-prescribe medicinal herbs. If you collect and use herbal medications, you must be an expert botanist or herbologist. If you buy them, you have the right to know everything about possible side effects, adverse reactions, toxicity and other dangers in using materials that are not subjected to rigid control procedures.

Medicinal herbs have been effectively used in Eastern medicine for thousands of years; however, only a small percentage have undergone rigorous scientific study.

The most important warnings:

- Don't use medicinal herbs for infants or children without guidance from an expert and your doctor's approval.
- Don't use medicinal herbs at all unless you know enough to use them safely.
- If you choose to use medicinal herbs, tell your doctor which ones you use and in what amounts when he or she asks if you take other medications. As you will see in the following charts, these substances could affect various medicines or courses of treatment your doctor may prescribe.
- Be cautious with the use of medicinal herbs during pregnancy or lactation—check with a knowledgeable health professional before taking.
- Lastly, it is most important to note that traditionally most medicinal herbs have been used in combination to treat the "whole" person rather than the single-symptom/single-herb approach more common to Western medicine.

For easy reference, the herbs in this book have been divided into two sections: COMMON HERBS and LESS COMMON HERBS.

Common Herbs

Astragalus (Huang-qi, Milk Vetch)

Basic Information

Biological name (genus and species):
Astragalus membranaceous

Parts used for medicinal purposes:
Root

Chemicals this herb contains:
- Asparagine
- Astragalosides
- Calcyosin
- Formononetin
- Kumatakenin
- Sterols

Known Effects

- Stimulates and protects the immune system
- Produces spontaneous sweating

Miscellaneous information:
Available as tea, fluid extract, capsules and dried root.

Possible Additional Effects

- May reduce fatigue/weakness
- Potential cold and flu treatment
- May increase stamina
- Potential treatment for immune-deficiency problems (AIDS, cancer)
- May reduce symptoms of chronic fatigue syndrome
- May improve appetite
- May alleviate diarrhea

Warnings and Precautions

Don't take if you are:
- Pregnant, think you may be pregnant or plan pregnancy in the near future
- Currently feverish

Consult your doctor if you:
- Take this herb for any medical problem that doesn't improve in 2 weeks (There may be safer, more effective treatments.)
- Take any medicinal drugs or herbs including aspirin, laxatives, cold and cough remedies, antacids, vitamins, minerals, amino acids, supplements, other prescription or nonprescription drugs

Pregnancy:
Use only on the advice of your physician.

Breastfeeding:
Use only on the advice of your physician.

Infants and children:
Treating infants and children under 2 with any herbal preparation is hazardous.

Storage:
- Store in cool, dry area away from direct light, but don't freeze.
- Store safely out of reach of children.
- Don't store in bathroom medicine cabinet. Heat and moisture may change the action of the herb.

Safe dosage:
Consult your doctor for the appropriate dose for your condition.

Toxicity

Comparative-toxicity rating is not available from standard references.

Adverse Reactions, Side Effects or Overdose Symptoms

None are expected.

MEDICINAL HERBS

Bilberry

 Basic Information

Biological name (genus and species):
Vaccinium myrtillus

Parts used for medicinal purposes:
Whole plant, especially fruits

Chemicals this herb contains:
- Anthocyanins
- Flavonoids
- Hydroquinone
- Loeanolic acid
- Neomyrtillin
- Sodium
- Tannins
- Ursolic acid

 Known Effects

- Acts as a diuretic
- Treats urinary tract infections
- Antioxidant
- Reduces acute diarrhea (dried berries only)
- Astringent

 Possible Additional Effects

- Potential anti-inflammatory
- May treat vision problems, including cataracts, diabetic retinopathy
- May reduce inflammation of oral cavity
- May treat hemorrhoids

 Warnings and Precautions

Don't take if you:
Are pregnant, think you may be pregnant or plan pregnancy in the near future.

Consult your doctor if you:
- Take this herb for any medical problem that doesn't improve in 2 weeks (There may be safer, more effective treatments.)
- Take any medicinal drugs or herbs including aspirin, laxatives, cold and cough remedies, antacids, vitamins, minerals, amino acids, supplements, other prescription or nonprescription drugs

Pregnancy:
Use only on the advice of your physician.

Breastfeeding:
Use only on the advice of your physician.

Infants and children:
Treating infants and children under 2 with any herbal preparation is hazardous.

Storage:
- Store in cool, dry area away from direct light, but don't freeze.
- Store safely out of reach of children.
- Don't store in bathroom medicine cabinet. Heat and moisture may change the action of the herb.

Safe dosage:
Consult your doctor for the appropriate dose for your condition.

 Toxicity

Comparative-toxicity rating is not available from standard references.

 Adverse Reactions, Side Effects or Overdose Symptoms

None are expected.

Calendula (Pot Marigold)

 Basic Information

Biological name (genus and species):
Calendula officinalis

Parts used for medicinal purposes:
- Flower
- Florets
- Petals

Chemicals this herb contains:
- Calenduline
- Chlorogenic acid
- Flavonoids
- Triterpenes
- Volatile oils (see Glossary)

 Known Effects

- Promotes wound healing by reducing inflammation and promoting new tissue growth
- Aids in the treatment of psoriasis, acne and eczema
- Antifungal properties to treat skin rashes including diaper rash and athlete's foot
- Anti-inflammatory

Miscellaneous information:
Available as lotions, ointments, oils, tinctures and fresh or dried leaves/florets.

 Possible Additional Effects

- May be good for gastritis, colitis and peptic ulcers
- May alleviate menstrual pain
- May treat gallbladder problems
- May treat canker sores

STOP Warnings and Precautions

Don't take if you:
Are pregnant, think you may be pregnant or plan pregnancy in the near future.

Consult your doctor if you:
- Take this herb for any medical problem that doesn't improve in 2 weeks (There may be safer, more effective treatments.)
- Take any medicinal drugs or herbs including aspirin, laxatives, cold and cough remedies, antacids, vitamins, minerals, amino acids, supplements, other prescription or nonprescription drugs
- Have a severe burn or deep wound

Pregnancy:
Don't use unless prescribed by your doctor.

Breastfeeding:
Don't use unless prescribed by your doctor.

Infants and children:
Treating infants and children under 2 with any herbal preparation is hazardous.

Storage:
- Store in cool, dry area away from direct light, but don't freeze.
- Store safely out of reach of children.
- Don't store in bathroom medicine cabinet. Heat and moisture may change the action of the herb.

Safe dosage:
Consult your doctor for the appropriate dose for your condition.

MEDICINAL HERBS

➜

Toxicity

Comparative-toxicity rating is not available from standard references.

 Adverse Reactions, Side Effects or Overdose Symptoms

None are expected.

Cascara Sagrada (Cascara Buckthorn)

 Basic Information

Biological name (genus and species):
Rhamnus purshiana

Parts used for medicinal purposes:
Bark

Chemicals this herb contains:
• Anthraquinone
• Cascarosides
• Volatile oils (see Glossary)

 Known Effects

• Used as a mild laxative
• Stimulant

Miscellaneous Information:

• Not recommended for prolonged use
• Standard medicinal product listed in the United States Pharmacopeia
• Available as extract or fluid extract dried into capsule form

 Possible Additional Effects

May treat intermittent constipation

 Warnings and Precautions

Don't take if you:
• Are pregnant, think you may be pregnant or plan pregnancy in the near future
• Have any chronic disease of the gastrointestinal tract, such as stomach or duodenal ulcers, reflux esophagitis, ulcerative colitis, spastic colitis, diverticulosis or diverticulitis

Consult your doctor if you:
• Take this herb for any medical problem that doesn't improve in 2 weeks (There may be safer, more effective treatments.)
• Take any medicinal drugs or herbs including aspirin, laxatives, cold and cough remedies, antacids, vitamins, minerals, amino acids, supplements, other prescription or nonprescription drugs

Pregnancy:
Don't use.

Breastfeeding:
Don't use.

Infants and children:
Treating infants and children under 2 with any herbal preparation is hazardous.

Others:

None are expected if you are beyond childhood, under 45, not pregnant, basically healthy, take it for only a short time and do not exceed manufacturer's recommended dose.

Storage:

- Store in cool, dry area away from direct light, but don't freeze.
- Store safely out of reach of children.
- Don't store in bathroom medicine cabinet. Heat and moisture may change the action of the herb.

Safe dosage:

Consult your doctor for the appropriate dose for your condition.

 Toxicity

Cascara sagrada is rated slightly dangerous, particularly in children, persons over 55 and those who take larger than appropriate quantities for extended periods of time.

It is for short-term use only. Long-term use can lead to lazy-bowel syndrome.

For symptoms of toxicity: See *Adverse Reactions, Side Effects or Overdose Symptoms* section below.

 Adverse Reactions, Side Effects or Overdose Symptoms

Signs and symptoms	What to do
With excessive dosage:	
Diarrhea, violent and watery	Discontinue. Call doctor immediately.
Nausea or vomiting	Discontinue. Call doctor immediately.
Stomach cramps	Discontinue. Call doctor immediately.

Cat's Claw (Una de Gato)

 Basic Information

Biological name (genus and species):
Uncaria tomentosa

Parts used for medicinal purposes:
- Root
- Bark

Chemicals this herb contains:
- Glycosides
- Oxindole alkaloids
- Polyphenols
- Proanthocyanidins
- Quinovic acid
- Triterpenes

 Known Effects

- Anti-inflammatory
- Stimulates the immune system (antiviral)

Miscellaneous information:

Commonly available in capsules, teas and liquid extracts.

 Possible Additional Effects

- May reduce symptoms of gastritis
- May help treat asthma
- May have antioxidant properties

MEDICINAL HERBS

- May provide relief from nausea and side effects of chemotherapy
- Being tested in conjunction with AZT to treat AIDS patients
- May promote healing of gastric ulcers
- May increase blood circulation
- May reduce bowel inflammation
- May promote normal bowel function
- Potential anticarcinogenic

 ## Warnings and Precautions

Don't take if you:

- Are pregnant, think you may be pregnant or plan pregnancy in the near future
- Are a tissue- or organ-transplant patient because of this herb's tendency to cause the immune system to reject foreign cells

Consult your doctor if you:

- Take this herb for any medical problem that doesn't improve in 2 weeks (There may be safer, more effective treatments.)
- Take any medicinal drugs or herbs including aspirin, laxatives, cold and cough remedies, antacids, vitamins, minerals, amino acids, supplements, other prescription or nonprescription drugs

Pregnancy:
Don't use.

Breastfeeding:
Don't use unless prescribed by your doctor.

Infants and children:
Treating infants and children under 2 with any herbal preparation is hazardous.

Storage:

- Store in cool, dry area away from direct light, but don't freeze.
- Store safely out of reach of children.
- Don't store in bathroom medicine cabinet. Heat and moisture may change the action of the herb.

Safe dosage:
Consult your doctor for the appropriate dose for your condition.

 ## Toxicity

Comparative-toxicity rating is not available from standard references.

For symptoms of toxicity: See *Adverse Reactions, Side Effects or Overdose Symptoms* section below.

 ## Adverse Reactions, Side Effects or Overdose Symptoms

Signs and symptoms	What to do
Diarrhea	Lower dose and monitor for 1 to 2 weeks. May occur for 1 to 2 weeks but should then resolve. Call doctor when convenient.

Cayenne (Capsicum)

Basic Information

Cayenne is also known as red-hot pepper, hot pepper, capsaicin, chili pepper, Africa pepper, American pepper, red pepper and Spanish pepper.

Biological name (genus and species): *Capsicum frutescens, Capsicum annuum*

Parts used for medicinal purposes: Berries/fruits

Chemicals this herb contains:
- Apsaicine
- Capsacutin
- Capsaicin
- Capsanthine
- Capsico
- Folic acid
- Vitamins A, B and C

Known Effects

- Provides counterirritation (see Glossary) when applied to skin overlying an inflamed or irritated joint
- Stimulant
- Antioxidant
- Reduces pain of diabetic neuropathy
- Treats cluster headache

Miscellaneous information:
- Available in powder form
- Available as oil capsules
- Available as fresh food
- Is used in small amounts as a condiment
- No effects are expected on the body, either good or bad, when herb is used in very small amounts to enhance the flavor of food

Possible Additional Effects

- May promote healing of oral lesions associated with chemotherapy, as well as canker sores
- May settle "upset stomach" and help relieve gas and indigestion
- Is used as external rub or poultice to relieve pain
- May reduce pain of arthritis
- May promote blood flow
- May influence healing of duodenal ulcers

Warnings and Precautions

Don't take if you:
- Are pregnant, think you may be pregnant or plan pregnancy in the near future
- Have any chronic disease of the gastrointestinal tract, such as stomach or duodenal ulcers, reflux esophagitis, ulcerative colitis, spastic colitis, diverticulosis or diverticulitis
- Have a bleeding problem

Consult your doctor if you:
- Take this herb for any medical problem that doesn't improve in 2 weeks (There may be safer, more effective treatments.)
- Take any medicinal drugs or herbs including aspirin, laxatives, cold and cough remedies, antacids, vitamins, minerals, amino acids, supplements, other prescription or nonprescription drugs

Pregnancy:
Problems in pregnant women taking small or usual amounts have not been proved, but the chance of problems does exist. Don't use unless prescribed by your doctor.

MEDICINAL HERBS

➜

Breastfeeding:
Problems in breastfed infants of lactating mothers taking small or usual amounts have not been proved, but the chance of problems does exist. Don't use unless prescribed by your doctor.

Infants and children:
Treating infants and children under 2 with any herbal preparation is hazardous.

Others:
Inhalation of cayenne can cause allergic alveolitis.

Storage:
• Store in cool, dry area away from direct light, but don't freeze.
• Store safely out of reach of children.
• Don't store in bathroom medicine cabinet. Heat and moisture may change the action of the herb.

Safe dosage:
Consult your doctor for the appropriate dose for your condition.

 Toxicity

• Cayenne is rated relatively safe when taken in appropriate quantities for short periods of time.
• Excessive intake may cause gastroenteritis, hepatic or renal damage.

For symptoms of toxicity: See *Adverse Reactions, Side Effects or Overdose Symptoms* section below.

 Adverse Reactions, Side Effects or Overdose Symptoms

Signs and symptoms	What to do
Diarrhea, regular or bloody	Discontinue. Call doctor immediately.
Nausea or vomiting	Discontinue. Call doctor immediately.
Vomiting blood	Seek emergency treatment.

Chamomile

 Basic Information

Biological name (genus and species):
Anthemis nobilis, A. flores

Parts used for medicinal purposes:
Various parts of the entire plant, frequently differing by country or culture

Chemicals this herb contains:
• Antheme
• Anthemic acid
• Anthesterol
• Apigenin
• Chamazulene
• Resin (see Glossary)
• Tannic acid
• Tiglic acid
• Volatile oils (see Glossary)

 Known Effects

• Decreases spasm of smooth or skeletal muscle
• Alleviates menstrual cramps
• Anti-inflammatory
• Mild sedative
• Interferes with absorption of iron and other minerals when taken internally

- Kills bacteria on skin
- Reduces stomach cramps, gas, indigestion

Miscellaneous information:

- Flowers are used to make extract and herbal tea.
- Chamomile is available as tea, tincture, oil, dried or fresh flowers.

 ## Possible Additional Effects

Internal use:

- Potential insomnia treatment
- Potential diarrhea treatment
- May treat bronchial infections
- Used as a gargle for gingivitis and sore throat
- May soothe sunburn, cuts and scrapes, sore or inflamed eyes

External use:

- Used as a poultice (see Glossary)
- May help medicate skin abscesses
- Potential hemorrhoid treatment

 ## Warnings and Precautions

Don't take if you:

- Are pregnant, think you may be pregnant or plan pregnancy in the near future
- Have any chronic disease of the gastrointestinal tract, such as stomach or duodenal ulcers, reflux esophagitis, ulcerative colitis, spastic colitis, diverticulosis or diverticulitis

Consult your doctor if you:

- Take this herb for any medical problem that doesn't improve in 2 weeks (There may be safer, more effective treatments.)

- Take any medicinal drugs or herbs including aspirin, laxatives, cold and cough remedies, antacids, vitamins, minerals, amino acids, supplements, other prescription or nonprescription drugs

Pregnancy:

Dangers outweigh any benefits. Don't use.

Breastfeeding:

Dangers outweigh any benefits. Don't use.

Infants and children:

Treating infants and children under 2 with any herbal preparation is hazardous.

Others:

Dangers outweigh any possible benefits. Don't use.

Storage:

- Store in cool, dry area away from direct light, but don't freeze.
- Store safely out of reach of children.
- Don't store in bathroom medicine cabinet. Heat and moisture may change the action of the herb.

Safe dosage:

Consult your doctor for the appropriate dose for your condition.

 ## Toxicity

Comparative-toxicity rating is not available from standard references.

For symptoms of toxicity: See *Adverse Reactions, Side Effects or Overdose Symptoms* section below.

MEDICINAL HERBS

→

Adverse Reactions, Side Effects or Overdose Symptoms

Signs and symptoms	What to do
Allergic reactions in individuals who are sensitive to ragweed pollens (rare)	Discontinue. Call doctor immediately.
Life-threatening anaphylaxis may follow injections— symptoms include immediate severe itching, paleness, low blood pressure, loss of consciousness, coma	Yell for help. Don't leave victim. Begin CPR (cardio-pulmonary resuscitation), mouth-to-mouth breathing and external cardiac massage. Have someone dial "0" (operator) or 911 (emergency). Don't stop CPR until help arrives.
Skin irritation	Discontinue. Call doctor when convenient.
Vomiting	Discontinue. Call doctor immediately.

Chickweed

Basic Information

Biological name (genus and species): *Stellaria media*

Parts used for medicinal purposes: Various parts of the entire plant, frequently differing by country or culture

Chemicals this herb contains:
• Ascorbic acid (vitamin C)
• Potash salts
• Rutin

Known Effects

Internal use:
• Protects scraped tissues
• Used as a vitamin-C supplement
• Relieves constipation

External use:
• Used as an ointment for rashes and sores
• Soothes cuts and wounds

Miscellaneous information:
• Due to high vitamin-C content, chickweed can treat scurvy.

• It is available as dried bulk, oil, ointment and tincture.

Possible Additional Effects

Internal use:
• May treat fatigue
• May treat bronchitis by reducing thickness of mucus in lungs
• May increase urine production

External use:
• May treat insect bites
• May treat eczema and itchy scalp conditions

Warnings and Precautions

Don't take if you:
Are pregnant, think you may be pregnant or plan pregnancy in the near future.

Consult your doctor if you:
• Take this herb for any medical problem that doesn't improve in 2 weeks (There may be safer, more effective treatments.)

- Take any medicinal drugs or herbs including aspirin, laxatives, cold and cough remedies, antacids, vitamins, minerals, amino acids, supplements, other prescription or nonprescription drugs

Pregnancy:
Don't use unless prescribed by your doctor.

Breastfeeding:
Don't use unless prescribed by your doctor.

Infants and children:
Treating infants and children under 2 with any herbal preparation is hazardous.

Others:
None are expected if you are beyond childhood, under 45, not pregnant, basically healthy, take it for only a short time and do not exceed manufacturer's recommended dose.

Storage:
- Store in cool, dry area away from direct light, but don't freeze.
- Store safely out of reach of children.
- Don't store in bathroom medicine cabinet. Heat and moisture may change the action of the herb.

Safe dosage:
Consult your doctor for the appropriate dose for your condition.

 Toxicity

Rated relatively safe when taken in appropriate quantities for short periods of time

For symptoms of toxicity: See *Adverse Reactions, Side Effects or Overdose Symptoms* section below.

 Adverse Reactions, Side Effects or Overdose Symptoms

Signs and symptoms	What to do
Temporary paralysis (large amounts only)	Seek emergency treatment.

Chicory

 Basic Information

Biological name (genus and species):
Cichorium intybus

Parts used for medicinal purposes:
Roots

Chemicals this herb contains:
- Ascorbic acid (vitamin C)
- Inulin
- Vitamin A

 Known Effects
- Laxative
- Mild diuretic

 Possible Additional Effects
- Potential dyspepsia treatment
- Potential jaundice treatment
- May treat rheumatism and gout
- May treat skin irritations as a compress

MEDICINAL HERBS

→

Warnings and Precautions

Don't take if you:
Are pregnant, think you may be pregnant or plan pregnancy in the near future.

Consult your doctor if you:
• Take this herb for any medical problem that doesn't improve in 2 weeks (There may be safer, more effective treatments.)
• Take any medicinal drugs or herbs including aspirin, laxatives, cold and cough remedies, antacids, vitamins, minerals, amino acids, supplements, other prescription or nonprescription drugs

Pregnancy:
Don't use unless prescribed by your doctor.

Breastfeeding:
Don't use unless prescribed by your doctor.

Infants and children:
Treating infants and children under 2 with any herbal preparation is hazardous.

Storage:
• Store in cool, dry area away from direct light, but don't freeze.
• Store safely out of reach of children.
• Don't store in bathroom medicine cabinet. Heat and moisture may change the action of the herb.

Safe dosage:
Consult your doctor for the appropriate dose for your condition.

 Toxicity

Comparative-toxicity rating is not available from standard references.

For symptoms of toxicity: See *Adverse Reactions, Side Effects or Overdose Symptoms* section below.

 Adverse Reactions, Side Effects or Overdose Symptoms

Signs and symptoms	What to do
Rapid heart rate	Seek medical care.
Red, swollen or irritated skin	Discontinue. Call doctor when convenient. Use gloves when handling.

Cinnamon (Camphor)

 Basic Information

Biological name (genus and species):
Cinnamomum camphora

Parts used for medicinal purposes:
• Leaves
• Roots
• Bark

Chemicals this herb contains:
• Camphor oil
• Cineole
• Cinnamic aldehyde
• Fatty acids
• Gum (see Glossary)
• Limonene
• Mannitol
• Safrole
• Tannins (see Glossary)
• Oils

Known Effects

- Helps expel gas from intestinal tract
- Acts as a mouthwash
- Relieves diarrhea

Miscellaneous information:

- Used to make celluloid, explosives and other chemicals
- Available as powder, pill and tincture

Possible Additional Effects

- Safrole is possible carcinogen
- May soothe indigestion
- May prevent ulcers
- May fight tooth decay
- Potential nausea relief
- May lessen menstrual cramps
- May help treat asthma
- May help treat loss of appetite

Warnings and Precautions

Don't take if you:

- Are pregnant, think you may be pregnant or plan pregnancy in the near future
- Have any chronic disease of the gastrointestinal tract, such as stomach or duodenal ulcers, reflux esophagitis, ulcerative colitis, spastic colitis, diverticulosis or diverticulitis

Consult your doctor if you:

- Take this herb for any medical problem that doesn't improve in 2 weeks (There may be safer, more effective treatments.)
- Take any medicinal drugs or herbs including aspirin, laxatives, cold and cough remedies, antacids, vitamins, minerals, amino acids, supplements, other prescription or nonprescription drugs

Pregnancy:
Don't use.

Breastfeeding:
Don't use.

Infants and children:
Treating infants and children under 2 with any herbal preparation is hazardous.

Others:
None are expected if you are beyond childhood, under 45, not pregnant, basically healthy, take it for only a short time and do not exceed manufacturer's recommended dose.

Storage:

- Store in cool, dry area away from direct light, but don't freeze.
- Store safely out of reach of children.
- Don't store in bathroom medicine cabinet. Heat and moisture may change the action of the herb.

Safe dosage:
Consult your doctor for the appropriate dose for your condition.

Toxicity

Rated dangerous, particularly in children, persons over 55 and those who take larger than appropriate quantities for extended periods of time

For symptoms of toxicity: See *Adverse Reactions, Side Effects or Overdose Symptoms* section below.

Adverse Reactions, Side Effects or Overdose Symptoms

Signs and symptoms	What to do
Convulsions	Seek emergency treatment.
Dizziness	Discontinue. Call doctor immediately.

→

MEDICINAL HERBS

| Hallucinations | Seek emergency treatment. |
| Large overdose (0.5ml/kg body weight) can cause coma or kidney damage | Seek emergency treatment. |

Nausea	Discontinue. Call doctor immediately.
Skin contact with oil can cause redness and burning sensation	Discontinue. Call doctor when convenient.
Vomiting	Discontinue. Call doctor immediately.

Cohosh, Black (Black Snakeroot, Rattle Root, Squaw Root)

Basic Information

Biological name (genus and species):
Cimicifuga racemosa

Parts used for medicinal purposes:
- Rhizomes
- Roots

Chemicals this herb contains:
- Glycosides
- Isoferulic acid
- Isoflavones
- Tannins (see Glossary)
- Volatile oils (see Glossary)

Known Effects
- Treats hot flashes and symptoms of menopause
- Treats PMS
- Treats dysmenorrhea

Possible Additional Effects
- May treat diarrhea
- Used as an antidote for rattlesnake poison
- May lower blood pressure

Warnings and Precautions

Don't take if you:
- Are pregnant, think you may be pregnant or plan pregnancy in the near future
- Have any chronic disease of the gastrointestinal tract, such as stomach or duodenal ulcers, reflux esophagitis, ulcerative colitis, spastic colitis, diverticulosis or diverticulitis

Consult your doctor if you:
- Take this herb for any medical problem that doesn't improve in 2 weeks (There may be safer, more effective treatments.)
- Take any medicinal drugs or herbs including aspirin, laxatives, cold and cough remedies, antacids, vitamins, minerals, amino acids, supplements, other prescription or nonprescription drugs

Pregnancy:
Don't use unless prescribed by your doctor.

Breastfeeding:
Don't use unless prescribed by your doctor.

Infants and children:
Treating infants and children under 2 with any herbal preparation is hazardous.

Others:
Limit use to six months.

Storage:
- Store in cool, dry area away from direct light, but don't freeze.
- Store safely out of reach of children.
- Don't store in bathroom medicine cabinet. Heat and moisture may change the action of the herb.

Safe dosage:
Consult your doctor for the appropriate dose for your condition.

 Toxicity

Rated slightly dangerous, particularly in children, persons over 55 and those who take larger than appropriate quantities for extended periods of time

For symptoms of toxicity: See *Adverse Reactions, Side Effects or Overdose Symptoms* section below.

 Adverse Reactions, Side Effects or Overdose Symptoms

Signs and symptoms	What to do
Gastroenteritis, characterized by stomach pain, nausea, diarrhea	Discontinue. Call doctor immediately.
Nausea or vomiting	Discontinue. Call doctor immediately.

Comfrey (Knitbone)

 Basic Information

Biological name (genus and species):
Symphytum officinale

Parts used for medicinal purposes:
- Leaves
- Roots

Chemicals this herb contains:
- Allantoin
- Consolidine
- Mucilage (see Glossary)
- Phosphorus
- Potassium
- Pyrrolizidine
- Starch
- Symphytocynglossine
- Tannins (see Glossary)
- Vitamins A and C

 Known Effects

- Reduces inflammation associated with injury
- Promotes healing of cuts, insect bites

Miscellaneous information:
- Taken internally, comfrey may cause liver damage.
- It may be toxic when applied to skin as well.

 Possible Additional Effects

- Used in poultices (see Glossary) to heal wounds and ulcers
- May protect scraped tissues
- May treat sunburns
- May treat psoriasis and skin rashes
- Potential dermatitis treatment
- May help body dispose of excess fluid by increasing the amount of urine produced

➔

Warnings and Precautions

Don't take if you:

Are pregnant, think you may be pregnant or plan pregnancy in the near future, because you need to restrict the potassium in your diet.

Consult your doctor if you:

- Take this herb for any medical problem that doesn't improve in 2 weeks (There may be safer, more effective treatments.)
- Take any medicinal drugs or herbs including aspirin, laxatives, cold and cough remedies, antacids, vitamins, minerals, amino acids, supplements, other prescription or nonprescription drugs

Pregnancy:

Do not use.

Breastfeeding:

Problems in breastfed infants of lactating mothers taking small or usual amounts have not been proved, but the chance of problems does exist. Don't use unless prescribed by your doctor.

Infants and children:

Treating infants and children under 2 with any herbal preparation is hazardous.

Others:

Do not take internally.

Storage:

- Store in cool, dry area away from direct light, but don't freeze.
- Store safely out of reach of children.
- Don't store in bathroom medicine cabinet. Heat and moisture may change the action of the herb.

Safe dosage:

Consult your doctor for the appropriate dose for your condition.

Toxicity

Comfrey is toxic if taken internally.

For symptoms of toxicity: See *Adverse Reactions, Side Effects or Overdose Symptoms* section below.

Adverse Reactions, Side Effects or Overdose Symptoms

Signs and symptoms	What to do
Coma	Seek emergency treatment.
Drowsiness	Discontinue. Call doctor immediately.
Lethargy	Discontinue. Call doctor immediately.
Rash	Call doctor when convenient.

Damiana

Basic Information

Biological name (genus and species):
Turnera diffusa

Parts used for medicinal purposes:
Leaves

Chemicals this herb contains:
- Arbutin
- Chlorophyll
- Damianian
- Resin (see Glossary)
- Starch
- Sugar
- Tannins (see Glossary)
- Volatile oils (see Glossary)

Known Effects

No proven medicinal qualities

Miscellaneous information:
- Tastes very bitter
- Used as food additive in baked goods and liqueurs

Possible Additional Effects

- Used as an aphrodisiac
- May alleviate headaches
- May reduce depression, anxiety or listlessness
- May improve sexual potency
- Used as a mild laxative

Warnings and Precautions

Don't take if you:
- Are pregnant, think you may be pregnant or plan pregnancy in the near future
- Have any chronic disease of the gastrointestinal tract, such as stomach or duodenal ulcers, reflux esophagitis, ulcerative colitis, spastic colitis, diverticulosis or diverticulitis
- Have kidney or urinary-tract disease

Consult your doctor if you:
- Take this herb for any medical problem that doesn't improve in 2 weeks (There may be safer, more effective treatments.)
- Take any medicinal drugs or herbs including aspirin, laxatives, cold and cough remedies, antacids, vitamins, minerals, amino acids, supplements, other prescription or nonprescription drugs

Pregnancy:
Don't use.

Breastfeeding:
Don't use.

Infants and children:
Treating infants and children under 2 with any herbal preparation is hazardous.

Others:
None are expected if you are beyond childhood, under 45, not pregnant, basically healthy, take it for only a short time and do not exceed manufacturer's recommended dose.

Storage:
- Store in cool, dry area away from direct light, but don't freeze.
- Store safely out of reach of children.
- Don't store in bathroom medicine cabinet. Heat and moisture may change the action of the herb.

MEDICINAL HERBS

→

Safe dosage:
Consult your doctor for the appropriate dose for your condition.

 Toxicity

Rated relatively safe when taken in appropriate quantities for short periods of time

For symptoms of toxicity: See *Adverse Reactions, Side Effects or Overdose Symptoms* section below.

 Adverse Reactions, Side Effects or Overdose Symptoms

Signs and symptoms	What to do
No documented cases reported. Theoretically:	
Change in urinary frequency	Discontinue. Call doctor when convenient.
Diarrhea	Discontinue. Call doctor immediately.
Headache	Discontinue. Call doctor immediately.
Insomnia	Discontinue. Call doctor immediately.
Nausea or vomiting	Discontinue. Call doctor immediately.

Dandelion

 Basic Information

Biological name (genus and species):
Taraxacum officinale

Parts used for medicinal purposes:
• Leaves
• Roots
• Young tops

Chemicals this herb contains:
• Bitters (see Glossary)
• Fats
• Gluten
• Gum (see Glossary)
• Inulin
• Iron
• Niacin
• Potash
• Proteins
• Resin (see Glossary)
• Taraxacerin
• Vitamins A, B, C and E

 Known Effects

No proven medicinal qualities

 Possible Additional Effects

• May treat dyspepsia
• May treat constipation
• May treat hepatitis
• May treat jaundice
• May treat rheumatism
• May treat anemia
• Potential diuretic
• May stimulate appetite

 Warnings and Precautions

Don't take if you:
Are pregnant, think you may be pregnant or plan pregnancy in the near future.

Consult your doctor if you:

- Take this herb for any medical problem that doesn't improve in 2 weeks (There may be safer, more effective treatments.)
- Take any medicinal drugs or herbs including aspirin, laxatives, cold and cough remedies, antacids, vitamins, minerals, amino acids, supplements, other prescription or nonprescription drugs

Pregnancy:
Don't use unless prescribed by your doctor.

Breastfeeding:
Don't use unless prescribed by your doctor.

Infants and children:
Treating infants and children under 2 with any herbal preparation is hazardous.

Others:
None are expected if you are beyond childhood, under 45, not pregnant, basically healthy, take it for only a short time and do not exceed manufacturer's recommended dose.

Storage:
- Store in cool, dry area away from direct light, but don't freeze.
- Store safely out of reach of children.
- Don't store in bathroom medicine cabinet. Heat and moisture may change the action of the herb.

Safe dosage:
Consult your doctor for the appropriate dose for your condition.

 Toxicity

Dandelion is generally regarded as safe when taken in appropriate quantities for short periods of time.

For symptoms of toxicity: See *Adverse Reactions, Side Effects or Overdose Symptoms* section below.

 Adverse Reactions, Side Effects or Overdose Symptoms

Signs and symptoms	What to do
Heartburn and diarrhea (rare)	Discontinue. Call doctor when convenient.

Dong Quai (Chinese Angelica, Dang Gui, Tank Kwei)

 Basic Information

Biological name (genus and species): *Angelica sinensis*

Parts used for medicinal purposes:
- Rhizomes
- Root

Chemicals this herb contains:
- Coumarins
- Vitamin B-12
- Volatile oils (see Glossary)

 Known Effects

- Treats menstrual irregularity
- Reduces pain of menstrual cramps

Miscellaneous information:
Available as teas, tablets and alcohol extracts.

MEDICINAL HERBS

→

Possible
Additional Effects

- May lower blood pressure
- Potential muscle relaxant
- May reduce menopausal symptoms, including hot flashes
- May improve circulation
- May relax bowel
- Potential anti-inflammatory
- May inhibit platelet aggregation, thus protecting against heart disease

 Warnings and
Precautions

Don't take if you:

- Are pregnant, think you may be pregnant or plan pregnancy in the near future
- Take medication for high blood pressure
- If you are prone to heavy menstrual flow
- Plan to have surgery in two weeks or less due to risk of increased bleeding time

Consult your doctor if you:

- Use this herb at all
- Take this herb for any medical problem that doesn't improve in 2 weeks (There may be safer, more effective treatments.)
- Take any medicinal drugs or herbs including aspirin, laxatives, cold and cough remedies, antacids, vitamins, minerals, amino acids, supplements, other prescription or nonprescription drugs

Pregnancy:
Don't use unless prescribed by your doctor.

Breastfeeding:
Don't use unless prescribed by your doctor.

Infants and children:
Treating infants and children under 2 with any herbal preparation is hazardous.

Others:
Use caution if taking with other blood-thinning medicines or herbs.

Storage:

- Store in cool, dry area away from direct light, but don't freeze.
- Store safely out of reach of children.
- Don't store in bathroom medicine cabinet. Heat and moisture may change the action of the herb.

Safe dosage:
4 to 7 grams (200 mg), three times daily between meals.

 Toxicity

Comparative-toxicity rating is not available from standard references.

For symptoms of toxicity: See *Adverse Reactions, Side Effects or Overdose Symptoms* section below.

 Adverse Reactions,
Side Effects or
Overdose Symptoms

Signs and symptoms	What to do
Diarrhea	Discontinue. Call doctor immediately.
Irritability, restlessness	Discontinue. Call doctor when convenient.
Nausea	Discontinue. Call doctor immediately.

Echinacea (Purple Coneflower)

 Basic Information

Biological name (genus and species):
Echinacea angustifolia, E. pallida

Parts used for medicinal purposes:
Various parts of the entire plant,
frequently differing by country or
culture

Chemicals this herb contains:
- Alkaloids
- Echinacoside
- Flavonoids
- Isobutyl amides
- Polyacetylenes
- Polysaccharides
- Volatile oils (see Glossary)

 Known Effects

Antibiotic

Miscellaneous information:
Another herb, *Rudbeckia laciniata,* is
also called *coneflower* and has been
reported to be toxic. If you take any
coneflower, be sure it is *Echinacea
angustifolia.*

 Possible
Additional Effects

- Potential natural antitoxin for
  internal and external infections
- May relieve symptoms of cold
  and flu
- May help heal wounds
- Possible antitumor activity
- May increase immune function after
  cancer treatment

 Warnings and
Precautions

Don't take if you:
- Are pregnant, think you may be
  pregnant or plan pregnancy in the
  near future
- Have tuberculosis, multiple sclerosis
  or collagen disease

Consult your doctor if you:
- Take this herb for any medical
  problem that doesn't improve in
  2 weeks (There may be safer, more
  effective treatments.)
- Take any medicinal drugs or
  herbs including aspirin, laxatives,
  cold and cough remedies, antacids,
  vitamins, minerals, amino acids,
  supplements, other prescription
  or nonprescription drugs
- Are a transplant patient

Pregnancy:
Don't use unless prescribed by
your doctor.

Breastfeeding:
Don't use unless prescribed by
your doctor.

Infants and children:
Treating infants and children under
2 with any herbal preparation
is hazardous.

Others:
None are expected if you are beyond
childhood, under 45, not pregnant,
basically healthy, take it for only a short
time and do not exceed manufacturer's
recommended dose.

Storage:
- Store in cool, dry area away from
  direct light, but don't freeze.

MEDICINAL HERBS

→

- Store safely out of reach of children.
- Don't store in bathroom medicine cabinet. Heat and moisture may change the action of the herb.

Safe dosage:
- Consult your doctor for the appropriate dose for your condition.
- Efficacy is improved if only used intermittently at first symptoms of an illness and only for six weeks or less.

 Toxicity

Comparative-toxicity rating is not available from standard references.

For symptoms of toxicity: See *Adverse Reactions, Side Effects or Overdose Symptoms* section below.

 Adverse Reactions, Side Effects or Overdose Symptoms

Signs and symptoms	What to do
Dermatitis (in sensitive patients)	Discontinue. Call doctor when convenient.

Evening Primrose

 Basic Information

Biological name (genus and species):
Oenothera biennis

Parts used for medicinal purposes:
Oil from seeds

Chemicals this herb contains:
Gamma-linolenic acid (GLA)

 Known Effects

- Anti-inflammatory
- Reduces high blood pressure
- Treats atopic eczema

 Possible Additional Effects

- Potential muscle relaxant
- May reduce effects of premenstrual syndrome (PMS)

- May lubricate hair, eyes, nails
- May treat eczema and other skin disorders
- Potential anticoagulant
- Potential astringent

 Warnings and Precautions

Don't take if you:
- Are pregnant, think you may be pregnant or plan pregnancy in the near future
- Take medication for high blood pressure
- Are prone to heavy menstrual flow

Consult your doctor if you:
- Take this herb for any medical problem that doesn't improve in 2 weeks (There may be safer, more effective treatments.)

• Take any medicinal drugs or herbs including aspirin, laxatives, cold and cough remedies, antacids, vitamins, minerals, amino acids, supplements, other prescription or nonprescription drugs

Pregnancy:
Don't use unless prescribed by your doctor.

Breastfeeding:
Don't use unless prescribed by your doctor.

Infants and children:
Treating infants and children under 2 with any herbal preparation is hazardous.

Storage:
• Store in cool, dry area away from direct light, but don't freeze.
• Store safely out of reach of children.
• Don't store in bathroom medicine cabinet. Heat and moisture may change the action of the herb.

Safe dosage:
Consult your doctor for the appropriate dose for your condition.

Toxicity

Comparative-toxicity rating is not available from standard references.

For symptoms of toxicity: See *Adverse Reactions, Side Effects or Overdose Symptoms* section below.

Adverse Reactions, Side Effects or Overdose Symptoms

Signs and symptoms	What to do
Abdominal discomfort	Discontinue. Call doctor when convenient.
Headache	Discontinue. Call doctor when convenient.
Nausea	Discontinue. Call doctor when convenient.
Skin rash	Discontinue. Call doctor when convenient.

Eyebright

Basic Information

Biological name (genus and species):
Euphrasia officinalis

Parts used for medicinal purposes:
Entire plant, except roots

Chemicals this herb contains:
• Bitters (see Glossary)
• Pantothenic acid
• Tannins (see Glossary)
• Vitamins A, B-12, C, E and D
• Volatile oils (see Glossary)

Known Effects

Reduces inflammation

Possible Additional Effects

Internal use:
• May treat nasal congestion
• May treat cough
• May treat sinusitis
• May treat allergies

MEDICINAL HERBS

➡

External use:
- Used as an eyewash to relieve discomfort caused from eyestrain or minor irritation
- May treat conjunctivitis

 Warnings and Precautions

Don't take if you:
Are pregnant, think you may be pregnant or plan pregnancy in the near future.

Consult your doctor if you:
- Take this herb for any medical problem that doesn't improve in 2 weeks (There may be safer, more effective treatments.)
- Take any medicinal drugs or herbs including aspirin, laxatives, cold and cough remedies, antacids, vitamins, minerals, amino acids, supplements, other prescription or nonprescription drugs

Pregnancy:
Don't use unless prescribed by your doctor.

Breastfeeding:
Don't use unless prescribed by your doctor.

Infants and children:
Treating infants and children under 2 with any herbal preparation is hazardous.

Others:
None are expected if you are beyond childhood, under 45, not pregnant,

basically healthy, take it for only a short time and do not exceed manufacturer's recommended dose.

Storage:
- Store in cool, dry area away from direct light, but don't freeze.
- Store safely out of reach of children.
- Don't store in bathroom medicine cabinet. Heat and moisture may change the action of the herb.

Safe dosage:
Consult your doctor for the appropriate dose for your condition.

 Toxicity

Rated relatively safe when taken in appropriate quantities for short periods of time

For symptoms of toxicity: See *Adverse Reactions, Side Effects or Overdose Symptoms* section below.

 Adverse Reactions, Side Effects or Overdose Symptoms

Signs and symptoms	What to do
Nausea	Discontinue. Call doctor immediately.
Skin rash	Discontinue. Call doctor when convenient.

Feverfew (Altamisa, Bachelor's Buttons)

Basic Information

Biological name (genus and species):
Tanacetum parthenium

Parts used for medicinal purposes:
- Bark
- Dried flowers
- Leaves

Chemicals this herb contains:
- Parthenolide
- Pyrethrins
- Santamarin
- Volatile oils (see Glossary)

Known Effects

- Decreases thickness and increases fluidity of mucus in lungs and bronchial tubes
- Lessens severity and reduces frequency of migraine attacks
- Antispasmodic

Possible Additional Effects

Leaves:
- May treat menstrual disorders
- May treat common cold
- May treat indigestion and diarrhea
- May stimulate appetite

Dried flowers:
- May treat intestinal parasites (worms)
- Potential aid in expelling gas from intestinal tract
- May relieve arthritis
- Potential anti-inflammatory
- May reduce fever

Warnings and Precautions

Don't take if you:
- Are allergic to pyrethrins
- Are pregnant, think you may be pregnant or plan pregnancy in the near future

Consult your doctor if you:
- Take this herb for any medical problem that doesn't improve in 2 weeks (There may be safer, more effective treatments.)
- Take any medicinal drugs or herbs including aspirin, laxatives, cold and cough remedies, antacids, vitamins, minerals, amino acids, supplements, other prescription or nonprescription drugs

Pregnancy:
Don't use.

Breastfeeding:
Don't use.

Infants and children:
Treating infants and children under 2 with any herbal preparation is hazardous.

Others:
Chewing leaves may cause mouth sores.

Storage:
- Store in cool, dry area away from direct light, but don't freeze.
- Store safely out of reach of children.
- Don't store in bathroom medicine cabinet. Heat and moisture may change the action of the herb.

MEDICINAL HERBS

Safe dosage:
- Consult your doctor for the appropriate dose for your condition.
- Pause occasionally in your treatment to enhance long-term efficacy.

Toxicity

Feverfew is generally regarded as safe when taken in very small quantities for short periods of time.

For symptoms of toxicity: See *Adverse Reactions, Side Effects or Overdose Symptoms* section below.

Adverse Reactions, Side Effects or Overdose Symptoms

Signs and symptoms	What to do
Abdominal pain	Seek medical care.
Internal mouth sores	Seek medical care.
Life-threatening anaphylaxis may follow injections— symptoms include immediate severe itching, paleness, low blood pressure, loss of consciousness, coma	Yell for help. Don't leave victim. Begin CPR (cardiopulmonary resuscitation), mouth-to-mouth breathing and external cardiac massage. Have someone dial 0 (operator) or 911 (emergency). Don't stop CPR until help arrives.

Flax (Linseed)

Basic Information

Biological name (genus and species):
Linum usitatissimum

Parts used for medicinal purposes:
- Oil
- Seeds

Chemicals this herb contains:
- Fixed oil (see Glossary)
- Glycosides
- Gum (see Glossary)
- Linamarin
- Linoleic acid
- Linolenic acid
- Mucilage (see Glossary)
- Protein
- Tannins (see Glossary)
- Wax (see Glossary)

Known Effects

- Treats skin disorders
- Forms bulk in intestinal tract
- Anti-inflammatory
- Laxative
- Contains essential fatty acids

Miscellaneous information:
- Purification has improved
- Increasingly being used in cereal, grain products
- Good for increasing fiber in your diet

Possible Additional Effects

- May ease symptoms of menopause
- May reduce cholesterol and triglyceride levels
- May soothe coughs
- Oil may soften or smooth skin
- Used for poultices (see Glossary) to apply to chest for colds and coughs

- May treat burns when applied externally
- May protect scraped tissues
- May reduce inflammation associated with arthritis
- May stimulate immune system

 Warnings and Precautions

Don't take if you:

Are pregnant, think you may be pregnant or plan pregnancy in the near future.

Consult your doctor if you:

- Take this herb for any medical problem that doesn't improve in 2 weeks (There may be safer, more effective treatments.)
- Take any medicinal drugs or herbs including aspirin, laxatives, cold and cough remedies, antacids, vitamins, minerals, amino acids, supplements, other prescription or nonprescription drugs

Pregnancy:

Dangers outweigh any possible benefits. Don't use.

Breastfeeding:

Dangers outweigh any possible benefits. Don't use.

Infants and children:

Treating infants and children under 2 with any herbal preparation is hazardous.

Others:

None are expected if you are beyond childhood, under 45, not pregnant, basically healthy, take it for only a short time and do not exceed manufacturer's recommended dose.

Storage:

- Store in cool, dry area away from direct light, but don't freeze.
- Store safely out of reach of children.
- Don't store in bathroom medicine cabinet. Heat and moisture may change the action of the herb.

Safe dosage:

Consult your doctor for the appropriate dose for your condition.

 Toxicity

Comparative-toxicity rating is not available from standard references.

 Adverse Reactions, Side Effects or Overdose Symptoms

None are expected.

Garlic

 Basic Information

Biological name (genus and species):
Allium sativum

Parts used for medicinal purposes:
Bulb

Chemicals this herb contains:

- Allicin
- Allyl disulfides
- Iron
- Magnesium
- Manganese
- Phytoncides
- Potassium
- Selenium
- Sulfur
- Unsaturated aldehydes
- Vitamins A, B-1 and C
- Volatile oils (see Glossary)

MEDICINAL HERBS

➡

Known Effects

- Protects against infection
- Relieves indigestion
- Decreases thickness and increases fluidity of mucus in lungs and bronchial tubes
- Helps body dispose of excess fluid by increasing amount of urine produced
- Promotes blood-pressure control
- Decreases cholesterol in hypercholesterolemic (see Glossary) males
- Antioxidant
- Antiviral and antibacterial
- Reduces platelet aggregation
- Anticoagulant

Miscellaneous information:
- Garlic is used as a condiment.
- Avoid using garlic as a medicinal herb in any amount with children!
- It is acceptable to use garlic as a flavoring in children's food.

Possible Additional Effects

- May treat cramping, abdominal pain in adults
- May inhibit certain forms of cancer
- May redden skin by increasing blood flow to it
- May treat sinusitis
- May improve circulation
- May treat burns when used externally as a moist pulp

Warnings and Precautions

Don't take if you:
Are being treated for any medical problem—consult your doctor first.

Consult your doctor if you:
- Take this herb for any medical problem that doesn't improve in 2 weeks (There may be safer, more effective treatments.)
- Take any medicinal drugs or herbs including aspirin, laxatives, cold and cough remedies, antacids, vitamins, minerals, amino acids, supplements, other prescription or nonprescription drugs

Pregnancy:
Don't use unless prescribed by your doctor.

Breastfeeding:
Don't use unless prescribed by your doctor.

Infants and children:
Treating infants and children under 2 with any herbal preparation is hazardous.

Storage:
- Store in cool, dry area away from direct light, but don't freeze.
- Store safely out of reach of children.
- Don't store in bathroom medicine cabinet. Heat and moisture may change the action of the herb.

Safe dosage:
- Limit intake to 5 cloves a day.
- 2-3 cloves of chopped fresh garlic daily are adequate to achieve therapeutic benefits.

Toxicity

Comparative-toxicity rating is not available from standard references.

For symptoms of toxicity: See *Adverse Reactions, Side Effects or Overdose Symptoms* section below.

Adverse Reactions, Side Effects or Overdose Symptoms

Signs and symptoms	What to do
Contact dermatitis	Wear gloves.
Gastrointestinal upset, nausea	Decrease dose.
Increased number of circulating white blood cells as determined by laboratory studies	Discontinue. Call doctor immediately.
Precipitous blood-pressure drop: symptoms include faintness, cold sweat, paleness, rapid pulse	Seek emergency treatment.
Skin eruptions	Discontinue. Call doctor when convenient.

Ginger (Ginger Rhizome)

Basic Information

Biological name (genus and species):
Zingiber officinale

Parts used for medicinal purposes:
Roots

Chemicals this herb contains:
• Bisabolene
• Borneal
• Camphene
• Choline
• Cineole
• Citral
• Sesquiterpene
• Volatile oils (see Glossary)
• Zingerone
• Zingiberene

Known Effects

• Helps expel gas from intestinal tract
• Provides counterirritation (see Glossary) when applied to skin overlying an inflamed or irritated joint
• Treats nausea and vomiting
• Treats motion sickness

Miscellaneous information:
• Ginger is used as a flavoring agent.
• No effects are expected on the body, either good or bad, when ginger is used in very small amounts to enhance the flavor of food.

Possible Additional Effects

• May treat indigestion
• May treat abdominal discomfort
• May reduce fever
• May treat migraine headache
• May act as an antioxidant
• May reduce pain of arthritis (anti-inflammatory)

Warnings and Precautions

Don't take if you:
• Are pregnant, think you may be pregnant or plan pregnancy in the near future

MEDICINAL HERBS

→

- Have any chronic disease of the gastrointestinal tract, such as stomach or duodenal ulcers, reflux esophagitis, ulcerative colitis, spastic colitis, diverticulosis or diverticulitis

Consult your doctor if you:
- Take this herb for any medical problem that doesn't improve in 2 weeks (There may be safer, more effective treatments.)
- Take any medicinal drugs or herbs including aspirin, laxatives, cold and cough remedies, antacids, vitamins, minerals, amino acids, supplements, other prescription or nonprescription drugs
- Have stomach or intestinal diseases

Pregnancy:
- Problems in pregnant women taking small or usual amounts have not been proved, but the chance of problems does exist. Don't use unless prescribed by your doctor.
- Do not use for morning sickness during pregnancy.

Breastfeeding:
Problems in breastfed infants of lactating mothers taking small or usual amounts have not been proved, but the chance of problems does exist. Don't use unless prescribed by your doctor.

Infants and children:
Treating infants and children under 2 with any herbal preparation is hazardous.

Others:
None are expected if you are beyond childhood, under 45, not pregnant, basically healthy, take it for only a short time and do not exceed manufacturer's recommended dose.

Storage:
- Store in cool, dry area away from direct light, but don't freeze.
- Store safely out of reach of children.
- Don't store in bathroom medicine cabinet. Heat and moisture may change the action of the herb.

Safe dosage:
Consult your doctor for the appropriate dose for your condition.

Toxicity

Comparative-toxicity rating is not available from standard references.

For symptoms of toxicity: See *Adverse Reactions, Side Effects or Overdose Symptoms* section below.

Adverse Reactions, Side Effects or Overdose Symptoms

Signs and symptoms	What to do
Diarrhea	Discontinue. Call doctor immediately.
Heartburn	Discontinue. Call doctor immediately.
Nausea or vomiting	Discontinue. Call doctor immediately.

Ginkgo Biloba

 Basic Information

Biological name (genus and species):
Ginkgoaceae, Ginkgo biloba

Parts used for medicinal purposes:
Leaf extract

Chemicals this herb contains:
- Bilobalide
- Ginkgolic acids
- Glycosides (quercetin and kaempferol)
- Isorhamnetin
- Terpene lactones (ginkgolides A, B and C)

 Known Effects

- Increases circulation to the brain and lower extremities
- Aids in treatment of memory loss associated with Alzheimer's disease
- Treats loss of concentration and emotional fatigue in the elderly

 Possible Additional Effects

- May treat tinnitus and vertigo
- May reduce vision loss due to aging
- May reduce symptoms associated with Raynaud's disease
- Potential aid in the treatment of peripheral vascular disease

 Warnings and Precautions

Don't take if you:
Have had a stroke or are prone to them.

Consult your doctor if you:
- Take this herb for any medical problem that doesn't improve in 2 weeks (There may be safer, more effective treatments.)
- Take any medicinal drugs or herbs including aspirin, laxatives, cold and cough remedies, antacids, vitamins, minerals, amino acids, supplements, other prescription or nonprescription drugs

Pregnancy:
Don't use unless prescribed by your doctor.

Breastfeeding:
Don't use unless prescribed by your doctor.

Infants and children:
Treating infants and children under 2 with any herbal preparation is hazardous.

Storage:
- Store in cool, dry area away from direct light, but don't freeze.
- Store safely out of reach of children.
- Don't store in bathroom medicine cabinet. Heat and moisture may change the action of the herb.

Safe dosage:
Consult your doctor for the appropriate dose for your condition.

 Toxicity

Comparative-toxicity rating is not available from standard references.

For symptoms of toxicity: See *Adverse Reactions, Side Effects or Overdose Symptoms* section below.

MEDICINAL HERBS

➜

Adverse Reactions, Side Effects or Overdose Symptoms

Signs and symptoms	What to do
Diarrhea	Discontinue. Call doctor immediately.
Headache	Discontinue. Call doctor immediately.
Irritability, restlessness	Discontinue. Call doctor when convenient.
Nausea	Discontinue. Call doctor immediately.

Ginseng

Basic Information

Ginseng is also known as Asian ginseng; panax ginseng; and American, Korean or Chinese ginseng.

Biological name (genus and species): *Panax quinquefolius*

Parts used for medicinal purposes: Roots

Chemicals this herb contains:
• Arabinose
• Camphor
• Ginsenosides
• Mucilage (see Glossary)
• Panaxosides
• Resin (see Glossary)
• Saponin (see Glossary)
• Starch

Known Effects
• Stimulates brain, heart, blood vessels
• Reduces stress and fatigue
• Increases secretion of histamine (see Glossary)
• Improves appetite and digestion
• Stimulant
• Antioxidant

Miscellaneous information:
• A favorite Chinese remedy used for almost everything
• A native plant in the U.S. state of Georgia

Possible Additional Effects
• Used as an aphrodisiac
• May increase mental and physical stamina
• May treat symptoms of menopause
• May reduce effects of radiation exposure
• May reduce blood glucose in diabetics
• May alleviate insomnia

Warnings and Precautions

Don't take if you:

- Are pregnant, think you may be pregnant or plan pregnancy in the near future
- Have any chronic disease of the gastrointestinal tract, such as stomach or duodenal ulcers, reflux esophagitis, ulcerative colitis, spastic colitis, diverticulosis or diverticulitis
- Have been diagnosed with cystic breast disease, breast cancer, heart disease or high blood pressure

Consult your doctor if you:

- Take this herb for any medical problem that doesn't improve in 2 weeks (There may be safer, more effective treatments.)
- Take any medicinal drugs or herbs including aspirin, laxatives, cold and cough remedies, antacids, vitamins, minerals, amino acids, supplements, other prescription or nonprescription drugs

Pregnancy:

Don't use unless prescribed by your doctor.

Breastfeeding:

Don't use unless prescribed by your doctor.

Infants and children:

Treating infants and children under 2 with any herbal preparation is hazardous.

Others:

None are expected if you are beyond childhood, under 45, not pregnant, basically healthy, take it for only a short time and do not exceed manufacturer's recommended dose.

Storage:

- Store in cool, dry area away from direct light, but don't freeze.
- Store safely out of reach of children.
- Don't store in bathroom medicine cabinet. Heat and moisture may change the action of the herb.

Safe dosage:

Consult your doctor for the appropriate dose for your condition.

 ## Toxicity

Generally regarded as safe when taken in appropriate quantities for short periods of time

For symptoms of toxicity: See *Adverse Reactions, Side Effects or Overdose Symptoms* section below.

 ## Adverse Reactions, Side Effects or Overdose Symptoms

Signs and symptoms	What to do
Diarrhea	Discontinue. Call doctor immediately.
Nausea or vomiting	Discontinue. Call doctor immediately.

Goldenseal

 Basic Information

Biological name (genus and species):
Hydrastis canadensis

Parts used for medicinal purposes:
• Rhizomes
• Roots

Chemicals this herb contains:
• Albumin
• Berberine
• Candine
• Fats
• Hydrastine
• Lignin
• Resin (see Glossary)
• Starch
• Sugar
• Volatile oils (see Glossary)

 Known Effects

• Antibiotic
• Decreases bleeding
• Large amounts stimulate central nervous system
• Depresses muscle tone of small blood vessels
• Laxative

Miscellaneous information:
Goldenseal has a very bitter taste.

 Possible Additional Effects

• May strengthen the immune system
• May treat trachoma
• May treat disorders of the liver
• May treat dyspepsia
• May increase appetite
• May treat and relieve sinusitis
• May treat infectious diarrhea

STOP Warnings and Precautions

Don't take if you:
• Are pregnant, think you may be pregnant or plan pregnancy in the near future
• Have any chronic disease of the gastrointestinal tract, such as stomach or duodenal ulcers, reflux esophagitis, ulcerative colitis, spastic colitis, diverticulosis or diverticulitis.
• Have heart disease, diabetes, glaucoma or high blood pressure
• Are taking coumadin, warfarin

Consult your doctor if you:
• Take this herb for any medical problem that doesn't improve in 2 weeks (There may be safer, more effective treatments.)
• Take any medicinal drugs or herbs including aspirin, laxatives, cold and cough remedies, antacids, vitamins, minerals, amino acids, supplements, other prescription or nonprescription drugs

Pregnancy:
Dangers outweigh any possible benefits. Don't use.

Breastfeeding:
Dangers outweigh any possible benefits. Don't use.

Infants and children:
Treating infants and children under 2 with any herbal preparation is hazardous.

Others:
None are expected if you are beyond childhood, under 45, not pregnant, basically healthy, take it for only a short time and do not exceed manufacturer's recommended dose.

Storage:

- Store in cool, dry area away from direct light, but don't freeze.
- Store safely out of reach of children.
- Don't store in bathroom medicine cabinet. Heat and moisture may change the action of the herb.

Safe dosage:

Consult your doctor for the appropriate dose for your condition.

 Toxicity

Rated slightly dangerous, particularly in children, persons over 55 and those who take larger than appropriate quantities for extended periods of time

For symptoms of toxicity: See *Adverse Reactions, Side Effects or Overdose Symptoms* section below.

 Adverse Reactions, Side Effects or Overdose Symptoms

Signs and symptoms	What to do
Breathing difficulties	Seek emergency treatment.
Convulsions	Seek emergency treatment.
Depression	Discontinue. Call doctor immediately.
Diarrhea	Discontinue. Call doctor immediately.
Mouth and throat irritation	Discontinue. Call doctor immediately.
Nausea or vomiting	Discontinue. Call doctor immediately.
Numbness of hands and feet	Discontinue. Call doctor immediately.
Weakness leading to paralysis of muscles	Seek emergency treatment.

Gotu Kola (Kola)

 Basic Information

Biological name (genus and species):
Centella asiatica

Parts used for medicinal purposes:
- Nuts
- Roots
- Seeds

Chemicals this herb contains:
- Caffeine
- Catechol
- Epicatechol
- Flavonoids
- Resins (see Glossary)
- Theobromine
- Triterpenoid compounds

 Known Effects

- Stimulates central nervous system
- Helps body dispose of excess fluid by increasing amount of urine produced
- Anti-inflammatory
- Treats skin disorders (burns, cellulite, scleroderma)

Miscellaneous information:

No effects are expected on the body, either good or bad, when this herb is used in very small amounts to enhance the flavor of food.

MEDICINAL HERBS

➜

Possible
Additional Effects

- May decrease fatigue
- May decrease anxiety
- May increase circulation in the legs
- May improve memory
- May help leprosy
- May lessen night cramps
- May decrease tingling/numbness of extremities
- May speed wound healing
- May treat eczema

 Warnings and Precautions

Don't take if you:

- Are pregnant, think you may be pregnant or plan pregnancy in the near future
- Have any chronic disease of the gastrointestinal tract, such as stomach or duodenal ulcers, reflux esophagitis, ulcerative colitis, spastic colitis, diverticulosis or diverticulitis

Consult your doctor if you:

- Take this herb for any medical problem that doesn't improve in 2 weeks (There may be safer, more effective treatments.)
- Take any medicinal drugs or herbs including aspirin, laxatives, cold and cough remedies, antacids, vitamins, minerals, amino acids, supplements, other prescription or nonprescription drugs

Pregnancy:
Don't use.

Breastfeeding:
Don't use.

Infants and children:
Treating infants and children under 2 with any herbal preparation is hazardous.

Others:
May cause contact dermatitis when applied topically.

Storage:

- Store in cool, dry area away from direct light, but don't freeze.
- Store safely out of reach of children.
- Don't store in bathroom medicine cabinet. Heat and moisture may change the action of the herb.

Safe dosage:
Consult your doctor for the appropriate dose for your condition.

 Toxicity

Rated relatively safe when taken in appropriate quantities for short periods of time

For symptoms of toxicity: See *Adverse Reactions, Side Effects or Overdose Symptoms* section below.

 Adverse Reaction, Side Effects or Overdose Symptoms

Signs and symptoms	What to do
Aggravated peptic ulcers in stomach, duodenum or esophagus	Discontinue. Call doctor immediately.
Inability to sleep	Discontinue. Call doctor when convenient.
Increased cholesterol	Discontinue. Call doctor immediately.
Nervousness	Discontinue. Call doctor when convenient.
Photosensitivity	Discontinue. Call doctor immediately.

Grape Seed Extract

Basic Information

Biological name (genus and species):
Vitis vinifera

Parts used for medicinal purposes:
Not applicable

Chemicals this herb contains:
- Essential fatty acids
- Proanthocyanidins
- Tocopherols

Known Effects

- Powerful antioxidant
- Helps prevent atherosclerosis
- Prevents free-radical (see Glossary) damage
- Improves circulation
- Anti-inflammatory

Possible Additional Effects

- May protect against effects of radiation
- May prevent retinopathy
- May reduce risk of varicose veins
- May help heal wounds
- May prevent dental cavities

Warnings and Precautions

Don't take if you:
Have any chronic disease, without consulting your doctor.

Consult your doctor if you:
- Take this herb for any medical problem that doesn't improve in 2 weeks (There may be safer, more effective treatments.)
- Take any medicinal drugs or herbs including aspirin, laxatives, cold and cough remedies, antacids, vitamins, minerals, amino acids, supplements, other prescription or nonprescription drugs

Pregnancy:
Don't use unless prescribed by your doctor.

Breastfeeding:
Don't use unless prescribed by your doctor.

Infants and children:
Treating infants and children under 2 with any herbal preparation is hazardous.

Others:
None are expected if you are beyond childhood, under 45, not pregnant, basically healthy, take it for only a short time and do not exceed manufacturer's recommended dose.

Storage:
- Store in cool, dry area away from direct light, but don't freeze.
- Store safely out of reach of children.
- Don't store in bathroom medicine cabinet. Heat and moisture may change the action of the herb.

Safe dosage:
Consult your doctor for the appropriate dose for your condition.

Toxicity

Comparative-toxicity rating is not available from standard references.

Adverse Reactions, Side Effects or Overdose Symptoms

None are expected.

Hawthorn

 Basic Information

Biological name (genus and species): *Crataegus oxyacantha*

Parts used for medicinal purposes:
- Berries
- Blossoms
- Leaves

Chemicals this herb contains:
- Acetylcholine
- Anthocyanin-type pigments
- Cardiotonic amines
- Choline
- Cratagolic acid
- Flavonoids
- Glycosides (see Glossary)
- Pectins
- Purines
- Saponins (see Glossary)
- Triterpene acids

 Known Effects

- Can depress respiration
- Increases blood flow to the heart
- Can depress heart rate
- Antiarrhythmic
- Coronary vasodilator (widens coronary blood vessels)

 Possible Additional Effects

- May treat high blood pressure
- May treat atherosclerosis
- May help treat circulatory disorders
- May lower cholesterol

 Warnings and Precautions

Don't take if you:
- Are pregnant, think you may be pregnant or plan pregnancy in the near future
- Have heart disease

Consult your doctor if you:
- Take this herb for any medical problem that doesn't improve in 2 weeks (There may be safer, more effective treatments.)
- Take any medicinal drugs or herbs including aspirin, laxatives, cold and cough remedies, antacids, vitamins, minerals, amino acids, supplements, other prescription or nonprescription drugs

Pregnancy:
Don't use.

Breastfeeding:
Don't use.

Infants and children:
Treating infants and children under 2 with any herbal preparation is hazardous.

Others:
- Do not attempt to self medicate. If you think you have heart problems, consult a physician immediately.

Storage:
- Store in cool, dry area away from direct light, but don't freeze.
- Store safely out of reach of children.
- Don't store in bathroom medicine cabinet. Heat and moisture may change the action of the herb.

Safe dosage:
Consult your doctor for the appropriate dose for your condition.

Toxicity

Comparative-toxicity rating is not available from standard references.

For symptoms of toxicity: See *Adverse Reactions, Side Effects or Overdose Symptoms* section below.

Adverse Reactions, Side Effects or Overdose Symptoms

Signs and symptoms	What to do
Breathing difficulties	Seek emergency treatment.
Heartbeat irregularities	Seek emergency treatment.

Hyssop

Basic Information

Biological name (genus and species):
Hyssopus officinalis

Parts used for medicinal purposes:
Aerial parts (those above ground)

• Essential oil
• Flowers
• Leaves

Chemicals this herb contains:

• Diosmine
• Flavonoids
• Hyssopin
• Isolic acid
• Marrubiin
• Oleonolic acid
• Resin (see Glossary)
• Tannins (see Glossary)
• Volatile oils (see Glossary)

Known Effects

Expectorant: stimulates coughing, relieves congestion

Miscellaneous information:
Available as tea, compress, tincture, dried or fresh.

Possible Additional Effects

• May treat bronchitis
• May have a mild sedative effect (antianxiety)
• Potential muscle relaxant
• Potential antiseptic: used externally, may treat small wounds and herpes simplex
• May have antiviral properties
• May reduce indigestion
• May help heal cold sores
• May decrease gastrointestinal gas production

Warnings and Precautions

Don't take if you:
Are pregnant, think you may be pregnant or are considering pregnancy.

Consult your doctor if you:
• Take this herb for any medical problem that doesn't improve in 2 weeks (There may be safer, more effective treatments.)
• Take any medicinal drugs or herbs including aspirin, laxatives, cold and cough remedies, antacids,

MEDICINAL HERBS

➜

vitamins, minerals, amino acids, supplements, other prescription or nonprescription drugs
• Plan to take hyssop at all—use only under medical supervision!

Pregnancy:
Don't use.

Breastfeeding:
Don't use unless prescribed by your doctor.

Infants and children:
Treating infants and children under 2 with any herbal preparation is hazardous.

Storage:
• Store in cool, dry area away from direct light, but don't freeze.
• Store safely out of reach of children.
• Don't store in bathroom medicine cabinet. Heat and moisture may change the action of the herb.

Safe dosage:
Consult your doctor for the appropriate dose for your condition.

 Toxicity

Comparative-toxicity rating is not available from standard references.

For symptoms of toxicity: See *Adverse Reactions, Side Effects or Overdose Symptoms* section below.

 Adverse Reactions, Side Effects or Overdose Symptoms

Signs and symptoms	What to do
Diarrhea	Discontinue. Call doctor if it persists.
Nausea	Discontinue. Call doctor if it persists.

Kava Kava

 Basic Information

Biological name (genus and species):
Piper methysticum

Parts used for medicinal purposes:
Roots

Chemicals this herb contains:
• Demethoxyyangonin
• Dihydrokawain
• Dihydromethysticin
• Flavorawin A
• Kawain
• Methysticin
• Starch
• Yangonin

 Known Effects
• Depresses the central nervous system
• Antianxiety

Miscellaneous information:
• Used to make a fermented liquor
• Sedative effect is mild
• Available in dry bulk, capsules, tinctures

 Possible Additional Effects
• Potential sedative for anxiety disorders
• May induce restful sleep

- May treat fatigue
- Potential genitourinary antiseptic (see Glossary)
- May treat coughs
- Potential muscle relaxant
- Potential analgesic

 ## Warnings and Precautions

Don't take if you:
- Are pregnant, think you may be pregnant or plan pregnancy in the near future
- Are driving or operating equipment (Large doses cause sedation.)

Consult your doctor if you:
- Take this herb for any medical problem that doesn't improve in 2 weeks (There may be safer, more effective treatments.)
- Take any medicinal drugs or herbs including aspirin, laxatives, cold and cough remedies, antacids, vitamins, minerals, amino acids, supplements, other prescription or nonprescription drugs

Pregnancy:
Problems in pregnant women taking small or usual amounts have not been proved, but the chance of problems does exist. Don't use unless prescribed by your doctor.

Breastfeeding:
Problems in breastfed infants of lactating mothers taking small or usual amounts have not been proved, but the chance of problems does exist. Don't use unless prescribed by your doctor.

Infants and children:
Treating infants and children under 2 with any herbal preparation is hazardous.

Others:
None are expected if you are beyond childhood, under 45, not pregnant, basically healthy, take it for only a short time and do not exceed manufacturer's recommended dose.

Storage:
- Store in cool, dry area away from direct light, but don't freeze.
- Store safely out of reach of children.
- Don't store in bathroom medicine cabinet. Heat and moisture may change the action of the herb.

Safe dosage:
Consult your doctor for the appropriate dose for your condition.

 ## Toxicity

Rated slightly dangerous, particularly in children, persons over 55 and those who take larger than appropriate quantities for extended periods of time

For symptoms of toxicity: See *Adverse Reactions, Side Effects or Overdose Symptoms* section below.

 ## Adverse Reactions, Side Effects or Overdose Symptoms

Signs and symptoms	What to do
Allergic skin reaction or shortness of breath	Discontinue. Call doctor immediately.
Gastrointestinal upset	Discontinue. Call doctor immediately.
Oversedation	Discontinue. Call doctor immediately.
Repeated small amounts may lead to undesirable skin and nail coloring, inflammation of the body and eyes	Discontinue. Call doctor immediately.

MEDICINAL HERBS

Milk Thistle (Mary Thistle, Wild Artichoke)

 Basic Information

Biological name (genus and species):
Silybum marianum

Parts used for medicinal purposes:
- Fruit
- Leaves
- Seeds

Chemicals this herb contains:
Silymarin

 Known Effects

- Protects the liver from chemical damage
- Increases the secretion and flow of bile
- Antioxidant
- Helps treat chronic inflammatory liver disease (hepatitis)

 Possible Additional Effects

- May reduce jaundice
- May reduce inflammation associated with hepatitis and cirrhosis
- May reduce gallbladder inflammation
- May help treat psoriasis

 Warnings and Precautions

Consult your doctor if you:
- Take this herb for any medical problem that doesn't improve in 2 weeks (There may be safer, more effective treatments.)
- Take any medicinal drugs or herbs including aspirin, laxatives, cold and cough remedies, antacids, vitamins, minerals, amino acids, supplements, other prescription or nonprescription drugs
- Have liver disease

Pregnancy:
Don't use unless prescribed by your doctor.

Breastfeeding:
Don't use unless prescribed by your doctor.

Infants and children:
Treating infants and children under 2 with any herbal preparation is hazardous.

Others:
You may develop loose stools during the first few days of use.

Storage:
- Store in cool, dry area away from direct light, but don't freeze.
- Store safely out of reach of children.
- Don't store in bathroom medicine cabinet. Heat and moisture may change the action of the herb.

Safe dosage:
Consult your doctor for the appropriate dose for your condition.

 Toxicity

Comparative-toxicity rating is not available from standard references.

For symptoms of toxicity: See *Adverse Reactions, Side Effects or Overdose Symptoms* section below.

 Adverse Reactions, Side Effects or Overdose Symptoms

Signs and symptoms	What to do
Loose stools	Discontinue. Call doctor when convenient.

Mullein

Basic Information

Biological name (genus and species):
Verbascum thapsiforme,
V. phlomoides, V. thapsus

Parts used for medicinal purposes:
• Flowers
• Leaves

Chemicals this herb contains:
Saponin (see Glossary)

Known Effects

• Covers and protects scraped tissues
• Softens and soothes irritated skin
• Treats throat irritations and coughs

Miscellaneous information:
Available as tea, compress
and inhalant.

Possible Additional Effects

• May relieve bronchial irritation when
smoked
• May treat sunburn, hemorrhoids,
injured skin and mucous membranes
when applied topically
• May treat stomach cramps
• May treat diarrhea

Warnings and Precautions

Don't take if you:
Are pregnant, think you may be
pregnant or plan pregnancy in the
near future.

Consult your doctor if you:
• Take this herb for any medical
problem that doesn't improve in
2 weeks (There may be safer, more
effective treatments.)
• Take any medicinal drugs or
herbs including aspirin, laxatives,
cold and cough remedies, antacids,
vitamins, minerals, amino acids,
supplements, other prescription
or nonprescription drugs

Pregnancy:
Don't use unless prescribed by
your doctor.

Breastfeeding:
Don't use unless prescribed by
your doctor.

Infants and children:
Treating infants and children under
2 with any herbal preparation
is hazardous.

Others:
None are expected if you are beyond
childhood, under 45, not pregnant,
basically healthy, take it for only a short
time and do not exceed manufacturer's
recommended dose.

Storage:
• Store in cool, dry area away from
direct light, but don't freeze.
• Store safely out of reach of children.
• Don't store in bathroom medicine
cabinet. Heat and moisture may
change the action of the herb.

Safe dosage:
Consult your doctor for the appropriate dose for your condition.

MEDICINAL HERBS

→

Toxicity

Comparative-toxicity rating is not available from standard references.

For symptoms of toxicity: See *Adverse Reactions, Side Effects or Overdose Symptoms* section below.

Adverse Reactions, Side Effects or Overdose Symptoms

Signs and symptoms	What to do
Mild stomach upset	Discontinue. Call doctor when convenient.

Myrrh

Basic Information

Biological name (genus and species): *Commiphora molmol*

Parts used for medicinal purposes:
• Leaves
• Resin from stems

Chemicals this herb contains:
• Acetic acid
• Formic acid
• Myrrholic acids
• Resin (see Glossary)
• Volatile oils (see Glossary)

Known Effects

Helps expel gas from intestinal tract

Miscellaneous information:
Primary use of myrrh is in perfumes and incense.

Possible Additional Effects

• May treat dyspepsia
• Used as mouthwash
• May treat bronchitis
• May treat sore and strep throat
• May treat canker sores
• May treat eczema

Warnings and Precautions

Don't take if you:
Are pregnant, think you may be pregnant or plan pregnancy in the near future.

Consult your doctor if you:
• Take this herb for any medical problem that doesn't improve in 2 weeks (There may be safer, more effective treatments.)
• Take any medicinal drugs or herbs including aspirin, laxatives, cold and cough remedies, antacids, vitamins, minerals, amino acids, supplements, other prescription or nonprescription drugs

Pregnancy:
Don't use unless prescribed by your doctor.

Breastfeeding:
Don't use unless prescribed by your doctor.

Infants and children:
Treating infants and children under 2 with any herbal preparation is hazardous.

Others:
None are expected if you are beyond childhood, under 45, not pregnant,

basically healthy, take it for only a short time and do not exceed manufacturer's recommended dose.

Storage:
- Store in cool, dry area away from direct light, but don't freeze.
- Store safely out of reach of children.
- Don't store in bathroom medicine cabinet. Heat and moisture may change the action of the herb.

Safe dosage:
Consult your doctor for the appropriate dose for your condition.

 Toxicity

Comparative-toxicity rating is not available from standard references. Myrrh may be toxic in high concentrations.

For symptoms of toxicity: See *Adverse Reactions, Side Effects or Overdose Symptoms* section below.

 Adverse Reactions, Side Effects or Overdose Symptoms

Signs and symptoms	What to do
Convulsions	Seek emergency treatment.
Drowsiness	Discontinue. Call doctor when convenient.
Lethargy	Discontinue. Call doctor when convenient.

Oats (Oat Beard)

 Basic Information

Biological name (genus and species):
Avena sativa

Parts used for medicinal purposes:
Seeds

Chemicals this herb contains:
- Albumin
- Gluten
- Gum oil
- Protein compound
- Salts
- Saponin (see Glossary)
- Starch
- Sugar

 Known Effects

- Aids sleep
- Decreases cholesterol
- Helps dry skin

Miscellaneous information:
- "Feeling his oats" refers to the stimulant effect of this herb on some animals, particularly horses.
- Fiber intake should be increased gradually.

 Possible Additional Effects

- May decrease depression
- May treat high cholesterol
- May relieve indigestion
- May treat insomnia

MEDICINAL HERBS

→

Warnings and Precautions

Don't take if you:
No proven contraindications
(see Glossary) exist.

Consult your doctor if you:
• Take this herb for any medical
problem that doesn't improve in
2 weeks (There may be safer, more
effective treatments.)
• Take any medicinal drugs or
herbs including aspirin, laxatives,
cold and cough remedies, antacids,
vitamins, minerals, amino acids,
supplements, other prescription
or nonprescription drugs

Pregnancy:
Pregnant women should experience
no problems taking usual amounts as
part of a balanced diet.

Breastfeeding:
Breastfed infants of lactating mothers
should experience no problems when
mother takes usual amounts as part of
a balanced diet.

Infants and children:
Treating infants and children under 2 with
any herbal preparation is hazardous.

Others:
None are expected if you are beyond
childhood and under 45, basically
healthy and take for only a short time.

Storage:
• Store in cool, dry area away from
direct light, but don't freeze.
• Store safely out of reach of children.
• Don't store in bathroom medicine
cabinet. Heat and moisture may
change the action of the herb.

Safe dosage:
Consult your doctor for the appropriate dose for your condition.

Toxicity

Comparative-toxicity rating is not available from standard references.

Adverse Reactions, Side Effects or Overdose Symptoms

None are expected.

Parsley

Basic Information

Biological name (genus and species):
Petroselinum crispum

Parts used for medicinal purposes:
• Berries/fruits
• Leaves
• Roots
• Stems

Chemicals this herb contains:
• Apiin (also called *parsley camphor*)
• Apiol
• Pinene
• Vitamins A and C
• Volatile oils (see Glossary)

Known Effects

- Reduces urinary tract inflammation
- Uterine stimulant
- Aids digestion
- Increases renal (see Glossary) function—it helps body dispose of excess fluid by increasing amounts of urine produced

Miscellaneous information:
- When fresh sprigs are eaten, no problems are expected.
- Parsley is available as tincture, leaves, seeds, stems and roots.
- It is a good source of vitamins C and A.

 Possible Additional Effects

- May treat painful menstruation and premenstrual syndrome (PMS)
- May treat dyspepsia
- May relieve gas
- May facilitate passage of kidney stones

 Warnings and Precautions

Don't take if you:
- Are pregnant, think you may be pregnant or plan pregnancy in the near future
- Have any chronic disease of the gastrointestinal tract, such as stomach or duodenal ulcers, reflux esophagitis, ulcerative colitis, spastic colitis, diverticulosis or diverticulitis

Consult your doctor if you:
- Take this herb for any medical problem that doesn't improve in 2 weeks (There may be safer, more effective treatments.)
- Take any medicinal drugs or herbs including aspirin, laxatives, cold and cough remedies, antacids, vitamins, minerals, amino acids, supplements, other prescription or nonprescription drugs

Pregnancy:
- Dangers outweigh any possible benefits. Avoid taking any herbal medication made from parsley.
- Fresh parsley as a condiment is all right to eat.

Breastfeeding:
- Dangers outweigh any possible benefits. Avoid taking any herbal medication made from parsley.
- Fresh parsley as a condiment is all right to eat.

Infants and children:
Treating infants and children under 2 with any herbal preparation is hazardous.

Others:
None are expected if you are beyond childhood, under 45, not pregnant, basically healthy, take it for only a short time and do not exceed manufacturer's recommended dose.

Storage:
- Store in cool, dry area away from direct light, but don't freeze.
- Store safely out of reach of children.
- Don't store in bathroom medicine cabinet. Heat and moisture may change the action of the herb.

Safe dosage:
Consult your doctor for the appropriate dose for your condition.

MEDICINAL HERBS

→

Toxicity

Rated relatively safe when taken in appropriate quantities for short periods of time

For symptoms of toxicity: See *Adverse Reactions, Side Effects or Overdose Symptoms* section below.

 Adverse Reactions, Side Effects or Overdose Symptoms

Signs and symptoms	What to do
Dizziness	Discontinue. Call doctor immediately.
Jaundice (yellow skin and eyes)	Discontinue. Call doctor immediately.
Nausea or vomiting	Discontinue. Call doctor immediately.
Photosensitivity	Avoid high sunlight exposure.

Pau D'Arco (Lapacho, Taheebo)

 Basic Information

Biological name (genus and species): *Tabebuia* (several species exist, including *avellanedae* and *impetiginosa*)

Parts used for medicinal purposes: Inner bark

Chemicals this herb contains:
Bioflavonoids
Naphthoquinones, especially lapachol

 Known Effects

• Antibiotic
• Antifungal
• Antiparasitic
• Relieves indigestion

Miscellaneous information:
• Prescribed as a cancer cure but no proven effects on cancer exist at this time.
• Pau d'arco is available as capsules, tinctures, tea and dried bark.

 Possible Additional Effects

• Potential anti-inflammatory
• May treat rheumatism

 Warnings and Precautions

Don't take if you:
Are pregnant, think you may be pregnant or plan pregnancy in the near future.

Consult your doctor if you:
• Take this herb for any medical problem that doesn't improve in 2 weeks (There may be safer, more effective treatments.)
• Take any medicinal drugs or herbs including aspirin, laxatives, cold and cough remedies, antacids, vitamins, minerals, amino acids, supplements, other prescription or nonprescription drugs

Pregnancy:
Don't use unless prescribed by your doctor.

Breastfeeding:
Don't use unless prescribed by your doctor.

Infants and children:
Treating infants and children under 2 with any herbal preparation is hazardous.

Others:
Extended use of this herb (more than 7–10 days) should be done only under the advice of your doctor.

Storage:
• Store in cool, dry area away from direct light, but don't freeze.
• Store safely out of reach of children.
• Don't store in bathroom medicine cabinet. Heat and moisture may change the action of the herb.

Safe dosage:
Consult your doctor for the appropriate dose for your condition. 250mg to 1 gram per day is average.

 Toxicity
Comparative-toxicity rating is not available from standard references.

 Adverse Reactions, Side Effects or Overdose Symptoms
None are expected.

Peppermint

 Basic Information

Biological name (genus and species):
Mentha piperita

Parts used for medicinal purposes:
• Flowering tops
• Leaves

Chemicals this herb contains:
• Menthol
• Menthone
• Methyl acetate
• Tannic acid
• Terpenes (see Glossary)
• Volatile oils (see Glossary)

 Known Effects
• Treats stomach discomfort
• Increases bile-acid flow for normal gallbladder function
• Stimulates gastrointestinal tract

Miscellaneous information:
• Peppermint is used to add flavor to medical and nonmedical preparations.
• No effects are expected on the body, either good or bad, when the herb is used in very small amounts to enhance the flavor of food.

 Possible Additional Effects
• May aid in expelling gas from intestinal tract
• May reduce insomnia
• Potential antibacterial

MEDICINAL HERBS

➔

Warnings and Precautions

Don't take if you:
• Are pregnant, think you may be pregnant or plan pregnancy in the near future
• Have any chronic disease of the gastrointestinal tract, such as stomach or duodenal ulcers, reflux esophagitis, ulcerative colitis, spastic colitis, diverticulosis or diverticulitis
• Have epilepsy or other neural disorders

Consult your doctor if you:
• Take this herb for any medical problem that doesn't improve in 2 weeks (There may be safer, more effective treatments.)
• Take any medicinal drugs or herbs including aspirin, laxatives, cold and cough remedies, antacids, vitamins, minerals, amino acids, supplements, other prescription or nonprescription drugs

Pregnancy:
Problems in pregnant women taking small or usual amounts have not been proved, but the chance of problems does exist. Don't use unless prescribed by your doctor.

Breastfeeding:
Problems in breastfed infants of lactating mothers taking small or usual amounts have not been proved, but the chance of problems does exist. Don't use unless prescribed by your doctor.

Infants and children:
Treating infants and children under 2 with any herbal preparation is hazardous.

Others:
None are expected if you are beyond childhood, under 45, not pregnant, basically healthy, take it for only a short time and do not exceed manufacturer's recommended dose.

Storage:
• Store in cool, dry area away from direct light, but don't freeze.
• Store safely out of reach of children.
• Don't store in bathroom medicine cabinet. Heat and moisture may change the action of the herb.

Safe dosage:
Consult your doctor for the appropriate dose for your condition.

 Toxicity

Comparative-toxicity rating is not available from standard references.

For symptoms of toxicity: See *Adverse Reactions, Side Effects or Overdose Symptoms* section below.

 Adverse Reactions, Side Effects or Overdose Symptoms

Signs and symptoms	What to do
Drowsiness	Discontinue. Call doctor when convenient.
Vomiting	Discontinue. Call doctor immediately.

Psyllium

 Basic Information

Biological name (genus and species):
Plantago psyllium

Parts used for medicinal purposes:
Seeds

Chemicals this herb contains:
- Glycosides (see Glossary)
- Mucilage (see Glossary)

 Known Effects

- Produces bulky bowel movements
- Softens stools
- Reduces risk of heart disease by removing excess cholesterol from blood

Miscellaneous information:
Psyllium is a popular product and available over-the-counter without prescription.

 Possible Additional Effects

May treat constipation

 Warnings and Precautions

Don't take if you:
Are pregnant, think you may be pregnant or plan pregnancy in the near future.

Consult your doctor if you:
- Take this herb for any medical problem that doesn't improve in 2 weeks (There may be safer, more effective treatments.)
- Take any medicinal drugs or herbs including aspirin, laxatives, cold and cough remedies, antacids, vitamins, minerals, amino acids, supplements, other prescription or nonprescription drugs

Pregnancy:
Problems in pregnant women taking small or usual amounts have not been proved, but the chance of problems does exist. Don't use unless prescribed by your doctor.

Breastfeeding:
Problems in breastfed infants of lactating mothers taking small or usual amounts have not been proved, but the chance of problems does exist. Don't use unless prescribed by your doctor.

Infants and children:
Treating infants and children under 2 with any herbal preparation is hazardous.

Others:
People with allergies to dust or grasses may have a reaction to psyllium.

Storage:
- Store in cool, dry area away from direct light, but don't freeze.
- Store safely out of reach of children.
- Don't store in bathroom medicine cabinet. Heat and moisture may change the action of the herb.

Safe dosage:
Consult your doctor for the appropriate dose for your condition.

 Toxicity

Comparative-toxicity rating is not available from standard references.

MEDICINAL HERBS

Adverse Reactions,
Side Effects or
Overdose Symptoms

None are expected.

Red Clover (Pavine Clover, Cowgrass)

 Basic Information

Biological name (genus and species):
Trifolium pratense

Parts used for medicinal purposes:
Flowers

Chemicals this herb contains:
- Folic acid
- Glycosides (see Glossary)
- Isoflavonoids

 Known Effects

- Decreases activity of central nervous system
- Expectorant

 Possible
Additional Effects

- May reduce upper abdominal cramps
- May treat indigestion
- May loosen secretions in bronchial tubes due to infections or chronic lung disease
- Contains antitumor compounds and may be used in combination with other drugs to treat some forms of cancer
- May reduce menopausal symptoms
- Potential aid for weakened immune systems

 Warnings and
Precautions

Don't take if you:
- Are pregnant, think you may be pregnant or plan pregnancy in the near future
- Have a history of heart disease or stroke

Consult your doctor if you:
- Take this herb for any medical problem that doesn't improve in 2 weeks (There may be safer, more effective treatments.)
- Take any medicinal drugs or herbs including aspirin, laxatives, cold and cough remedies, antacids, vitamins, minerals, amino acids, supplements, other prescription or nonprescription drugs

Pregnancy:
Don't use unless prescribed by your doctor. Red clover has some estrogen-like properties.

Breastfeeding:
Don't use unless prescribed by your doctor.

Infants and children:
Treating infants and children under 2 with any herbal preparation is hazardous.

Others:
None are expected if you are beyond childhood, under 45, not pregnant,

basically healthy, take it for only a short time and do not exceed manufacturer's recommended dose.

Storage:
- Store in cool, dry area away from direct light, but don't freeze.
- Store safely out of reach of children.
- Don't store in bathroom medicine cabinet. Heat and moisture may change the action of the herb.

Safe dosage:
Consult your doctor for the appropriate dose for your condition.

 Toxicity

Generally regarded as safe when taken in appropriate quantities for short periods of time

 Adverse Reactions, Side Effects or Overdose Symptoms

None are expected.

Saffron (Saffron Crocus)

 Basic Information

Biological name (genus and species): *Crocus sativus*

Parts used for medicinal purposes: Berries/fruits

Chemicals this herb contains:
- Glycosides (see Glossary)
- Volatile oils (see Glossary)

 Known Effects

- Reduces irritation of gastrointestinal tract
- Increases perspiration
- Increases fluidity of bronchial secretions

Miscellaneous information:
- No effects are expected on the body, good or bad, when this herb is used in very small amounts to enhance the flavor of food; however, in large amounts saffron is highly toxic—use only recommended doses.
- Saffron is very expensive.

 Possible Additional Effects

- May stimulate respiration in those with asthma, whooping cough
- May reduce cholesterol
- May relieve indigestion
- May help control blood pressure

 Warnings and Precautions

Don't take if you:
- Are pregnant, think you may be pregnant or plan pregnancy in the near future
- Have any chronic disease of the gastrointestinal tract, such as stomach or duodenal ulcers, reflux esophagitis, ulcerative colitis, spastic colitis, diverticulosis or diverticulitis

Consult your doctor if you:
- Take this herb for any medical problem that doesn't improve in 2 weeks (There may be safer, more effective treatments.)

MEDICINAL HERBS

→

- Take any medicinal drugs or herbs including aspirin, laxatives, cold and cough remedies, antacids, vitamins, minerals, amino acids, supplements, other prescription or nonprescription drugs

Pregnancy:
Don't use.

Breastfeeding:
Don't use.

Infants and children:
Treating infants and children under 2 with any herbal preparation is hazardous.

Others:
None are expected if you are beyond childhood, under 45, not pregnant, basically healthy, take it for only a short time and do not exceed manufacturer's recommended dose.

Storage:
- Store in cool, dry area away from direct light, but don't freeze.
- Store safely out of reach of children.
- Don't store in bathroom medicine cabinet. Heat and moisture may change the action of the herb.

Safe dosage:
Consult your doctor for the appropriate dose for your condition.

 Toxicity

Rated relatively safe when taken in appropriate quantities for short periods of time

For symptoms of toxicity: See *Adverse Reactions, Side Effects or Overdose Symptoms* section below.

 Adverse Reactions, Side Effects or Overdose Symptoms

Signs and symptoms	What to do
Diarrhea	Discontinue. Call doctor immediately.
Dizziness	Discontinue. Call doctor immediately.
Nosebleeds	Discontinue. Call doctor when convenient.
Slow heart rate	Seek emergency treatment.
Stupor	Seek emergency treatment.
Vomiting	Discontinue. Call doctor immediately.

Sage

 Basic Information

Biological name (genus and species):
Salvia officinalis

Parts used for medicinal purposes:
Leaves

Chemicals this herb contains:

- Camphor
- Flavonoids
- Resin (see Glossary)
- Salvene
- Saponin (see Glossary)
- Tannins (see Glossary)
- Terpene (see Glossary)
- Thujone
- Volatile oils (see Glossary)

 Known Effects

- Depresses fever-control center in brain
- Relieves spasm in skeletal or smooth muscle

- Stimulates gastrointestinal tract
- Stimulates central nervous system
- Interferes with absorption of iron and other minerals when taken internally

Miscellaneous information:
- Sage is used as a flavoring agent and in perfume.
- Salvia is *not* the brush sage of the desert or red sage.
- No effects are expected on the body, either good or bad, when this herb is used in very small amounts to enhance the flavor of food; however, prolonged use of large amounts can cause seizures and unconsciousness.
- Sage is available dried, fresh or as tincture or tea.

Possible Additional Effects

- May help expel gas from intestinal tract
- May repel insects
- May treat throat and mouth infections when used as mouthwash
- May reduce night sweats associated with menopause
- May relieve insect bites when applied externally

Warnings and Precautions

Don't take if you:
Are pregnant, think you may be pregnant or plan pregnancy in the near future.

Consult your doctor if you:
- Take this herb for any medical problem that doesn't improve in 2 weeks (There may be safer, more effective treatments.)
- Take any medicinal drugs or herbs including aspirin, laxatives, cold and cough remedies, antacids, vitamins, minerals, amino acids, supplements, other prescription or nonprescription drugs

Pregnancy:
Don't use unless prescribed by your doctor.

Breastfeeding:
Sage may reduce milk flow. Don't use.

Infants and children:
Treating infants and children under 2 with any herbal preparation is hazardous.

Others:
None are expected if you are beyond childhood, under 45, not pregnant, basically healthy, take it for only a short time and do not exceed manufacturer's recommended dose.

Storage:
- Store in cool, dry area away from direct light, but don't freeze.
- Store safely out of reach of children.
- Don't store in bathroom medicine cabinet. Heat and moisture may change the action of the herb.

Safe dosage:
Consult your doctor for the appropriate dose for your condition.

Toxicity

Generally regarded as safe when taken in appropriate quantities for short periods of time

For symptoms of toxicity: See *Adverse Reactions, Side Effects or Overdose Symptoms* section below.

Adverse Reactions, Side Effects or Overdose Symptoms

Signs and symptoms	What to do
Dry mouth	Discontinue. Call doctor when convenient.
Swelling of lips	Drinking tea can result in swelling of lips. Discontinue. Call doctor when convenient.

➜

St. John's Wort (Klamath Weed)

Basic Information

Biological name (genus and species):
Hypericum perforatum

Parts used for medicinal purposes:
- Flowers
- Petals
- Stems

Chemicals this herb contains:
- Hypericin
- Resin (see Glossary)
- Tannins (see Glossary)
- Volatile oils (see Glossary)

Known Effects

- Reduces depressive moods (mild to moderate)
- Relieves anxiety
- Slightly depresses central nervous system
- Acts as an antibacterial to help heal wounds

Possible Additional Effects

- Potential antiviral
- May treat seasonal affective disorder (SAD)
- Used externally for mild burns

Warnings and Precautions

Don't take if you:
- Are pregnant, think you may be pregnant or plan pregnancy in the near future
- Are taking other antidepressive medicines

Consult your doctor if you:
- Take this herb for any medical problem that doesn't improve in 2 weeks (There may be safer, more effective treatments.)
- Take any medicinal drugs or herbs including aspirin, laxatives, cold and cough remedies, antacids, vitamins, minerals, amino acids, supplements, other prescription or nonprescription drugs

Pregnancy:
Don't use unless prescribed by your doctor.

Breastfeeding:
Don't use unless prescribed by your doctor.

Infants and children:
Treating infants and children under 2 with any herbal preparation is hazardous.

Others:
- Do not take in combination with prescription antidepressants, unless prescribed by your doctor.
- If you believe you are depressed, seek medical treatment prior to using St. John's Wort.
- In large doses, St. John's Wort may cause sensitivity to sunlight.

Storage:
- Store in cool, dry area away from direct light, but don't freeze.
- Store safely out of reach of children.
- Don't store in bathroom medicine cabinet. Heat and moisture may change the action of the herb.

Safe dosage:
Consult your doctor for the appropriate dose for your condition.

Toxicity

Rated slightly dangerous, particularly in children, persons over 55 and those who take larger than appropriate quantities for extended periods of time

For symptoms of toxicity: See *Adverse Reactions, Side Effects or Overdose Symptoms* section below.

Adverse Reactions, Side Effects or Overdose Symptoms

Signs and symptoms	What to do
Abdominal upset	Discontinue. Call doctor when convenient.
Abnormal skin coloring	Discontinue. Call doctor when convenient.
Sun sensitivity	Discontinue. Call doctor when convenient.

Sassafras

Basic Information

Biological name (genus and species):
Sassafras albidum

Parts used for medicinal purposes:
• Bark
• Roots

Chemicals this herb contains:
• Cadinene
• Camphor
• Eugenol
• Phellandrene
• Pinene
• Safrole

Known Effects

• Depresses central nervous system
• Irritates mucous membranes
• No proven medical efficacy shown

Miscellaneous information:
Banned in United States as a flavoring agent because of proved carcinogenic potential.

Possible Additional Effects

• Used as a "tonic" that exerts a restorative or nourishing action on the body
• May treat syphilis

Warnings and Precautions

Don't take if you:
• Are pregnant, think you may be pregnant or plan pregnancy in the near future
• Have any chronic disease of the gastrointestinal tract, such as stomach or duodenal ulcers, reflux esophagitis, ulcerative colitis, spastic colitis, diverticulosis or diverticulitis.

Consult your doctor if you:
• Take this herb for any medical problem that doesn't improve in 2 weeks (There may be safer, more effective treatments.)
• Take any medicinal drugs or herbs including aspirin, laxatives, cold and cough remedies, antacids, vitamins, minerals, amino acids, supplements, other prescription or nonprescription drugs

MEDICINAL HERBS

➜

Pregnancy:
Risks outweigh potential benefits.
Don't use.

Breastfeeding:
Risks outweigh potential benefits.
Don't use.

Infants and children:
Treating infants and children under
2 with any herbal preparation
is hazardous.

Others:
None are expected if you are beyond
childhood, under 45, not pregnant,
basically healthy, take it for only a short
time and do not exceed manufacturer's
recommended dose.

Storage:
• Store in cool, dry area away from
  direct light, but don't freeze.
• Store safely out of reach of children.
• Don't store in bathroom medicine
  cabinet. Heat and moisture may
  change the action of the herb.

Safe dosage:
Consult your doctor for the appropriate dose for your condition.

Toxicity

Sassafras has carcinogenic potential.
Don't use. It is felt to be unsafe and
ineffective.

For symptoms of toxicity: See
*Adverse Reactions, Side Effects or
Overdose Symptoms* section below.

Adverse Reactions, Side Effects or Overdose Symptoms

Signs and symptoms	What to do
Breathing difficulties	Seek emergency treatment.
Coma	Seek emergency treatment.
Dilated pupils	Discontinue. Call doctor immediately.
Fainting	Discontinue. Call doctor immediately.
Heart, liver, kidney damage characterized by swelling of extremities, shortness of breath, jaundice (yellow skin and eyes), blood in urine	Seek emergency treatment.
Nausea or vomiting	Discontinue. Call doctor immediately.
Nosebleeds (frequent)	Discontinue. Call doctor when convenient.

Saw Palmetto (Sabal)

Basic Information

Biological name (genus and species):
Serenoa repens

Parts used for medicinal purposes:
• Berries
• Seeds

Chemicals this herb contains:
• Capric acids
• Caproic acids
• Caprylic acids
• Lauric acids
• Oleic acids
• Palmitic acids
• Resin (see Glossary)

Known Effects

• Improves urination in men with benign prostate hyperplasia (see Glossary)
• Treats symptoms of enlarged prostate (consult your doctor)
• Irritates mucous membranes

Miscellaneous information:
Berries are edible but don't taste good.

Possible Additional Effects

• May treat chronic cystitis
• May treat urethritis and other inflammations of male genitourinary tract, including prostatitis
• May stimulate appetite
• Potential anti-inflammatory
• Potential immune stimulant

Warnings and Precautions

Don't take if you:
• Are pregnant, think you may be pregnant or plan pregnancy in the near future
• Have any chronic disease of the gastrointestinal tract, such as stomach or duodenal ulcers, reflux esophagitis, ulcerative colitis, spastic colitis, diverticulosis or diverticulitis

Consult your doctor if you:
• Take this herb for any medical problem that doesn't improve in 2 weeks (There may be safer, more effective treatments.)
• Take any medicinal drugs or herbs including aspirin, laxatives, cold and cough remedies, antacids, vitamins, minerals, amino acids, supplements, other prescription or nonprescription drugs
• Have enlarged prostate

Pregnancy:
Don't use unless prescribed by your doctor.

Breastfeeding:
Don't use unless prescribed by your doctor.

Infants and children:
Treating infants and children under 2 with any herbal preparation is hazardous.

Others:
None are expected if you are beyond childhood, under 45, not pregnant, basically healthy, take it for only a short time and do not exceed manufacturer's recommended dose.

MEDICINAL HERBS

→

Storage:
- Store in cool, dry area away from direct light, but don't freeze.
- Store safely out of reach of children.
- Don't store in bathroom medicine cabinet. Heat and moisture may change the action of the herb.

Safe dosage:
Consult your doctor for the appropriate dose for your condition.

 Toxicity

Rated relatively safe when taken in appropriate quantities for short periods of time

For symptoms of toxicity: See *Adverse Reactions, Side Effects or Overdose Symptoms* section below.

 Adverse Reactions, Side Effects or Overdose Symptoms

Signs and symptoms	What to do
Diarrhea	Discontinue. Call doctor when convenient.
Headaches	Discontinue. Call doctor when convenient.
Nausea	Discontinue. Call doctor when convenient.
Vomiting	Discontinue. Call doctor immediately.

Slippery Elm (Red Elm)

 Basic Information

Biological name (genus and species):
Ulmus rubra, U. fulva

Parts used for medicinal purposes:
Inner bark

Chemicals this herb contains:
- Bioflavonoids
- Calcium
- Calcium oxalate
- Mucilage (see Glossary)
- Phosphorus
- Polysaccharide
- Starch
- Tannins (see Glossary)

 Known Effects

- Decreases thickness and increases fluidity of mucus in lungs and bronchial tubes

- Soothes sore throats
- Decreases discomfort of cough

Miscellaneous information:
Available as tea, lozenge, poultice (see Glossary).

 Possible Additional Effects

- May treat ulcers
- May be useful for diarrhea
- May soothe and heal cuts and scrapes when used externally

 Warnings and Precautions

Don't take if you:
Are pregnant, think you may be pregnant or plan pregnancy in the near future.

Consult your doctor if you:

- Take this herb for any medical problem that doesn't improve in 2 weeks (There may be safer, more effective treatments.)
- Take any medicinal drugs or herbs including aspirin, laxatives, cold and cough remedies, antacids, vitamins, minerals, amino acids, supplements, other prescription or nonprescription drugs

Pregnancy:

Dangers outweigh any possible benefits. Don't use.

Breastfeeding:

Dangers outweigh any possible benefits. Don't use.

Infants and children:

Treating infants and children under 2 with any herbal preparation is hazardous.

Others:

None are expected if you are beyond childhood, under 45, not pregnant, basically healthy, take it for only a short time and do not exceed manufacturer's recommended dose.

Storage:

- Store in cool, dry area away from direct light, but don't freeze.
- Store safely out of reach of children.
- Don't store in bathroom medicine cabinet. Heat and moisture may change the action of the herb.

Safe dosage:

Consult your doctor for the appropriate dose for your condition.

 Toxicity

Rated relatively safe when taken in appropriate quantities for short periods of time

For symptoms of toxicity: See *Adverse Reactions, Side Effects or Overdose Symptoms* section below.

 Adverse Reactions, Side Effects or Overdose Symptoms

Signs and symptoms	What to do
Allergic response	Discontinue. Call doctor immediately.
Skin rash	Discontinue. Call doctor when convenient.

Tea Tree Oil

 Basic Information

Biological name (genus and species): *Melaleuca alternifolia*

Parts used for medicinal purposes: Essential oil

Chemicals this herb contains:
- Germicidal agents
- Terpene hydrocarbons

 Known Effects

- Works well as a disinfectant for cuts and abrasions
- Has antibacterial and antifungal properties
- Helps treat insect bites

MEDICINAL HERBS

➜

Possible
Additional Effects

- May reduce teenage acne
- Used in flea shampoo for pets
- May treat athlete's foot
- May help soothe tonsils with tonsillitis
- May help treat bladder infections
- May reduce cold/flu symptoms

 Warnings and
Precautions

Don't take if you:
Are pregnant, think you may be pregnant or plan pregnancy in the near future.

Consult your doctor if you:
- Take this herb for any medical problem that doesn't improve in 2 weeks (There may be safer, more effective treatments.)
- Take any medicinal drugs or herbs including aspirin, laxatives, cold and cough remedies, antacids, vitamins, minerals, amino acids, supplements, other prescription or nonprescription drugs

Pregnancy:
Don't use unless prescribed by your doctor.

Breastfeeding:
Don't use unless prescribed by your doctor.

Infants and children:
Treating infants and children under 2 with any herbal preparation is hazardous.

Others:
- Irritation may occur on persons with very sensitive skin. If this happens, try diluting the oil with distilled water or vitamin-E oil or consult your physician.
- Tea tree oil is safe for use as a topical antiseptic but not recommended for oral ingestion.

Storage:
- Store in cool, dry area away from direct light, but don't freeze.
- Store safely out of reach of children.
- Don't store in bathroom medicine cabinet. Heat and moisture may change the action of the herb.

Safe dosage:
Consult your doctor for the appropriate dose for your condition.

 Toxicity

Comparative-toxicity rating is not available from standard references.

For symptoms of toxicity: See *Adverse Reactions, Side Effects or Overdose Symptoms* section below.

 Adverse Reactions,
Side Effects or
Overdose Symptoms

Signs and symptoms	What to do
Skin irritation	Discontinue. Call doctor when convenient.

Valerian (Garden Heliotrope, Tobacco Root)

Basic Information

Biological name (genus and species):
Valeriana edulis, V. officinalis

Parts used for medicinal purposes:
- Rhizomes
- Roots

Chemicals this herb contains:
- Acetic acid
- Butyric acid
- Camphene
- Chatinine
- Formic acid
- Glycosides (see Glossary)
- Pinene
- Resin (see Glossary)
- Valeric acid
- Valerine
- Volatile oils (see Glossary)

Known Effects

- Depresses central nervous system
- Treats hypertension
- Treats insomnia
- Causes sedation/calming effect

Miscellaneous information:
- Cats are attracted to this herb.
- Do not use with sedatives or tranquilizers because of the combined effect.
- Avoid driving when taking this herb.
- Valerian is available as tea or dried rhizome/roots.

Possible Additional Effects

- May relieve menstrual cramps
- May treat irritable bowel syndrome
- May treat anxiety

Warnings and Precautions

Don't take if you:
Are pregnant, think you may be pregnant or plan pregnancy in the near future.

Consult your doctor if you:
- Take this herb for any medical problem that doesn't improve in 2 weeks (There may be safer, more effective treatments.)
- Take any medicinal drugs or herbs including aspirin, laxatives, cold and cough remedies, antacids, vitamins, minerals, amino acids, supplements, other prescription or nonprescription drugs

Pregnancy:
Don't use unless prescribed by your doctor.

Breastfeeding:
Don't use unless prescribed by your doctor.

Infants and children:
Treating infants and children under 2 with any herbal preparation is hazardous.

Others:
None are expected if you are beyond childhood, under 45, not pregnant, basically healthy, take it for only a short time and do not exceed manufacturer's recommended dose.

Storage:
- Store in cool, dry area away from direct light, but don't freeze.
- Store safely out of reach of children.
- Don't store in bathroom medicine cabinet. Heat and moisture may change the action of the herb.

MEDICINAL HERBS

- Use fresh material only. Dried valerian loses potency.

Safe dosage:
Consult your doctor for the appropriate dose for your condition.

Toxicity

Rated relatively safe when taken in appropriate quantities for short periods of time

For symptoms of toxicity: See *Adverse Reactions, Side Effects or Overdose Symptoms* section below.

Adverse Reactions, Side Effects or Overdose Symptoms

Signs and symptoms	What to do
Diarrhea	Discontinue. Call doctor immediately.
Nausea or vomiting	Discontinue. Call doctor immediately.

Vervain (European Vervaine, Verbena)

Basic Information

Biological name (genus and species):
Verbena officinalis

Parts used for medicinal purposes:
Roots

Chemicals this herb contains:
Verbenaline

Known Effects

- Stimulates gastrointestinal tract
- Stimulates parasympathetic (see Glossary) branch of autonomic nervous system

Possible Additional Effects

- May treat coughs
- May treat upper abdominal pain
- May induce vomiting
- May treat headache

Warnings and Precautions

Don't take if you:
- Are pregnant, think you may be pregnant or plan pregnancy in the near future
- Have any chronic disease of the gastrointestinal tract, such as stomach or duodenal ulcers, reflux esophagitis, ulcerative colitis, spastic colitis, diverticulosis or diverticulitis

Consult your doctor if you:
- Take this herb for any medical problem that doesn't improve in 2 weeks (There may be safer, more effective treatments.)
- Take any medicinal drugs or herbs including aspirin, laxatives, cold and cough remedies, antacids, vitamins, minerals, amino acids, supplements, other prescription or nonprescription drugs

Pregnancy:
Don't use unless prescribed by your doctor.

Breastfeeding:

Don't use unless prescribed by your doctor.

Infants and children:

Treating infants and children under 2 with any herbal preparation is hazardous.

Others:

None are expected if you are beyond childhood, under 45, not pregnant, basically healthy, take it for only a short time and do not exceed manufacturer's recommended dose.

Storage:

- Store in cool, dry area away from direct light, but don't freeze.
- Store safely out of reach of children.
- Don't store in bathroom medicine cabinet. Heat and moisture may change the action of the herb.

Safe dosage:

Consult your doctor for the appropriate dose for your condition.

Toxicity

Generally regarded as safe when taken in appropriate quantities for short periods of time

For symptoms of toxicity: See *Adverse Reactions, Side Effects or Overdose Symptoms* section below.

Adverse Reactions, Side Effects or Overdose Symptoms

Signs and symptoms	What to do
Diarrhea	Discontinue. Call doctor immediately.
Nausea or vomiting	Discontinue. Call doctor immediately.

Yohimbe

Basic Information

Biological name (genus and species): *Corynanthe yohimbe, Pausinystalia yohimbe*

Parts used for medicinal purposes: Bark

Chemicals this herb contains: Yohimbine (also called *quebrachine* and *aphrodine*)

Known Effects

- Blocks responses of parts of autonomic nervous system
- Increases blood pressure
- Inhibits monoamine oxidase and may cause alarming blood-pressure rise, even strokes, when taken with cheese, red wine or other foods or supplements containing tyramines
- Arouses or enhances sexual desire

Miscellaneous information:

- Yohimbe can produce severe anxiety when given intravenously.

MEDICINAL HERBS

- It is not available over-the-counter in the United States and has a high number of side effects and low potential benefit.

Possible Additional Effects

- May treat impotency/erectile dysfunction
- May treat painful menstrual cramps
- May treat chest pain due to coronary artery disease (angina)
- May treat arteriosclerosis

Warnings and Precautions

Don't take if you:
- Are pregnant, think you may be pregnant or plan pregnancy in the near future
- Have kidney or liver disease

Consult your doctor if you:
- Take this herb for any medical problem that doesn't improve in 2 weeks (There may be safer, more effective treatments.)
- Take any medicinal drugs or herbs including aspirin, laxatives, cold and cough remedies, antacids, vitamins, minerals, amino acids, supplements, other prescription or nonprescription drugs
- Are considering taking yohimbe

Pregnancy:
Don't use.

Breastfeeding:
Don't use.

Infants and children:
Treating infants and children under 2 with any herbal preparation is hazardous.

Others:
This product will not help you and may cause toxic symptoms.

Storage:
- Store in cool, dry area away from direct light, but don't freeze.
- Store safely out of reach of children.
- Don't store in bathroom medicine cabinet. Heat and moisture may change the action of the herb.

Safe dosage:
Consult your doctor for the appropriate dose for your condition.

Toxicity

Rated dangerous, particularly in children, persons over 55 and those who take larger than appropriate quantities for extended periods of time

For symptoms of toxicity: See *Adverse Reactions, Side Effects or Overdose Symptoms* section below.

Adverse Reactions, Side Effects or Overdose Symptoms

Signs and symptoms	What to do
Abdominal pain	Discontinue. Call doctor when convenient.
Agitation	Discontinue. Call doctor immediately.
Anxiety	Discontinue. Call doctor when convenient.
Fatigue	Discontinue. Call doctor when convenient.
Hallucinations	Seek emergency treatment.
High blood pressure	Discontinue. Call doctor immediately.
Increased heart rate	Discontinue. Call doctor immediately.
Insomnia	Discontinue. Call doctor when convenient.
Muscle paralysis	Seek emergency treatment.
Nausea or vomiting	Discontinue. Call doctor immediately.
Weakness	Discontinue. Call doctor immediately.

Less Common Herbs

Aconite (Blue Rocket, Fu-Tzu, Monkshood)

 ## Basic Information

Biological name (genus and species):
Aconitum napellus

Parts used for medicinal purposes:
• Leaves
• Roots

Chemicals this herb contains:
• Aconine
• Aconitine
• Benzoylamine
• Neopelline
• Picraconitine

 ## Known Effects

• Small amounts stimulate central nervous system and peripheral nerves.
• Large amounts depress central nervous system and peripheral nerves—dangerous.
• Normalizes heartbeat irregularities.
• A dose as low as 5ml (about 1 teaspoon) of the root can be lethal.
• Anti-inflammatory.

Miscellaneous information:
Used for centuries as an arrow poison.

 ## Possible Additional Effects

• May decrease fever
• May reduce heartbeat irregularities
• May soothe sore throats and laryngitis
• May reduce pain of rheumatoid arthritis and gout
• May help treat croup and bronchitis

 ## Warnings and Precautions

Don't take if you:
• Are pregnant, think you may be pregnant or plan pregnancy in the near future
• Have any chronic disease of the gastrointestinal tract, such as stomach or duodenal ulcers, reflux esophagitis, ulcerative colitis, spastic colitis, diverticulosis or diverticulitis

Consult your doctor if you:
• Take this herb for any medical problem that doesn't improve in 2 weeks (There may be safer, more effective treatments.)
• Take any medicinal drugs or herbs including aspirin, laxatives, cold and cough remedies, antacids, vitamins, minerals, amino acids, supplements, other prescription or nonprescription drugs

Pregnancy:
Don't use.

Breastfeeding:
Don't use.

Infants and children:
Treating infants and children under 2 with any herbal preparation is hazardous.

Others:
Dangers outweigh any possible benefits. Don't use.

Storage:
• Store in cool, dry area away from direct light, but don't freeze.
• Store safely out of reach of children.

- Don't store in bathroom medicine cabinet. Heat and moisture may change the action of the herb.

Safe dosage:
Consult your doctor for the appropriate dose for your condition.

Toxicity

Rated dangerous, particularly in children, persons over 55 and those who take larger than appropriate quantities for extended periods of time

For symptoms of toxicity: See *Adverse Reactions, Side Effects or Overdose Symptoms* section below.

Adverse Reactions, Side Effects or Overdose Symptoms

Signs and symptoms	What to do
Burning or numbness of tongue and lips	Discontinue. Call doctor immediately.
Difficulty swallowing	Discontinue. Call doctor immediately.
Irritability	Discontinue. Call doctor when convenient.
Nausea or vomiting	Discontinue. Call doctor immediately.
Restlessness	Discontinue. Call doctor when convenient.
Speech difficulties	Discontinue. Call doctor immediately.
Vision doubled or blurred	Discontinue. Call doctor immediately.

Agave

Basic Information

Biological name (genus and species):
Agave lecheguilla

Parts used for medicinal purposes:
- Leaves
- Roots
- Sap

Chemicals this herb contains:
- Diosgenin
- Photosensitizing pigment (see Glossary)
- Steroidal chemicals (see Glossary)
- Vitamin C

Known Effects

- Causes disintegration of red blood cells
- Irritates skin
- Irritates lining of gastrointestinal tract
- Small amounts depress central nervous system
- Damages cells (dissolves membranes of red blood cells and changes tissue permeability)

Miscellaneous information:
- Agave is used to make mescal, an alcoholic beverage.
- Fibers are used for rope.
- Sap is used as a syrup.
- Roots and leaves contain active chemicals.

→

Possible Additional Effects

- Roots and leaves are used to relieve toothache
- May provide nutrition
- Potential hormone replacement
- May produce immunosuppressive effects on body
- May cause abortion or miscarriage
- May treat dysentery
- May relieve pain of sprains

 ## Warnings and Precautions

Don't take if you:
- Are pregnant, think you may be pregnant or plan pregnancy in the near future
- Have symptoms of a disease caused by a hormone deficiency
- Have any chronic disease of the gastrointestinal tract, such as stomach or duodenal ulcers, reflux esophagitis, ulcerative colitis, spastic colitis, diverticulosis or diverticulitis

Consult your doctor if you:
- Have stomach problems
- Take cortisone, ACTH, testosterone or androgenic steroids

Pregnancy:
Don't use unless prescribed by your doctor.

Breastfeeding:
Don't use unless prescribed by your doctor.

Infants and children:
Treating infants and children under 2 with any herbal preparation is hazardous.

Others:
None are expected if you are beyond childhood, under 45, not pregnant, basically healthy, take it for only a short time and do not exceed manufacturer's recommended dose.

Storage:
- Store in cool, dry area away from direct light, but don't freeze.
- Store safely out of reach of children.
- Don't store in bathroom medicine cabinet. Heat and moisture may change the action of the herb.

Safe dosage:
Consult your doctor for the appropriate dose for your condition.

 ## Toxicity

Comparative-toxicity rating is not available from standard references.

For symptoms of toxicity: See *Adverse Reactions, Side Effects or Overdose Symptoms* section below.

 ## Adverse Reactions, Side Effects or Overdose Symptoms

Signs and symptoms	What to do
Abortion (remote possibility if taken in large amounts)	Seek emergency treatment.
Diarrhea	Discontinue. Call doctor immediately.
Increased sensitivity to sunlight	Discontinue. Call doctor when convenient.
Jaundice (yellow skin and eyes)	Discontinue. Call doctor immediately.
Nausea or vomiting	Discontinue. Call doctor immediately.
Skin itching and rash	Discontinue. Call doctor when convenient.
Unusual bleeding	Discontinue. Call doctor immediately.

Alder, Black (Alder Buckthorn)

 Basic Information

Biological name (genus and species):
Alnus glutinosa, Rhamnus frangula, Frangula

Parts used for medicinal purposes:
Various parts of the entire plant, frequently differing by country and culture

Chemicals this herb contains:
- Anthraquinone glycosides
- Emodin
- Rhamnose

 Known Effects

- Irritates gastrointestinal tract
- Causes vomiting

Miscellaneous information:
- Alder is used in veterinary medicine for its cathartic properties.
- Emetic action (causing vomiting) is less when plant is dried for 1 year or more.

 Possible Additional Effects

May temporarily relieve constipation

 Warnings and Precautions

Don't take if you:
- Are pregnant, think you may be pregnant or plan pregnancy in the near future
- Have any chronic disease of the gastrointestinal tract, such as stomach or duodenal ulcers, reflux esophagitis, ulcerative colitis, spastic colitis, diverticulosis or diverticulitis

Consult your doctor if you:
- Take this herb for any medical problem that doesn't improve in 2 weeks (There may be safer, more effective treatments.)
- Take any medicinal drugs or herbs including aspirin, laxatives, cold and cough remedies, antacids, vitamins, minerals, amino acids, supplements, other prescription or nonprescription drugs

Pregnancy:
Don't use unless prescribed by your doctor.

Breastfeeding:
Don't use unless prescribed by your doctor.

Infants and children:
Treating infants and children under 2 with any herbal preparation is hazardous.

Others:
None are expected if you are beyond childhood, under 45, not pregnant, basically healthy, take it for only a short time and do not exceed manufacturer's recommended dose.

Storage:
- Store in cool, dry area away from direct light, but don't freeze.
- Store safely out of reach of children.
- Don't store in bathroom medicine cabinet. Heat and moisture may change the action of the herb.

Safe dosage:
Consult your doctor for the appropriate dose for your condition.

MEDICINAL HERBS

Toxicity

Rated slightly dangerous, particularly in children, persons over 55 and those who take larger than appropriate quantities for extended periods of time

For symptoms of toxicity: See *Adverse Reactions, Side Effects or Overdose Symptoms* section below.

 ## Adverse Reactions, Side Effects or Overdose Symptoms

Signs and symptoms	What to do
Abdominal cramps (severe)	Discontinue. Call doctor immediately.
Abdominal pain	Discontinue. Call doctor when convenient.
Nausea or vomiting	Discontinue. Call doctor immediately.

Alfalfa

 ## Basic Information

Biological name (genus and species): *Medicago sativa*

Parts used for medicinal purposes:
- Leaves
- Petals/flower
- Sprouts

Chemicals this herb contains:
- Proteins
- Saponin (see Glossary)
- Vitamins A, B, D, K

 ## Known Effects

- Provides useful proteins and vitamins for dietary use
- Stimulates menstruation
- Stimulates milk production in lactating women
- Has antifungal properties

Miscellaneous information:
Alfalfa is usually compressed into capsules or brewed as tea.

 ## Possible Additional Effects

- May treat arthritis
- May treat unusual bleeding
- May lower cholesterol
- May relieve constipation
- May treat morning sickness

 ## Warnings and Precautions

Don't take if you:
- Take anticoagulants such as warfarin sodium (coumadin) or heparin
- Have lupus erythematosus

Consult your doctor if you:
Have any bleeding disorder.

Pregnancy:
Pregnant women should experience no problems taking usual amounts as part of a balanced diet. Other products extracted from this herb have not been proved to cause problems.

Breastfeeding:

Breastfed infants of lactating mothers should experience no problems when mother takes usual amounts as part of a balanced diet. Other products extracted from this herb have not been proved to cause problems.

Infants and children:

Treating infants and children under 2 with any herbal preparation is hazardous.

Others:

- None are expected if you are beyond childhood, under 45, not pregnant, basically healthy, take it for only a short time and do not exceed manufacturer's recommended dose.
- Alfalfa sprouts eaten in large amounts may cause a form of anemia.

Storage:

- Store in cool, dry area away from direct light, but don't freeze.
- Store safely out of reach of children.
- Don't store in bathroom medicine cabinet. Heat and moisture may change the action of the herb.

Safe dosage:

Consult your doctor for the appropriate dose for your condition.

Toxicity

Generally regarded as safe when taken in appropriate quantities for short periods of time

For symptoms of toxicity: See *Adverse Reactions, Side Effects or Overdose Symptoms* section below.

Adverse Reactions, Side Effects or Overdose Symptoms

Signs and symptoms	What to do
Abdominal cramps	Discontinue. Call doctor immediately.
Diarrhea	Discontinue. Call doctor when convenient.

Allspice (Clove Pepper, Jamaican Pepper)

Basic Information

Biological name (genus and species):
Pimenta dioica

Parts used for medicinal purposes:
Berries/fruits

Chemicals this herb contains:

- Acid-fixed oil
- Eugenol
- Resin (see Glossary)
- Tannic acid
- Volatile oils (see Glossary)

Known Effects

- Irritates mucous membranes, including lining of gastrointestinal tract
- Aids in expelling gas from intestines to relieve colic or griping

Miscellaneous information:

- Active chemicals are in berries
- Provides flavor in toothpaste and other products
- Used as an aromatic spice in foods

MEDICINAL HERBS

➔

Possible
Additional Effects

May relieve diarrhea

 Warnings and
Precautions

Don't take if you:

• Are pregnant, think you may be pregnant or plan pregnancy in the near future
• Have any chronic disease of the gastrointestinal tract, such as stomach or duodenal ulcers, reflux esophagitis, ulcerative colitis, spastic colitis, diverticulosis or diverticulitis

Consult your doctor if you:

• Take this herb for any medical problem that doesn't improve in 2 weeks (There may be safer, more effective treatments.)
• Take any medicinal drugs or herbs including aspirin, laxatives, cold and cough remedies, antacids, vitamins, minerals, amino acids, supplements, other prescription or nonprescription drugs

Pregnancy:

Don't use unless prescribed by your doctor.

Breastfeeding:

Don't use unless prescribed by your doctor.

Infants and children:

Treating infants and children under 2 with any herbal preparation is hazardous.

Others:

None are expected if you are beyond childhood, under 45, not pregnant, basically healthy, take it for only a short time and do not exceed manufacturer's recommended dose.

Storage:

• Store in cool, dry area away from direct light, but don't freeze.
• Store safely out of reach of children.
• Don't store in bathroom medicine cabinet. Heat and moisture may change the action of the herb.

Safe dosage:

Consult your doctor for the appropriate dose for your condition.

 Toxicity

Rated relatively safe when taken in appropriate quantities for short periods of time

For symptoms of toxicity: See *Adverse Reactions, Side Effects or Overdose Symptoms* section below.

 Adverse Reactions,
Side Effects or
Overdose Symptoms

Signs and symptoms	What to do
Excess of 5 ml (about 1 teaspoon) of eugenol (a volatile oil found in allspice) may cause convulsions, nausea, vomiting	Discontinue. Call doctor immediately.

Aloe

Basic Information

Aloe is also called Mediterranean aloe, Barbados aloe, Curacao aloe and aloe vera.

Biological name (genus and species): *Aloe vera, A. barbadensis, A. officinalis*

Parts used for medicinal purposes: Leaves

Chemicals this herb contains:
• Aloectin B
• Anthraquinones
• Polysaccharides
• Resins (see Glossary)
• Tannins (see Glossary)

Known Effects

• Milky secretion (not dried preparations) from leaves helps reduce inflammation and hasten recovery in first- and second-degree burns.
• Acts as cathartic, but whether this is beneficial or dangerous depends on many factors.
• Treats X-ray or radiation burns.
• Interferes with absorption of iron and other minerals when taken internally.
• Has antibacterial and antiviral activity.
• General wound healing.
• Heals skin ulcers.

Miscellaneous information:

• Not useful for clearing intestinal tract before surgery because only cleanses small intestine
• Used as an ingredient in many over-the-counter laxatives
• Used as an ingredient in some cosmetics

Possible Additional Effects

• May kill *Pseudomonas aeruginosa*, a bacterium, when applied to skin, but probably does not promote healing
• May treat amenorrhea (lack of menstrual periods) when taken internally
• May relieve headache when applied to head

Warnings and Precautions

Don't take if you:
• Have gastric ulcers
• Have small-bowel problems, such as regional enteritis
• Have ulcerative colitis
• Have diverticulosis or diverticulitis
• Have proctitis or hemorrhoids

Consult your doctor if you:
• Have any digestive disorder
• Intend to take it internally

Pregnancy:
Don't use unless prescribed by your doctor.

Breastfeeding:
Don't use unless prescribed by your doctor.

Infants and children:
Treating infants and children under 2 with any herbal preparation is hazardous.

Others:
Healing properties of aloe taken internally are still tentative and need more study.

MEDICINAL HERBS

Storage:
- Store in cool, dry area away from direct light, but don't freeze.
- Store safely out of reach of children.
- Don't store in bathroom medicine cabinet. Heat and moisture may change the action of the herb.

Safe dosage:

Consult your doctor for the appropriate dose for your condition.

 Toxicity

Generally regarded as safe when taken in appropriate quantities for short periods of time

For symptoms of toxicity: See *Adverse Reactions, Side Effects or Overdose Symptoms* section below.

 Adverse Reactions, Side Effects or Overdose Symptoms

Signs and symptoms	What to do
Abdominal cramps	Discontinue. Call doctor when convenient.
Bloody diarrhea, shock (with high doses)	Seek emergency treatment.
Bowel irritation	Discontinue. Call doctor when convenient.
Diarrhea	Discontinue. Call doctor immediately.
Minor skin irritation	Cleanse skin with clear water. Do not apply (with external applications) aloe again.
Nausea or vomiting	Discontinue. Call doctor immediately.
Red urine	Discontinue. Call doctor when convenient.
Increased urinary frequency, backache pain on urination with long continued use	Discontinue. Call doctor immediately.

Alum Root (American Sanicle)

 Basic Information

Biological name (genus and species): *Heuchera*

Parts used for medicinal purposes: Roots

Chemicals this herb contains: Tannins (see Glossary)

 Known Effects

- Shrinks tissues
- Prevents secretion of fluids

Miscellaneous information:
- Used externally and internally by some tribes of North American Indians for many disorders
- Used as a douche

 Possible Additional Effects

- May treat heart disease
- May prevent infection in injured skin

Warnings and Precautions

Don't take if you:

• Have liver or kidney disease
• Are pregnant, think you may be pregnant or plan pregnancy in the near future
• Have any chronic disease of the gastrointestinal tract, such as stomach or duodenal ulcers, reflux esophagitis, ulcerative colitis, spastic colitis, diverticulosis or diverticulitis

Consult your doctor if you:

• Take this herb for any medical problem that doesn't improve in 2 weeks (There may be safer, more effective treatments.)
• Take any medicinal drugs or herbs including aspirin, laxatives, cold and cough remedies, antacids, vitamins, minerals, amino acids, supplements, other prescription or nonprescription drugs

Pregnancy:

Don't use unless prescribed by your doctor.

Breastfeeding:

Don't use unless prescribed by your doctor.

Infants and children:

Treating infants and children under 2 with any herbal preparation is hazardous.

Others:

Toxic effects greatly outweigh any possible benefits. Don't take this herb internally!

Storage:

• Store in cool, dry area away from direct light, but don't freeze.
• Store safely out of reach of children.
• Don't store in bathroom medicine cabinet. Heat and moisture may change the action of the herb.

Safe dosage:

Consult your doctor for the appropriate dose for your condition.

 Toxicity

Comparative-toxicity rating is not available from standard references. However, it is believed toxic effects greatly outweigh any possible benefits.

For symptoms of toxicity: See *Adverse Reactions, Side Effects or Overdose Symptoms* section below.

 Adverse Reactions, Side Effects or Overdose Symptoms

Signs and symptoms	What to do
Burning indigestion	Discontinue. Call doctor when convenient.
Edema (swelling of hands and feet)	Discontinue. Call doctor when convenient.
Jaundice (yellow skin and eyes)	Discontinue. Call doctor immediately.
Nausea or vomiting	Discontinue. Call doctor immediately.

MEDICINAL HERBS

American Dogwood (American Boxwood, Dogwood)

Basic Information

Biological name (genus and species):
Cornus florida

Parts used for medicinal purposes:
Bark

Chemicals this herb contains:
• Betulic acid
• Cornin

Known Effects

• Irritates gastrointestinal tract and acts as a cathartic
• Causes uterine contractions

Possible Additional Effects

• May reduce fever
• May kill bacteria in boils, carbuncles, infected skin rashes, insect bites
• May treat malaria

Warnings and Precautions

Don't take if you:
Are pregnant. It may cause miscarriage.

Consult your doctor if you:
Take this herb for any medical problem that doesn't improve in 2 weeks (There may be safer, more effective treatments.)

Pregnancy:
Dangers outweigh any possible benefits. Don't use.

Breastfeeding:
Dangers outweigh any possible benefits. Don't use.

Infants and children:
Treating infants and children under 2 with any herbal preparation is hazardous.

Storage:
• Store in cool, dry area away from direct light, but don't freeze.
• Store safely out of reach of children.
• Don't store in bathroom medicine cabinet. Heat and moisture may change the action of the herb.

Safe dosage:
Consult your doctor for the appropriate dose for your condition.

Toxicity

Rated relatively safe when taken in appropriate quantities for short periods of time

For symptoms of toxicity: See *Adverse Reactions, Side Effects or Overdose Symptoms* section below.

Adverse Reactions, Side Effects or Overdose Symptoms

Signs and symptoms	What to do
Abortion	Seek emergency treatment.
Dermatitis	Discontinue. Call doctor when convenient.

Angelica (European Angelica, Garden Angelica)

Basic Information

Biological name (genus and species):
Angelica archangelica

Parts used for medicinal purposes:
Entire plant

Chemicals this herb contains:
• Angelic acid
• Resin (see Glossary)
• Volatile oils (see Glossary)

Known Effects

Volatile oil gives angelica the following effects:

• Decreases thickness and increases fluidity of mucus in lungs and bronchial tubes
• Increases perspiration

Possible Additional Effects

• Seeds and roots used to reduce odor and volume of intestinal gases
• May bring on menstruation
• May ease intestinal colic and flatulence

Warnings and Precautions

Don't take if you:
• Are pregnant, think you may be pregnant or plan pregnancy in the near future
• Have any chronic disease of the gastrointestinal tract, such as stomach or duodenal ulcers, reflux esophagitis, ulcerative colitis, spastic colitis, diverticulosis or diverticulitis

Consult your doctor if you:
• Take this herb for any medical problem that doesn't improve in 2 weeks (There may be safer, more effective treatments.)
• Take any medicinal drugs or herbs including aspirin, laxatives, cold and cough remedies, antacids, vitamins, minerals, amino acids, supplements, other prescription or nonprescription drugs

Pregnancy:
Dangers outweigh any possible benefits. Don't use.

Breastfeeding:
Dangers outweigh any possible benefits. Don't use.

Infants and children:
Treating infants and children under 2 with any herbal preparation is hazardous.

Others:
None are expected if you are beyond childhood, under 45, not pregnant, basically healthy, take it for only a short time and do not exceed manufacturer's recommended dose.

Storage:
• Store in cool, dry area away from direct light, but don't freeze.
• Store safely out of reach of children.
• Don't store in bathroom medicine cabinet. Heat and moisture may change the action of the herb.

Safe dosage:
Consult your doctor for the appropriate dose for your condition.

MEDICINAL HERBS

Toxicity

Rated relatively safe when taken in appropriate quantities for short periods of time

Adverse Reactions, Side Effects or Overdose Symptoms

None are expected.

Anise

Basic Information

Biological name (genus and species):
Pimpinella anisum

Parts used for medicinal purposes:
Seeds

Chemicals this herb contains:
• Anethole
• Creosol
• Dianethole
• Essential oils (see Glossary)
• Flavonoids
• Proteins
• Sterols
• Terpene (see Glossary)

Known Effects

• Helps expel gas from intestinal tract
• Helps body dispose of excess fluid by increasing amount of urine produced
• Reduces cough

Miscellaneous information:
• Anise is also used in perfumes, soaps, beverages, baked goods, liqueur and as a flavoring.
• It is available as a tincture or tea.

Possible Additional Effects

• May relieve indigestion
• May decrease colic
• May kill body lice when applied externally
• May treat bronchitis

Warnings and Precautions

Don't take if you:
• Are pregnant, think you may be pregnant or plan pregnancy in the near future
• Have any chronic disease of the gastrointestinal tract, such as stomach or duodenal ulcers, reflux esophagitis, ulcerative colitis, spastic colitis, diverticulosis or diverticulitis

Consult your doctor if you:
• Take this herb for any medical problem that doesn't improve in 2 weeks (There may be safer, more effective treatments.)
• Take any medicinal drugs or herbs including aspirin, laxatives, cold and cough remedies, antacids, vitamins, minerals, amino acids, supplements, other prescription or nonprescription drugs

Pregnancy:
Dangers outweigh any possible benefits. Don't use.

Breastfeeding:
Dangers outweigh any possible benefits. Don't use.

Infants and children:
Treating infants and children under 2 with any herbal preparation is hazardous.

Storage:
• Store in cool, dry area away from direct light, but don't freeze.
• Store safely out of reach of children.
• Don't store in bathroom medicine cabinet. Heat and moisture may change the action of the herb.

Safe dosage:
Consult your doctor for the appropriate dose for your condition.

Toxicity

• Rated relatively safe when taken in appropriate quantities for short periods of time

• Japan: Poisonous Japeneses anise *(Illicium anisatum)*—do not mistake the two

For symptoms of toxicity: See *Adverse Reactions, Side Effects or Overdose Symptoms* section below.

Adverse Reactions, Side Effects or Overdose Symptoms

Signs and symptoms	What to do
Oil may cause	
Diarrhea	Discontinue. Call doctor immediately.
Difficulty breathing	Seek emergency treatment.
Nausea or vomiting	Discontinue. Call doctor immediately.
Seizures	Seek emergency treatment.
Skin irritation, when applied to skin	Discontinue. Call doctor when convenient.

Asafetida (Devil's Dung)

Basic Information

Biological name (genus and species):
Ferula assafoetida, F. foetida

Parts used for medicinal purposes:
Roots

Chemicals this herb contains:
• Gum (see Glossary)
• Resin (see Glossary)
• Volatile oils (see Glossary)

Known Effects

Irritates lining of gastrointestinal tract and produces laxative effect

Miscellaneous information:
• Introduced by Arab physicians to European medical practitioners
• Has garlic-like odor and bitter taste, which may result in good placebo effect because it is so disagreeable
• Used in sack around the neck by some people to repel evil

➜

MEDICINAL HERBS

- Used as a condiment
- Provides flavor as an ingredient in Worcestershire sauce

Possible Additional Effects

- May decrease thickness and increase fluidity of mucus in lungs and bronchial tubes
- May treat colic (see Glossary)
- May temporarily relieve constipation
- May treat nerve disorders

Warnings and Precautions

Don't take if you:

- Are pregnant, think you may be pregnant or plan pregnancy in the near future
- Have any chronic disease of the gastrointestinal tract, such as stomach or duodenal ulcers, reflux esophagitis, ulcerative colitis, spastic colitis, diverticulosis or diverticulitis

Consult your doctor if you:

- Take this herb for any medical problem that doesn't improve in 2 weeks (There may be safer, more effective treatments.)
- Take any medicinal drugs or herbs including aspirin, laxatives, cold and cough remedies, antacids, vitamins, minerals, amino acids, supplements, other prescription or nonprescription drugs

Pregnancy:

Dangers outweigh any possible benefits. Don't use.

Breastfeeding:

Dangers outweigh any possible benefits. Don't use.

Infants and children:

Treating infants and children under 2 with any herbal preparation is hazardous.

Others:

None are expected if you are beyond childhood, under 45, not pregnant, basically healthy, take it for only a short time and do not exceed manufacturer's recommended dose.

Storage:

- Store in cool, dry area away from direct light, but don't freeze.
- Store safely out of reach of children.
- Don't store in bathroom medicine cabinet. Heat and moisture may change the action of the herb.

Safe dosage:

Consult your doctor for the appropriate dose for your condition.

Toxicity

Rated relatively safe when taken in appropriate quantities for short periods of time

For symptoms of toxicity: See
Adverse Reactions, Side Effects or Overdose Symptoms section below.

Adverse Reactions, Side Effects or Overdose Symptoms

Signs and symptoms	What to do
Diarrhea	Discontinue. Call doctor immediately.

Barberry (European Barberry)

 Basic Information

Biological name (genus and species):
Berberis vulgaris

Parts used for medicinal purposes:
- Berries/fruits
- Rootbark

Chemicals this herb contains:
- Berbamine
- Berberine
- Berberrubine
- Columbamine
- Hydrastine
- Jatrorrhizine
- Oxyacanthine
- Palmatine

 Known Effects

- Dilates blood vessels
- Decreases heart rate
- Stimulates intestinal movement, helps relieve constipation
- Reduces bronchial constriction

Miscellaneous information:
- Fruit is made into jelly.
- Roots are used to dye wool.

 Possible Additional Effects

- May reduce diarrhea
- May reduce dyspepsia, indigestion, heartburn
- May treat skin infections
- May reduce symptoms of hepatitis, liver disease, jaundice
- May treat hangover

STOP Warnings and Precautions

Don't take if you:
Are pregnant, think you may be pregnant or plan pregnancy in the near future.

Consult your doctor if you:
- Take this herb for any medical problem that doesn't improve in 2 weeks (There may be safer, more effective treatments.)
- Take any medicinal drugs or herbs including aspirin, laxatives, cold and cough remedies, antacids, vitamins, minerals, amino acids, supplements, other prescription or nonprescription drugs

Pregnancy:
Dangers outweigh any possible benefits. Don't use.

Breastfeeding:
Dangers outweigh any possible benefits. Don't use.

Infants and children:
Treating infants and children under 2 with any herbal preparation is hazardous.

Others:
None are expected if you are beyond childhood, under 45, not pregnant, basically healthy, take it for only a short time and do not exceed manufacturer's recommended dose.

Storage:
- Store in cool, dry area away from direct light, but don't freeze.
- Store safely out of reach of children.
- Don't store in bathroom medicine cabinet. Heat and moisture may change the action of the herb.

MEDICINAL HERBS

→

Safe dosage:
Consult your doctor for the appropriate dose for your condition.

 Toxicity

Rated slightly dangerous, particularly in children, persons over 55 and those who take larger than appropriate quantities for extended periods of time

For symptoms of toxicity: See *Adverse Reactions, Side Effects or Overdose Symptoms* section below.

 Adverse Reactions, Side Effects or Overdose Symptoms

Signs and symptoms	What to do
Change in heart rate	Discontinue use. Call doctor immediately.
Convulsions	Discontinue use. Call doctor immediately.
Nausea, vomiting	Discontinue use. Call doctor immediately.
Upset stomach, diarrhea	Discontinue use. Call doctor when convenient.

Barley

 Basic Information

Biological name (genus and species): *Hordeum distichon*

Parts used for medicinal purposes: Various parts of the entire plant, frequently differing by country and culture

Chemicals this herb contains:
• Ash
• Cellulose
• Hordenine
• Invert sugar (see Glossary)
• Lignin
• Malt
• Nitrogen
• Pectin
• Pentosan
• Protein
• Starch
• Sucrose

 Known Effects

Provides nutrition to body

Miscellaneous information:
Barley is a grain and primarily contains nutrients.

 Possible Additional Effects

Used as a "restorative" following stomach and intestinal irritation

 Warnings and Precautions

Don't take if you:
Are allergic or sensitive to barley or gluten.

Consult your doctor if you:
• Take this herb for any medical problem that doesn't improve in

2 weeks (There may be safer, more effective treatments.)
- Take any medicinal drugs or herbs including aspirin, laxatives, cold and cough remedies, antacids, vitamins, minerals, amino acids, supplements, other prescription or nonprescription drugs

Pregnancy:
Don't use unless prescribed by your doctor.

Breastfeeding:
Don't use unless prescribed by your doctor.

Infants and children:
Treating infants and children under 2 with any herbal preparation is hazardous.

Others:
Barley infested with fungus can cause poisoning in animals.

Storage:
- Store in cool, dry area away from direct light, but don't freeze.
- Store safely out of reach of children.
- Don't store in bathroom medicine cabinet. Heat and moisture may change the action of the herb.

Safe dosage:
Consult your doctor for the appropriate dose for your condition.

 Toxicity

Comparative-toxicity rating is not available from standard references.

 Adverse Reactions, Side Effects or Overdose Symptoms

None are expected.

Bayberry (Wax Myrtle)

 Basic Information

Biological name (genus and species):
Myrica cerifera

Parts used for medicinal purposes:
- Bark
- Berries/fruits
- Leaves

Chemicals this herb contains:
- Albumin
- Berberine
- Essential oil (see Glossary)
- Flavonoids
- Gallic acid
- Gum
- Myricitrin
- Myricinic acid, related to saponin
- Palmitin
- Resin (see Glossary)
- Starch
- Sucrose
- Tannic acid
- Triterpenes

 Known Effects

- Reduces nasal congestion
- Reduces fever
- Interferes with absorption of iron and other minerals when taken internally

Miscellaneous information:
- Injections of bark extract have caused cancer in laboratory animals.
- Bayberry is frequently used as a basic ingredient in cosmetics, pharmaceuticals and candles.

➜

MEDICINAL HERBS

Possible Additional Effects

Internal use:
- May cause vomiting
- May treat the common cold
- May treat diarrhea
- May treat jaundice

External use:
- May heal ulcers
- May treat gum problems
- May reduce varicose veins
- May increase circulation

Warnings and Precautions

Don't take if you:
- Are pregnant, think you may be pregnant or plan pregnancy in the near future
- Have a history of cancer (not recommended due to high tannin content)

Consult your doctor if you:
- Take this herb for any medical problem that doesn't improve in 2 weeks (There may be safer, more effective treatments.)
- Take any medicinal drugs or herbs including aspirin, laxatives, cold and cough remedies, antacids, vitamins, minerals, amino acids, supplements, other prescription or nonprescription drugs

Pregnancy:
Don't use unless prescribed by your doctor.

Breastfeeding:
Don't use unless prescribed by your doctor.

Infants and children:
Treating infants and children under 2 with any herbal preparation is hazardous.

Others:
- None expected if you are beyond childhood, under 45, not pregnant, basically healthy, take it for only a short time and do not exceed manufacturer's recommended dose
- Can effect electrolyte balance by increasing sodium but decreasing potassium, which can lead to high blood pressure and edema

Storage:
- Store in cool, dry area away from direct light, but don't freeze.
- Store safely out of reach of children.
- Don't store in bathroom medicine cabinet. Heat and moisture may change the action of the herb.

Safe dosage:
Consult your doctor for the appropriate dose for your condition.

Toxicity

Rated relatively safe when taken in appropriate quantities for short periods of time

Adverse Reactions, Side Effects or Overdose Symptoms

None are expected.

Bearberry (Uva-ursi)

Basic Information

Biological name (genus and species):
Arctostaphylos uva-ursi

Parts used for medicinal purposes:
Leaves

Chemicals this herb contains:
- Arbutin
- Chlorine
- Ellagic acid
- Ericolin
- Gallic acid
- Hydroquinone
- Malic acid
- Myricetin
- Quercetin
- Tannins (see Glossary)
- Ursolic acid
- Volatile oils (see Glossary)

Known Effects

- Shrinks urinary tissues
- Prevents secretion of fluids
- Relieves urinary pain
- Helps body dispose of excess fluid by increasing amount of urine produced
- Antibacterial
- Interferes with absorption of iron and other minerals when taken internally

Miscellaneous information:
- Bearberry turns urine green.
- It was used extensively for urinary tract infections before the development of more effective drugs.

Possible Additional Effects

Boiled, bruised leaves:
- May be good for kidney infections
- Potential sedative
- May relieve nausea
- May decrease ringing in ears
- May treat breathing problems

Warnings and Precautions

Don't take if you:
Are pregnant, think you may be pregnant or plan pregnancy in the near future

Consult your doctor if you:
- Take this herb for any medical problem that doesn't improve in 2 weeks (There may be safer, more effective treatments.)
- Take any medicinal drugs or herbs including aspirin, laxatives, cold and cough remedies, antacids, vitamins, minerals, amino acids, supplements, other prescription or nonprescription drugs

Pregnancy:
Don't use unless prescribed by your doctor.

Breastfeeding:
Don't use unless prescribed by your doctor.

Infants and children:
Treating infants and children under 2 with any herbal preparation is hazardous.

MEDICINAL HERBS

→

Others:

None are expected if you are beyond childhood, under 45, not pregnant, basically healthy, take it for only a short time and do not exceed manufacturer's recommended dose.

Storage:

- Store in cool, dry area away from direct light, but don't freeze.
- Store safely out of reach of children.
- Don't store in bathroom medicine cabinet. Heat and moisture may change the action of the herb.

Safe dosage:

Consult your doctor for the appropriate dose for your condition.

 Toxicity

Rated relatively safe when taken in appropriate quantities for short periods of time (no more than one week)

 Adverse Reactions, Side Effects or Overdose Symptoms

None are expected.

Birch

 Basic Information

Biological name (genus and species):
Betula alba, B. lenta

Parts used for medicinal purposes:
- Bark
- Leaves

Chemicals this herb contains:
- Betulin
- Methyl salicylate (similar to aspirin)
- Resin (see Glossary)
- Tar (creosol, phenol, creosote, guaiacol)

 Known Effects

- Provides counterirritation (see Glossary) when applied to skin overlying an inflamed or irritated joint
- Decreases inflammation in tissues

Miscellaneous information:
- Leaves have an agreeable aromatic odor but bitter taste.
- When treating urinary tract infections, drink plenty of water.

 Possible Additional Effects

- May treat rheumatism and congestive heart failure when steeped to extract its medicinal properties
- May treat skin disorders when applied topically
- May shrink tissues
- May treat arthritis
- May prevent secretion of fluids

 Warnings and Precautions

Don't take if you:

Are pregnant, think you may be pregnant or plan pregnancy in the near future.

Consult your doctor if you:

- Take this herb for any medical problem that doesn't improve in 2 weeks (There may be safer, more effective treatments.)
- Take any medicinal drugs or herbs including aspirin, laxatives, cold and cough remedies, antacids, vitamins, minerals, amino acids, supplements, other prescription or nonprescription drugs

Pregnancy:
Don't use unless prescribed by your doctor.

Breastfeeding:
Don't use unless prescribed by your doctor.

Infants and children:
Treating infants and children under 2 with any herbal preparation is hazardous.

Others:
None are expected if you are beyond childhood, under 45, not pregnant, basically healthy, take it for only a short time and do not exceed manufacturer's recommended dose.

Storage:

- Store in cool, dry area away from direct light, but don't freeze.
- Store safely out of reach of children.
- Don't store in bathroom medicine cabinet. Heat and moisture may change the action of the herb.

Safe dosage:
Consult your doctor for the appropriate dose for your condition.

Toxicity

Comparative-toxicity rating is not available from standard references.

Adverse Reactions, Side Effects or Overdose Symptoms

None are expected.

Birthroot (Bethroot)

Basic Information

Biological name (genus and species):
Trillium erectum, T. pendulum

Parts used for medicinal purposes:
Various parts of the entire plant, frequently differing by country and culture

Chemicals this herb contains:

- Resin (see Glossary)
- Saponin (see Glossary)
- Starch
- Tannins (see Glossary)
- Volatile oils (see Glossary)

Known Effects

- Irritates mucous membranes
- Treats gastrointestinal upsets

→

MEDICINAL HERBS

Miscellaneous information:
• The name "birthroot" resulted from pioneers using this herb to stop bleeding after childbirth.
• It is used as an aphrodisiac by Indians in the southeastern United States.
• It is also used as an astringent poultice (see Glossary).

Possible Additional Effects

May treat menstrual irregularity or increased menstrual frequency

Warnings and Precautions

Don't take if you:
Are pregnant, think you may be pregnant or plan pregnancy in the near future.

Consult your doctor if you:
• Take this herb for any medical problem that doesn't improve in 2 weeks (There may be safer, more effective treatments.)
• Take any medicinal drugs or herbs including aspirin, laxatives, cold and cough remedies, antacids, vitamins, minerals, amino acids, supplements, other prescription or nonprescription drugs

Pregnancy:
Don't use unless prescribed by your doctor.

Breastfeeding:
Don't use unless prescribed by your doctor.

Infants and children:
Treating infants and children under 2 with any herbal preparation is hazardous.

Others:
None are expected if you are beyond childhood, under 45, not pregnant, basically healthy, take it for only a short time and do not exceed manufacturer's recommended dose.

Storage:
• Store in cool, dry area away from direct light, but don't freeze.
• Store safely out of reach of children.
• Don't store in bathroom medicine cabinet. Heat and moisture may change the action of the herb.

Safe dosage:
Consult your doctor for the appropriate dose for your condition.

Toxicity

Comparative-toxicity rating is not available from standard references.

Adverse Reactions, Side Effects or Overdose Symptoms

None are expected.

Bistort (Snakeweed)

 Basic Information

Biological name (genus and species):
Polygonum bistorta

Parts used for medicinal purposes:
Various parts of the entire plant,
frequently differing by country
and culture

Chemicals this herb contains:
Tannins (see Glossary)

 Known Effects

Roots are used for astringent gargle.

 Possible Additional Effects

Roots may cause vomiting.

STOP **Warnings and Precautions**

Don't take if you:
• Are pregnant, think you may be
  pregnant or plan pregnancy in the
  near future
• Have any chronic disease of the
  gastrointestinal tract, such as
  stomach or duodenal ulcers, reflux
  esophagitis, ulcerative colitis, spastic
  colitis, diverticulosis or diverticulitis

Consult your doctor if you:
• Take this herb for any medical
  problem that doesn't improve in
  2 weeks (There may be safer, more
  effective treatments.)
• Take any medicinal drugs or herbs
  including aspirin, laxatives, cold and
  cough remedies, antacids, vitamins,
  minerals, amino acids, supplements,
  other prescription or
  nonprescription drugs

Pregnancy:
Dangers outweigh any possible
benefits. Don't use.

Breastfeeding:
Dangers outweigh any possible
benefits. Don't use.

Infants and children:
Treating infants and children under
2 with any herbal preparation
is hazardous.

Others:
None are expected if you are beyond
childhood, under 45, not pregnant,
basically healthy, take it for only a short
time and do not exceed manufacturer's
recommended dose.

Storage:
• Store in cool, dry area away from
  direct light, but don't freeze.
• Store safely out of reach of children.
• Don't store in bathroom medicine
  cabinet. Heat and moisture may
  change the action of the herb.

Safe dosage:
Consult your doctor for the appropriate dose for your condition.

 Toxicity

Comparative-toxicity rating is not available from standard references.

For symptoms of toxicity: See
*Adverse Reactions, Side Effects or
Overdose Symptoms* section below.

MEDICINAL HERBS

Adverse Reactions, Side Effects or Overdose Symptoms

Signs and symptoms	What to do
Bleeding from stomach characterized by vomiting bright red blood or material that looks like coffee grounds	Discontinue. Call doctor immediately.
Kidney damage characterized by blood in urine, decreased urine flow, swelling of hands and feet	Seek emergency treatment.
Nausea or vomiting	Discontinue. Call doctor immediately.

Bitter Lettuce (Prickly Lettuce)

Basic Information

Biological name (genus and species):
Lactuca virosa, L. scariola

Parts used for medicinal purposes:
Latex, which exudes from stem of flower stalks

Chemicals this herb contains:
- Caoutchouc
- Hyoscyamine
- Lactucerol
- Lactucic acid
- Lactucin
- Mannite
- Nitrates
- Volatile oils (see Glossary)

Known Effects

Depresses central nervous system

Possible Additional Effects

- Potential sedative to relieve anxiety or nervous disorders
- May treat coughs
- May treat chest pain due to coronary artery disease (angina)
- May cause a "high" when smoked

Warnings and Precautions

Don't take if you:
Are pregnant, think you may be pregnant or plan pregnancy in the near future.

Consult your doctor if you:

- Take this herb for any medical problem that doesn't improve in 2 weeks (There may be safer, more effective treatments.)
- Take any medicinal drugs or herbs including aspirin, laxatives, cold and cough remedies, antacids, vitamins, minerals, amino acids, supplements, other prescription or nonprescription drugs

Pregnancy:

Dangers outweigh any possible benefits. Don't use.

Breastfeeding:

Dangers outweigh any possible benefits. Don't use.

Infants and children:

Treating infants and children under 2 with any herbal preparation is hazardous.

Others:

Use only under medical supervision.

Storage:

- Store in cool, dry area away from direct light, but don't freeze.
- Store safely out of reach of children.
- Don't store in bathroom medicine cabinet. Heat and moisture may change the action of the herb.

Safe dosage:

Consult your doctor for the appropriate dose for your condition.

Toxicity

Rated relatively safe when taken in appropriate quantities for short periods of time

For symptoms of toxicity: See *Adverse Reactions, Side Effects or Overdose Symptoms* section below.

Adverse Reactions, Side Effects or Overdose Symptoms

Signs and symptoms	What to do
Breathing difficulties	Seek emergency treatment.

Bitter Root (Rheumatism Weed, Spreading Dogbane, Wild Ipecac)

Basic Information

Biological name (genus and species): *Apocynum androsaemifolium*

Parts used for medicinal purposes:
- Bark
- Petals/flower
- Rhizomes
- Roots

Chemicals this herb contains:
- Apocynein
- Apocynin
- Cymarin
- Saponin (see Glossary)

Known Effects

- Slows heartbeat
- Helps body dispose of excess fluid by increasing amount of urine produced
- Causes vomiting

➜

MEDICINAL HERBS

Miscellaneous information:
- Bitter root has a marked effect on the heart. Prescribed FDA-approved digitalis preparations are far superior in treating heart disorders such as congestive heart failure and heartbeat irregularities.
- Many plants of varying potency and toxicity are called by this name. Be sure you know what you buy and take.
- You will need increased potassium if you take this herb. Take potassium supplements or eat more food high in potassium, such as apricots, citrus fruits and bananas.

Possible Additional Effects

- May help treat congestive heart failure
- May help treat palpitations
- May help treat gallstones
- May "correct" bile flow
- May restore normal tone to tissues or stimulate appetite when roots and rhizomes are used to make a medicinal preparation

Warnings and Precautions

Don't take if you:
- Are pregnant, think you may be pregnant or plan pregnancy in the near future
- Have any chronic disease of the gastrointestinal tract, such as stomach or duodenal ulcers, reflux esophagitis, ulcerative colitis, spastic colitis, diverticulosis or diverticulitis

Consult your doctor if you:
- Take this herb for any medical problem that doesn't improve in 2 weeks (There may be safer, more effective treatments.)
- Take any medicinal drugs or herbs including aspirin, laxatives, cold and cough remedies, antacids, vitamins, minerals, amino acids, supplements, other prescription or nonprescription drugs

Pregnancy:
Don't use unless prescribed by your doctor.

Breastfeeding:
Don't use unless prescribed by your doctor.

Infants and children:
Treating infants and children under 2 with any herbal preparation is hazardous.

Others:
Use only under medical supervision.

Storage:
- Store in cool, dry area away from direct light, but don't freeze.
- Store safely out of reach of children.
- Don't store in bathroom medicine cabinet. Heat and moisture may change the action of the herb.

Safe dosage:
Consult your doctor for the appropriate dose for your condition.

Toxicity

Rated slightly dangerous, particularly in children, persons over 55 and those who take larger than appropriate quantities for extended periods of time

For symptoms of toxicity: See *Adverse Reactions, Side Effects or Overdose Symptoms* section below.

Adverse Reactions, Side Effects or Overdose Symptoms

Signs and symptoms	What to do
Precipitous blood-pressure drop: symptoms include faintness, cold sweat, paleness, rapid pulse	Seek emergency treatment.
Gastritis	Discontinue. Call doctor when convenient.
Heartbeat irregularities	Seek emergency treatment.
Vomiting	Discontinue. Call doctor immediately.

Bittersweet (Bitter Nightshade, European Bittersweet)

Basic Information

Biological name (genus and species):
Solanum dulcamara

Parts used for medicinal purposes:
• Leaves
• Roots

Chemicals this herb contains:
• Dulcamarin
• Saponins (see Glossary)
• Solanidine
• Solanine

Known Effects

Depresses central nervous system

Miscellaneous information:
Bittersweet is a potentially dangerous herb. Toxic amounts depress the nervous system and cause drowsiness. Berries are poisonous.

Possible Additional Effects

• May treat eczema (see Glossary)
• May reduce pain
• Potential aphrodisiac

MEDICINAL HERBS

Warnings and Precautions

Don't take if you:

- Are pregnant, think you may be pregnant or plan pregnancy in the near future
- Have any chronic disease of the gastrointestinal tract, such as stomach or duodenal ulcers, reflux esophagitis, ulcerative colitis, spastic colitis, diverticulosis or diverticulitis

Consult your doctor if you:

- Take this herb for any medical problem that doesn't improve in 2 weeks (There may be safer, more effective treatments.)
- Take any medicinal drugs or herbs including aspirin, laxatives, cold and cough remedies, antacids, vitamins, minerals, amino acids, supplements, other prescription or nonprescription drugs

Pregnancy:

Dangers outweigh any possible benefits. Don't use.

Breastfeeding:

Dangers outweigh any possible benefits. Don't use.

Infants and children:

Treating infants and children under 2 with any herbal preparation is hazardous.

Others:

Dangers outweigh any possible benefits. Don't use.

Storage:

- Store in cool, dry area away from direct light, but don't freeze.
- Store safely out of reach of children.
- Don't store in bathroom medicine cabinet. Heat and moisture may change the action of the herb.

Safe dosage:

Consult your doctor for the appropriate dose for your condition.

 ## Toxicity

Rated slightly dangerous, particularly in children, persons over 55 and those who take larger than appropriate quantities for extended periods of time

For symptoms of toxicity: See *Adverse Reactions, Side Effects or Overdose Symptoms* section below.

 ## Adverse Reactions, Side Effects or Overdose Symptoms

Signs and symptoms	What to do
Toxins are mostly in unripe fruit, which cause the following symptoms:	
Burning throat	Discontinue. Call doctor when convenient.
Coma	Seek emergency treatment.
Dilated pupils	Discontinue. Call doctor immediately.
Dizziness	Discontinue. Call doctor immediately.
Headache	Discontinue. Call doctor when convenient.
Muscle weakness	Discontinue. Call doctor immediately.
Nausea or vomiting	Discontinue. Call doctor immediately.
Slow pulse	Seek emergency treatment.

Black Walnut

Basic Information

Biological name (genus and species):
Juglans nigra

Parts used for medicinal purposes:
- Husks
- Inner bark
- Leaves
- Nuts

Chemicals this herb contains:
- Ellagic acid
- Juglone
- Mucin

Known Effects

- Reduces constipation
- Reduces intestinal parasites

Miscellaneous information:
- Nut husks yield brown dye for hair and clothing.
- Black walnut is available as tincture, extract, dried bark or leaves and fruit rind.

Possible Additional Effects

- May treat fungal infections of skin
- May treat poison ivy and warts
- May treat herpes and cold sores
- May treat athlete's foot and jock itch
- May relieve toxic blood conditions
- May help treat acne
- May help treat fungal infections
- May help treat mouth canker sores

Warnings and Precautions

Don't take if you:
- Are pregnant, think you may be pregnant or plan pregnancy in the near future
- Have any chronic disease of the gastrointestinal tract, such as stomach or duodenal ulcers, reflux esophagitis, ulcerative colitis, spastic colitis, diverticulosis or diverticulitis

Consult your doctor if you:
- Take this herb for any medical problem that doesn't improve in 2 weeks (There may be safer, more effective treatments.)
- Take any medicinal drugs or herbs including aspirin, laxatives, cold and cough remedies, antacids, vitamins, minerals, amino acids, supplements, other prescription or nonprescription drugs

Pregnancy:
Don't use unless prescribed by your doctor.

Breastfeeding:
Don't use unless prescribed by your doctor.

Infants and children:
Treating infants and children under 2 with any herbal preparation is hazardous.

Others:
None are expected if you are beyond childhood, under 45, not pregnant, basically healthy, take it for only a short time and do not exceed manufacturer's recommended dose.

MEDICINAL HERBS

➡

Storage:
- Store in cool, dry area away from direct light, but don't freeze.
- Store safely out of reach of children.
- Don't store in bathroom medicine cabinet. Heat and moisture may change the action of the herb.

Safe dosage:

Consult your doctor for the appropriate dose for your condition.

Toxicity

Comparative-toxicity rating is not available from standard references.

For symptoms of toxicity: See *Adverse Reactions, Side Effects or Overdose Symptoms* section below.

Adverse Reactions, Side Effects or Overdose Symptoms

Signs and symptoms	What to do
Mild laxative effect	Discontinue. Call doctor when convenient.
Nausea	Discontinue. Call doctor immediately.
Upper abdominal pain	Discontinue. Call doctor when convenient.

Bladderwrack

Basic Information

Biological name (genus and species):
Fuycus vesiculosus

Parts used for medicinal purposes:
Various parts of the entire plant, frequently differing by country and culture

Chemicals this herb contains:
- Alginic acid
- Bromine iodine
- Fucodin
- Laminarin

Known Effects

Absorbs water in intestines to form bulk

Possible Additional Effects

- May treat obesity
- May increase thyroid activity
- May kill intestinal parasites

Warnings and Precautions

Don't take if you:

Are pregnant, think you may be pregnant or plan pregnancy in the near future.

Consult your doctor if you:
- Take this herb for any medical problem that doesn't improve in 2 weeks (There may be safer, more effective treatments.)
- Take any medicinal drugs or herbs including aspirin, laxatives, cold and cough remedies, antacids,

vitamins, minerals, amino acids, supplements, other prescription or nonprescription drugs

Pregnancy:
Don't use unless prescribed by your doctor.

Breastfeeding:
Don't use unless prescribed by your doctor.

Infants and children:
Treating infants and children under 2 with any herbal preparation is hazardous.

Others:
None are expected if you are beyond childhood, under 45, not pregnant, basically healthy, take it for only a short time and do not exceed manufacturer's recommended dose.

Storage:
• Store in cool, dry area away from direct light, but don't freeze.

• Store safely out of reach of children.
• Don't store in bathroom medicine cabinet. Heat and moisture may change the action of the herb.

Safe dosage:
Consult your doctor for the appropriate dose for your condition.

Toxicity

Comparative-toxicity rating is not available from standard references.

Adverse Reactions, Side Effects or Overdose Symptoms

None are expected.

Blessed Thistle

Basic Information

Biological name (genus and species):
Cnicus benedictus

Parts used for medicinal purposes:
Various parts of the entire plant, frequently differing by country and culture

Chemicals this herb contains:
• Cincin
• Volatile oils (see Glossary)

Known Effects

• Stimulates milk production in lactating women
• Antibacterial
• Anti-inflammatory
• Coagulant

Miscellaneous information:
• Applied to skin overlying a joint to cause an irritant to relieve another irritant
• Effects have not been studied to any great extent
• Careful handling necessary to avoid toxic effects on skin

➜

Possible
Additional Effects

- May help reduce fever
- May reduce headache
- May regulate menses
- May induce vomiting
- May treat cuts, bruises and wounds when applied externally

 Warnings and Precautions

Don't take if you:

- Are pregnant, think you may be pregnant or plan pregnancy in the near future
- Have any chronic disease of the gastrointestinal tract, such as stomach or duodenal ulcers, reflux esophagitis, ulcerative colitis, spastic colitis, diverticulosis or diverticulitis

Consult your doctor if you:

- Take this herb for any medical problem that doesn't improve in 2 weeks (There may be safer, more effective treatments.)
- Take any medicinal drugs or herbs including aspirin, laxatives, cold and cough remedies, antacids, vitamins, minerals, amino acids, supplements, other prescription or nonprescription drugs

Pregnancy:
Don't use unless prescribed by your doctor.

Breastfeeding:
Don't use unless prescribed by your doctor.

Infants and children:
Treating infants and children under 2 with any herbal preparation is hazardous.

Others:
None are expected if you are beyond childhood, under 45, not pregnant, basically healthy, take it for only a short time and do not exceed manufacturer's recommended dose.

Storage:

- Store in cool, dry area away from direct light, but don't freeze.
- Store safely out of reach of children.
- Don't store in bathroom medicine cabinet. Heat and moisture may change the action of the herb.

Safe dosage:
Consult your doctor for the appropriate dose for your condition.

 Toxicity

Comparative-toxicity rating is not available from standard references.

For symptoms of toxicity: See *Adverse Reactions, Side Effects or Overdose Symptoms* section below.

 Adverse Reactions, Side Effects or Overdose Symptoms

Signs and symptoms	What to do
Vomiting	Discontinue. Call doctor immediately.

Blueberry

 Basic Information

Biological name (genus and species):
Vaccinium (many species exist)

Parts used for medicinal purposes:
- Leaves
- Stems

Chemicals this herb contains:
- Fatty acids (see Glossary)
- Hydroquinone
- Loeanolic acid
- Neomyrtillin
- Tannins (see Glossary)
- Ursolic acid

 Known Effects

- Decreases blood sugar
- Interferes with absorption of iron and other minerals when taken internally
- Treats diarrhea

 Possible Additonal Effects

- May treat ulcers
- May treat gastroenteritis
- May help body dispose of excess fluid by increasing amount of urine produced
- May treat and prevent scurvy

 Warnings and Precautions

Don't take if you:
Are pregnant, think you may be pregnant or plan pregnancy in the near future.

Consult your doctor if you:
- Take this herb for any medical problem that doesn't improve in 2 weeks (There may be safer, more effective treatments.)
- Take any medicinal drugs or herbs including aspirin, laxatives, cold and cough remedies, antacids, vitamins, minerals, amino acids, supplements, other prescription or nonprescription drugs

Pregnancy:
Don't use unless prescribed by your doctor.

Breastfeeding:
Don't use unless prescribed by your doctor.

Infants and children:
Treating infants and children under 2 with any herbal preparation is hazardous.

Others:
None are expected if you are beyond childhood, under 45, not pregnant, basically healthy, take it for only a short time and do not exceed manufacturer's recommended dose.

Storage:
- Store in cool, dry area away from direct light, but don't freeze.
- Store safely out of reach of children.
- Don't store in bathroom medicine cabinet. Heat and moisture may change the action of the herb.

Safe dosage:
Consult your doctor for the appropriate dose for your condition.

MEDICINAL HERBS

Toxicity

Comparative-toxicity rating is not available from standard references.

Adverse Reactions, Side Effects or Overdose Symptoms

None are expected.

Boneset (Ague Weed, Richweed, White Snakeroot)

Basic Information

Biological name (genus and species):
Eupatorium perfoliatum, E. rugosum

Parts used for medicinal purposes:
- Leaves
- Petals/flower

Chemicals this herb contains:
- Eupatorin
- Resin (see Glossary)
- Sugar
- Tremetone
- Volatile oils (see Glossary)
- Wax (see Glossary)

Known Effects

- Can produce "milk sickness" in humans, an acute disease characterized by trembling, vomiting and severe abdominal pain caused by eating dairy products or beef from cattle poisoned by eating boneset
- Causes vomiting

Miscellaneous information:
Tremetone can accumulate slowly in animal bodies and cause toxic symptoms. It may do the same in humans.

Possible Additional Effects

- May decrease blood sugar
- May treat malaria
- May treat fever
- May treat flu and colds, coughs
- Potential anti-inflammatory
- May treat arthritis

Warnings and Precautions

Don't take if you:
- Are pregnant, think you may be pregnant or plan pregnancy in the near future
- Have any chronic disease of the gastrointestinal tract, such as stomach or duodenal ulcers, reflux esophagitis, ulcerative colitis, spastic colitis, diverticulosis or diverticulitis

Consult your doctor if you:
- Take this herb for any medical problem that doesn't improve in 2 weeks (There may be safer, more effective treatments.)
- Take any medicinal drugs or herbs including aspirin, laxatives, cold and cough remedies, antacids, vitamins, minerals, amino acids, supplements, other prescription or nonprescription drugs

Pregnancy:
Dangers outweigh any possible benefits. Don't use.

Breastfeeding:
Dangers outweigh any possible benefits. Don't use.

Infants and children:
Treating infants and children under 2 with any herbal preparation is hazardous.

Others:
Dangers outweigh any possible benefits. Don't use.

Storage:
• Store in cool, dry area away from direct light, but don't freeze.
• Store safely out of reach of children.
• Don't store in bathroom medicine cabinet. Heat and moisture may change the action of the herb.

Safe dosage:
Consult your doctor for the appropriate dose for your condition.

Toxicity

Comparative-toxicity rating is not available from standard references.

For symptoms of toxicity: See *Adverse Reactions, Side Effects or Overdose Symptoms* section below.

Adverse Reactions, Side Effects or Overdose Symptoms

Signs and symptoms	What to do
Breathing difficulties	Seek emergency treatment.
Coma	Seek emergency treatment.
Diarrhea	Discontinue. Call doctor immediately.
Drooling	Discontinue. Call doctor when convenient.
Muscle trembling	Discontinue. Call doctor immediately.
Nausea or vomiting	Discontinue. Call doctor immediately.
Stiffness	Discontinue. Call doctor when convenient.
Weakness	Discontinue. Call doctor when convenient.

MEDICINAL HERBS

Buchu (Honey Buchu, Short-leaf Mountain Buchu)

Basic Information

Biological name (genus and species):
Barosma betulina

Parts used for medicinal purposes:
Leaves

Chemicals this herb contains:
- Camphor
- Diosmine
- Hesperidin
- Isomenthone
- Mucilage (see Glossary)
- Resin (see Glossary)
- Volatile oils (see Glossary)

Known Effects

- Helps body dispose of excess fluid by increasing amount of urine produced
- Works as a urinary antiseptic
- Helps expel gas from intestinal tract

Miscellaneous information:
Buchu has a peppermint-like odor.

Possible Additional Effects

- May treat bladder irritation
- May treat urethral irritation
- May treat bloating associated with premenstrual syndrome (PMS)
- Potential diuretic

Warnings and Precautions

Don't take if you:
- Are pregnant, think you may be pregnant or plan pregnancy in the near future
- Have any chronic disease of the gastrointestinal tract, such as stomach or duodenal ulcers, reflux esophagitis, ulcerative colitis, spastic colitis, diverticulosis or diverticulitis

Consult your doctor if you:
- Take this herb for any medical problem that doesn't improve in 2 weeks (There may be safer, more effective treatments.)
- Take any medicinal drugs or herbs including aspirin, laxatives, cold and cough remedies, antacids, vitamins, minerals, amino acids, supplements, other prescription or nonprescription drugs

Pregnancy:
Dangers outweigh any possible benefits. Don't use.

Breastfeeding:
Dangers outweigh any possible benefits. Don't use.

Infants and children:
Treating infants and children under 2 with any herbal preparation is hazardous.

Others:
None are expected if you are beyond childhood, under 45, not pregnant, basically healthy, take it for only a short time and do not exceed manufacturer's recommended dose.

Storage:
- Store in cool, dry area away from direct light, but don't freeze.
- Store safely out of reach of children.
- Don't store in bathroom medicine cabinet. Heat and moisture may change the action of the herb.

Safe dosage:
Consult your doctor for the appropriate dose for your condition.

Toxicity

Rated relatively safe when taken in appropriate quantities for short periods of time

For symptoms of toxicity: See *Adverse Reactions, Side Effects or Overdose Symptoms* section below.

 Adverse Reactions, Side Effects or Overdose Symptoms

Signs and symptoms	What to do
Diarrhea	Discontinue. Call doctor when convenient.
Nausea or vomiting	Discontinue. Call doctor immediately.

Buckthorn

 Basic Information

Biological name (genus and species): *Rhamnus cathartica*

Parts used for medicinal purposes:
• Bark
• Berries/fruits

Chemicals this herb contains:
• Anthraquinone
• Emodin

 Known Effects

• Irritates gastrointestinal tract and may cause watery, explosive bowel movements
• Used to treat constipation short term

Miscellaneous information:
• Several dyes are made from the juice of the berries.
• Children can have toxic symptoms after eating as few as 20 berries.
• The syrup of buckthorn is made from berries.

 Possible Additional Effects

Potential laxative

 Warnings and Precautions

Don't take if you:
• Are pregnant, think you may be pregnant or plan pregnancy in the near future
• Have any chronic disease of the gastrointestinal tract, such as stomach or duodenal ulcers, reflux esophagitis, ulcerative colitis, spastic colitis, diverticulosis or diverticulitis

Consult your doctor if you:
• Take this herb for any medical problem that doesn't improve in 2 weeks (There may be safer, more effective treatments.)
• Take any medicinal drugs or herbs including aspirin, laxatives, cold and cough remedies, antacids, vitamins, minerals, amino acids, supplements, other prescription or nonprescription drugs

MEDICINAL HERBS

➔

Pregnancy:
Dangers outweigh any possible benefits. Don't use.

Breastfeeding:
Dangers outweigh any possible benefits. Don't use.

Infants and children:
Treating infants and children under 2 with any herbal preparation is hazardous.

Others:
• None are expected if you are beyond childhood, under 45, not pregnant, basically healthy, take it for only a short time and do not exceed manufacturer's recommended dose.
• Do not use in combination with other laxatives.

Storage:
• Store in cool, dry area away from direct light, but don't freeze.
• Store safely out of reach of children.
• Don't store in bathroom medicine cabinet. Heat and moisture may change the action of the herb.

Safe dosage:
Consult your doctor for the appropriate dose for your condition.

 Toxicity

Comparative-toxicity rating is not available from standard references.

For symptoms of toxicity: See *Adverse Reactions, Side Effects or Overdose Symptoms* section below.

 Adverse Reactions, Side Effects or Overdose Symptoms

Signs and symptoms	What to do
Diarrhea, severe and watery	Discontinue. Call doctor immediately.
Diarrhea, violent	Seek emergency treatment if uncontrollable.
Kidney damage (with large amounts over long period of time) characterized by blood in urine, decreased urine flow, swelling of hands and feet	Seek emergency treatment.
Nausea or vomiting	Discontinue. Call doctor immediately.
Stomach cramps	Discontinue. Call doctor immediately.

Burdock (Edible Burdock, Great Burdock, Lappa)

 Basic Information

Biological name (genus and species):
Arctium lappa

Parts used for medicinal purposes:
• Roots
• Seeds

Chemicals this herb contains:
• Arctiin
• Inulin
• Tannins (see Glossary)
• Vitamins B and E
• Volatile oils (see Glossary)

Known Effects

Stimulates the immune system

 Possible Additional Effects

• May treat skin disorders
• May treat gout
• May relieve urinary tract infections
• May treat fungal and bacterial infections
• May treat arthritis and rheumatism

 Warnings and Precautions

Don't take if you:
Are pregnant, think you may be pregnant or plan pregnancy in the near future.

Consult your doctor if you:
• Take this herb for any medical problem that doesn't improve in 2 weeks (There may be safer, more effective treatments.)
• Take any medicinal drugs or herbs including aspirin, laxatives, cold and cough remedies, antacids, vitamins, minerals, amino acids, supplements, other prescription or nonprescription drugs

Pregnancy:
Dangers outweigh any possible benefits. Don't use.

Breastfeeding:
Dangers outweigh any possible benefits. Don't use.

Infants and children:
Treating infants and children under 2 with any herbal preparation is hazardous.

Storage:
• Store in cool, dry area away from direct light, but don't freeze.
• Store safely out of reach of children.
• Don't store in bathroom medicine cabinet. Heat and moisture may change the action of the herb.

Safe dosage:
Consult your doctor for the appropriate dose for your condition.

 Toxicity

Rated relatively safe when taken in appropriate quantities for short periods of time

For symptoms of toxicity: See *Adverse Reactions, Side Effects or Overdose Symptoms* section below.

 Adverse Reactions, Side Effects or Overdose Symptoms

Signs and symptoms	What to do
Dilated pupils	Discontinue. Call doctor immediately.
Dry mouth	Discontinue. Call doctor when convenient.
Hallucinations	Seek emergency treatment.
Stomach discomfort	Discontinue. Call doctor immediately.

MEDICINAL HERBS

Calamus Root

Basic Information

Calamus root is also called sweet root, acore, rat root, sweet flag, sweet myrtle, sweet cane, sweet sedge, flagroot and calamus.

Biological name (genus and species): *Acorus calamus*

Parts used for medicinal purposes: Roots

Chemicals this herb contains:
- Asarone
- Beta-asarone
- Camphene
- Caryophyllene
- Eugenol
- Pinene
- Volatile oils (see Glossary)

Known Effects

- Aids in expelling gas from the intestinal tract
- Depresses central nervous system
- Causes hallucinations

Miscellaneous information:
- Calamus root is used primarily in India for many illnesses.
- Essential oil extracted from the root causes cancer in rats. The FDA has banned all varieties of this plant for human use.

Possible Additional Effects

- May treat asthma
- May treat coughs
- May treat dyspepsia
- May treat convulsions
- May treat epilepsy
- May treat hysteria
- May treat insanity
- May treat intestinal parasites
- Potential aphrodisiac
- May reduce fever

Warnings and Precautions

Don't take if you:
Are pregnant, think you may be pregnant or plan pregnancy in the near future.

Consult your doctor if you:
- Take this herb for any medical problem that doesn't improve in 2 weeks (There may be safer, more effective treatments.)
- Take any medicinal drugs or herbs including aspirin, laxatives, cold and cough remedies, antacids, vitamins, minerals, amino acids, supplements, other prescription or nonprescription drugs

Pregnancy:
Don't use unless prescribed by your doctor.

Breastfeeding:
Don't use unless prescribed by your doctor.

Infants and children:
Treating infants and children under 2 with any herbal preparation is hazardous.

Others:
None are expected if you are beyond childhood, under 45, not pregnant, basically healthy, take it for only a short time and do not exceed manufacturer's recommended dose.

Storage:
- Store in cool, dry area away from direct light, but don't freeze.
- Store safely out of reach of children.
- Don't store in bathroom medicine cabinet. Heat and moisture may change the action of the herb.

Safe dosage:
Consult your doctor for the appropriate dose for your condition.

 Toxicity

Rated dangerous, particularly in children, persons over 55 and those who take larger than appropriate quantities for extended periods of time

For symptoms of toxicity: See *Adverse Reactions, Side Effects or Overdose Symptoms* section below.

 Adverse Reactions, Side Effects or Overdose Symptoms

Signs and symptoms	What to do
Drowsiness	Discontinue. Call doctor when convenient.
Hallucinations	Seek emergency treatment.

California Poppy

 Basic Information

Biological name (genus and species):
Eschscholzia californica

Parts used for medicinal purposes:
Entire plant, except roots

Chemicals this herb contains:
- Coptisine
- Sanguinarine

 Known Effects

- Feeble narcotic action
- Increases perspiration
- Depresses central nervous system

Miscellaneous information:
California poppy does not contain any narcotic derivatives, such as morphine or codeine. The poppy plant that has

narcotic properties is different from this one.

 Possible Additional Effects

Used by drug abusers for sedative or mind-altering effects

 Warnings and Precautions

Don't take if you:
Are pregnant, think you may be pregnant or plan pregnancy in the near future.

Consult your doctor if you:
- Take this herb for any medical problem that doesn't improve in 2 weeks (There may be safer, more effective treatments.)

MEDICINAL HERBS

→

- Take any medicinal drugs or herbs including aspirin, laxatives, cold and cough remedies, antacids, vitamins, minerals, amino acids, supplements, other prescription or nonprescription drugs

Pregnancy:
Don't use unless prescribed by your doctor.

Breastfeeding:
Don't use unless prescribed by your doctor.

Infants and children:
Treating infants and children under 2 with any herbal preparation is hazardous.

Others:
None are expected if you are beyond childhood, under 45, not pregnant, basically healthy, take it for only a short time and do not exceed manufacturer's recommended dose.

Storage:
- Store in cool, dry area away from direct light, but don't freeze.
- Store safely out of reach of children.

- Don't store in bathroom medicine cabinet. Heat and moisture may change the action of the herb.

Safe dosage:
Consult your doctor for the appropriate dose for your condition.

Toxicity

Rated slightly dangerous, particularly in children, persons over 55 and those who take larger than appropriate quantities for extended periods of time

For symptoms of toxicity: See *Adverse Reactions, Side Effects or Overdose Symptoms* section below.

Adverse Reactions, Side Effects or Overdose Symptoms

Signs and symptoms	What to do
Change in heart rate	Discontinue. Call doctor immediately.
Drowsiness	Discontinue. Call doctor immediately.

Caraway

Basic Information

Biological name (genus and species):
Carum carvi

Parts used for medicinal purposes:
- Leaves
- Seeds

Chemicals this herb contains:
- Calcium oxalate
- Carveol
- Carvone, a volatile oil (see Glossary)

- Dihydrocarvone
- Fatty acids (see Glossary)
- Proteins

Known Effects
- Aromatic (see Glossary)
- Helps expel gas from intestinal tract

Miscellaneous information:
- Caraway is used as a flavoring agent in baking.
- The oil is used in making ice cream.
- No effects are expected on the body,

either good or bad, when this herb is used in very small amounts to enhance the flavor of food.

 Possible Additional Effects

- May reduce flatulence in infants
- May treat abdominal cramping
- May treat nausea
- May treat scabies

 Warnings and Precautions

Don't take if you:

- Are pregnant, think you may be pregnant or plan pregnancy in the near future
- Have any chronic disease of the gastrointestinal tract, such as stomach or duodenal ulcers, reflux esophagitis, ulcerative colitis, spastic colitis, diverticulosis or diverticulitis

Consult your doctor if you:

- Take this herb for any medical problem that doesn't improve in 2 weeks (There may be safer, more effective treatments.)
- Take any medicinal drugs or herbs including aspirin, laxatives, cold and cough remedies, antacids, vitamins, minerals, amino acids, supplements, other prescription or nonprescription drugs

Pregnancy:

Don't use unless prescribed by your doctor.

Breastfeeding:

Don't use unless prescribed by your doctor.

Infants and children:

Treating infants and children under 2 with any herbal preparation is hazardous.

Others:

None are expected if you are beyond childhood, under 45, not pregnant, basically healthy, take it for only a short time and do not exceed manufacturer's recommended dose.

Storage:

- Store in cool, dry area away from direct light, but don't freeze.
- Store safely out of reach of children.
- Don't store in bathroom medicine cabinet. Heat and moisture may change the action of the herb.

Safe dosage:

Consult your doctor for the appropriate dose for your condition.

 Toxicity

Comparative-toxicity rating is not available from standard references.

For symptoms of toxicity: See *Adverse Reactions, Side Effects or Overdose Symptoms* section below.

 Adverse Reactions, Side Effects or Overdose Symptoms

Signs and symptoms	What to do
In very large amounts only:	
Central-nervous-system depression	Seek emergency treatment.
Nausea or vomiting	Discontinue. Call doctor immediately.

MEDICINAL HERBS

Cardamom Seed

Basic Information

Biological name (genus and species):
Ellettaria cardamonum

Parts used for medicinal purposes:
Seeds

Chemicals this herb contains:
- Fixed oil (see Glossary)
- Gum (see Glossary)
- Limonene
- Starch
- Terpene alcohol
- Terpinene
- Volatile oils (see Glossary)
- Yellow coloring

Known Effects

- Helps expel gas from intestinal tract
- Causes explosive watery diarrhea

Miscellaneous information:
Provides flavor in foods.

Possible Additional Effects

- May treat bronchitis
- May treat urinary incontinence

Don't take if you:
- Are pregnant, think you may be pregnant or plan pregnancy in the near future
- Have any chronic disease of the gastrointestinal tract, such as stomach or duodenal ulcers, reflux esophagitis, ulcerative colitis, spastic colitis, diverticulosis or diverticulitis

Consult your doctor if you:
- Take this herb for any medical problem that doesn't improve in 2 weeks (There may be safer, more effective treatments.)
- Take any medicinal drugs or herbs including aspirin, laxatives, cold and cough remedies, antacids, vitamins, minerals, amino acids, supplements, other prescription or nonprescription drugs

Pregnancy:
Don't use unless prescribed by your doctor.

Breastfeeding:
Don't use unless prescribed by your doctor.

Infants and children:
Treating infants and children under 2 with any herbal preparation is hazardous.

Others:
None are expected if you are beyond childhood, under 45, not pregnant, basically healthy, take it for only a short time and do not exceed manufacturer's recommended dose.

Storage:
- Store in cool, dry area away from direct light, but don't freeze.
- Store safely out of reach of children.
- Don't store in bathroom medicine cabinet. Heat and moisture may change the action of the herb.

Safe dosage:
Consult your doctor for the appropriate dose for your condition.

Toxicity

Comparative-toxicity rating is not available from standard references.

For symptoms of toxicity: See *Adverse Reactions, Side Effects or Overdose Symptoms* section below.

 Adverse Reactions, Side Effects or Overdose Symptoms

Signs and symptoms	What to do
Diarrhea	Discontinue. Call doctor immediately.
Nausea or vomiting	Discontinue. Call doctor immediately.

Catalpa

 Basic Information

Biological name (genus and species):
Catalpa bignonioides

Parts used for medicinal purposes:
Various parts of the entire plant, frequently differing by country and culture

Chemicals this herb contains:
• Catalpin
• Catalposide

 Known Effects

Irritates gastrointestinal tract

 Possible Additional Effects

May treat asthma

 Warnings and Precautions

Don't take if you:
• Are pregnant, think you may be pregnant or plan pregnancy in the near future

• Have any chronic disease of the gastrointestinal tract, such as stomach or duodenal ulcers, reflux esophagitis, ulcerative colitis, spastic colitis, diverticulosis or diverticulitis

Consult your doctor if you:
• Take this herb for any medical problem that doesn't improve in 2 weeks (There may be safer, more effective treatments.)
• Take any medicinal drugs or herbs including aspirin, laxatives, cold and cough remedies, antacids, vitamins, minerals, amino acids, supplements, other prescription or nonprescription drugs

Pregnancy:
Dangers outweigh any possible benefits. Don't use.

Breastfeeding:
Dangers outweigh any possible benefits. Don't use.

Infants and children:
Treating infants and children under 2 with any herbal preparation is hazardous.

Others:
Dangers outweigh any possible benefits. Don't use.

MEDICINAL HERBS

→

Storage:
- Store in cool, dry area away from direct light, but don't freeze.
- Store safely out of reach of children.
- Don't store in bathroom medicine cabinet. Heat and moisture may change the action of the herb.

Safe dosage:
Consult your doctor for the appropriate dose for your condition.

 Toxicity

Comparative-toxicity rating is not available from standard references.

For symptoms of toxicity: See *Adverse Reactions, Side Effects or Overdose Symptoms* section below.

 Adverse Reactions, Side Effects or Overdose Symptoms

Signs and symptoms	What to do
Cold, clammy skin	Discontinue. Call doctor when convenient.
Diarrhea	Discontinue. Call doctor immediately.
Nausea or vomiting	Discontinue. Call doctor immediately.
Precipitous blood-pressure drop: symptoms include faintness, cold sweat, paleness, rapid pulse	Seek emergency treatment.
Rapid, weak pulse	Seek emergency treatment.

Catechu, Black

 Basic Information

Biological name (genus and species): *Acacia catechu*

Parts used for medicinal purposes: Various parts of the entire plant, frequently differing by country and culture

Chemical this herb contains: Tannins (see Glossary)

 Known Effects

- Shrinks tissues
- Prevents secretion of fluids
- Interferes with absorption of iron and other minerals when taken internally

 Possible Additional Effects

- May decrease unusual bleeding
- May treat chronic diarrhea
- Used as gargle for sore throat

 Warnings and Precautions

Don't take if you:
- Are pregnant, think you may be pregnant or plan pregnancy in the near future
- Have any chronic disease of the gastrointestinal tract, such as stomach or duodenal ulcers, reflux esophagitis, ulcerative colitis, spastic colitis, diverticulosis or diverticulitis

Consult your doctor if you:

- Take this herb for any medical problem that doesn't improve in 2 weeks (There may be safer, more effective treatments.)
- Take any medicinal drugs or herbs including aspirin, laxatives, cold and cough remedies, antacids, vitamins, minerals, amino acids, supplements, other prescription or nonprescription drugs

Pregnancy:

Dangers outweigh any possible benefits. Don't use.

Breastfeeding:

Dangers outweigh any possible benefits. Don't use.

Infants and children:

Treating infants and children under 2 with any herbal preparation is hazardous.

Others:

None are expected if you are beyond childhood, under 45, not pregnant, basically healthy, take it for only a short time and do not exceed manufacturer's recommended dose.

Storage:

- Store in cool, dry area away from direct light, but don't freeze.
- Store safely out of reach of children.

- Don't store in bathroom medicine cabinet. Heat and moisture may change the action of the herb.

Safe dosage:

Consult your doctor for the appropriate dose for your condition.

 Toxicity

Comparative-toxicity rating is not available from standard references.

For symptoms of toxicity: See *Adverse Reactions, Side Effects or Overdose Symptoms* section below.

 Adverse Reactions, Side Effects or Overdose Symptoms

Signs and symptoms	What to do
Diarrhea	Discontinue. Call doctor immediately.
Kidney damage characterized by blood in urine, decreased urine flow, swelling of hands and feet	Seek emergency treatment.
Vomiting	Discontinue. Call doctor immediately.

Catha (Khat plant)

 Basic Information

Biological name (genus and species): *Catha edulis*

Parts used for medicinal purposes: Leaves

Chemicals this herb contains:

- Cathidine
- Cathine (a form of ephedrine)
- Cathinone
- Celastrin
- Choline
- Katine
- Tannins (see Glossary)

MEDICINAL HERBS

→

Known Effects

- Stimulates brain and spinal cord through synapses
- Interferes with absorption of iron and other minerals when taken internally

Miscellaneous information:

Can be habit forming—addicts become talkative then depressed and apathetic.

Possible Additional Effects

- May treat fatigue when leaves are chewed or steeped to make tea
- May suppress appetite

Warnings and Precautions

Don't take if you:

- Are pregnant, think you may be pregnant or plan pregnancy in the near future
- Have heart trouble
- Have high blood pressure

Consult your doctor if you:

- Take this herb for any medical problem that doesn't improve in 2 weeks (There may be safer, more effective treatments.)
- Take any medicinal drugs or herbs including aspirin, laxatives, cold and cough remedies, antacids, vitamins, minerals, amino acids, supplements, other prescription or nonprescription drugs

Pregnancy:

Dangers outweigh any possible benefits. Don't use.

Breastfeeding:

Dangers outweigh any possible benefits. Don't use.

Infants and children:

Treating infants and children under 2 with any herbal preparation is hazardous.

Storage:

- Store in cool, dry area away from direct light, but don't freeze.
- Store safely out of reach of children.
- Don't store in bathroom medicine cabinet. Heat and moisture may change the action of the herb.

Safe dosage:

Consult your doctor for the appropriate dose for your condition.

Toxicity

Rated slightly dangerous, particularly in children, persons over 55 and those who take larger than appropriate quantities for extended periods of time

For symptoms of toxicity: See *Adverse Reactions, Side Effects or Overdose Symptoms* section below.

Adverse Reactions, Side Effects or Overdose Symptoms

Signs and symptoms	What to do
Large amounts:	
Breathing difficulties	Seek emergency treatment.
Depression	Discontinue. Call doctor when convenient.
Euphoria	Discontinue. Call doctor when convenient.
Increased blood pressure	Discontinue. Call doctor immediately.
Increased heart rate	Seek emergency treatment.
Paralysis	Seek emergency treatment.
Stomach irritation, with bleeding	Discontinue. Call doctor immediately.

Catnip (Catmint, Catnep)

Basic Information

Biological name (genus and species):
Nepeta cataria

Parts used for medicinal purposes:
Leaves

Chemicals this herb contains:
• Acetic acid
• Buteric acid
• Citral
• Dipentene
• Lifronella
• Limonene
• Nepetalic acid
• Tannins (see Glossary)
• Terpene (see Glossary)
• Valeric acid
• Volatile oils (see Glossary)

Known Effects

• Affects central nervous system
• Relieves spasm in skeletal or smooth muscle
• Relieves indigestion

Miscellaneous information:
Catnip is not a psychedelic or euphoria-producing drug, despite several reports to the contrary.

Possible Additional Effects

• May increase sweating to reduce fevers when leaves are steeped
• May treat colic (see Glossary) when leaves used as snuff
• May treat insomnia
• May treat colds and flu
• May relieve bronchial congestion

STOP Warnings and Precautions

Don't take if you:
Are pregnant, think you may be pregnant or plan pregnancy in the near future.

Consult your doctor if you:
• Take this herb for any medical problem that doesn't improve in 2 weeks (There may be safer, more effective treatments.)
• Take any medicinal drugs or herbs including aspirin, laxatives, cold and cough remedies, antacids, vitamins, minerals, amino acids, supplements, other prescription or nonprescription drugs

Pregnancy:
Don't use unless prescribed by your doctor.

Breastfeeding:
Don't use unless prescribed by your doctor.

Infants and children:
Treating infants and children under 2 with any herbal preparation is hazardous.

Others:
None are expected if you are beyond childhood, under 45, not pregnant, basically healthy, take it for only a short time and do not exceed manufacturer's recommended dose.

Storage:
• Store in cool, dry area away from direct light, but don't freeze.
• Store safely out of reach of children.
• Don't store in bathroom medicine cabinet. Heat and moisture may change the action of the herb.

MEDICINAL HERBS

Safe dosage:
Consult your doctor for the appropriate dose for your condition.

Toxicity

Generally regarded as safe when taken in appropriate quantities for short periods of time

For symptoms of toxicity: See *Adverse Reactions, Side Effects or Overdose Symptoms* section below.

Adverse Reactions, Side Effects or Overdose Symptoms

Signs and symptoms	What to do
Upset stomach	Discontinue. Call doctor immediately.

Celery Fruit (Celery)

Basic Information

Biological name (genus and species):
Apium graveolens

Parts used for medicinal purposes:
- Juice
- Roots
- Seeds

Chemicals this herb contains:
- D-limonene
- Nitrates
- Resin (see Glossary)
- Sedanoic anhydrides
- Sedanolide
- Volatile oils (see Glossary)

Known Effects

- Relieves spasm in skeletal or smooth muscle
- Causes uterine contractions, whether pregnant or not
- Reduces blood pressure, when in juice form
- Reduces gas in gastrointestinal tract

Miscellaneous information:
- No effects are expected on the body, either good or bad, when this herb is used in very small amounts to enhance the flavor of food or when eaten as a common food.
- Workers in celery fields may develop skin rashes.

Possible Additional Effects

- Potential antioxidant (seeds)
- Potential sedative
- May treat dysmenorrhea (menstrual cramps)
- May treat arthritis
- Potential aphrodisiac (roots)

Warnings and Precautions

Don't take if you:
Are in your third trimester of a pregnancy.

Consult your doctor if you:
- Take this herb for any medical problem that doesn't improve in 2 weeks (There may be safer, more effective treatments.)
- Take any medicinal drugs or herbs including aspirin, laxatives, cold and cough remedies, antacids, vitamins, minerals, amino acids, supplements, other prescription or nonprescription drugs

Pregnancy:
Pregnant women should experience no problems taking usual amounts as part of a balanced diet. Don't drink large quantities of celery juice.

Breastfeeding:
Breastfed infants of lactating mothers should experience no problems when mother takes usual amounts as part of a balanced diet. Other products extracted from this herb have not been proved to cause problems.

Infants and children:
Treating infants and children under 2 with any herbal preparation is hazardous.

Others:
None are expected if you are beyond childhood, under 45, not pregnant, basically healthy, take it for only a short time and do not exceed manufacturer's recommended dose.

Storage:
- Store in cool, dry area away from direct light, but don't freeze.
- Store safely out of reach of children.
- Don't store in bathroom medicine cabinet. Heat and moisture may change the action of the herb.

Safe dosage:
Consult your doctor for the appropriate dose for your condition.

 Toxicity

Rated relatively safe when taken in appropriate quantities for short periods of time

For symptoms of toxicity: See *Adverse Reactions, Side Effects or Overdose Symptoms* section below.

 Adverse Reactions, Side Effects or Overdose Symptoms

Signs and symptoms	What to do
Deep sedation (with large amounts)	Seek emergency treatment.
Premature labor	Seek emergency treatment.

MEDICINAL HERBS

Centaury (Minor Centaury)

Basic Information

Biological name (genus and species):
Centaurium erythraea,
C. umbellatum

Parts used for medicinal purposes:
Petals/flower

Chemicals this herb contains:
- Amarogentin
- Erytaurin
- Erythrocentaurin
- Gentiopicrin
- Gentisin

Known Effects

- Reduces indigestion
- May stimulate appetite

Possible Additional Effects

No additional effects are known.

Warnings and Precautions

Don't take if you:
- Are pregnant, think you may be pregnant or plan pregnancy in the near future
- Have any chronic disease of the gastrointestinal tract, such as stomach or duodenal ulcers, reflux esophagitis, ulcerative colitis, spastic colitis, diverticulosis or diverticulitis

Consult your doctor if you:
- Take this herb for any medical problem that doesn't improve in 2 weeks (There may be safer, more effective treatments.)
- Take any medicinal drugs or herbs including aspirin, laxatives, cold and cough remedies, antacids, vitamins, minerals, amino acids, supplements, other prescription or nonprescription drugs

Pregnancy:
Don't use unless prescribed by your doctor.

Breastfeeding:
Don't use unless prescribed by your doctor.

Infants and children:
Treating infants and children under 2 with any herbal preparation is hazardous.

Others:
None are expected if you are beyond childhood, under 45, not pregnant, basically healthy, take it for only a short time and do not exceed manufacturer's recommended dose.

Storage:
- Store in cool, dry area away from direct light, but don't freeze.
- Store safely out of reach of children.
- Don't store in bathroom medicine cabinet. Heat and moisture may change the action of the herb.

Safe dosage:
Consult your doctor for the appropriate dose for your condition.

Toxicity

Comparative-toxicity rating is not available from standard references.

For symptoms of toxicity: See *Adverse Reactions, Side Effects or Overdose Symptoms* section below.

 Adverse Reactions, Side Effects or Overdose Symptoms

Signs and symptoms	What to do
Only with very large amounts or accidental overdose:	
Nausea or vomiting	Discontinue. Call doctor immediately.

Chinese Rhubarb (Canton Rhubarb)

 Basic Information

Biological name (genus and species):
Rheum officinalis, R. palmatum

Parts used for medicinal purposes:
• Roots
• Dried rhizomes

Chemicals this herb contains:
• Aloe-emodin
• Anthraquinone
• Chrysophanol
• Emodin
• Tannins (see Glossary)

 Known Effects

• Irritates mucous membranes of intestinal tract
• Strong laxative

Miscellaneous information:
This is not the garden variety of rhubarb.

 Possible Additional Effects

Additional effects are unknown.

 Warnings and Precautions

Don't take if you:
• Are pregnant, think you may be pregnant or plan pregnancy in the near future
• Have any chronic disease of the gastrointestinal tract, such as stomach or duodenal ulcers, reflux esophagitis, ulcerative colitis, spastic colitis, diverticulosis or diverticulitis

Consult your doctor if you:
• Take this herb for any medical problem that doesn't improve in 2 weeks (There may be safer, more effective treatments.)
• Take any medicinal drugs or herbs including aspirin, laxatives, cold and cough remedies, antacids, vitamins, minerals, amino acids, supplements, other prescription or nonprescription drugs

Pregnancy:
Avoid overeating this herb.

Breastfeeding:
Avoid overeating this herb.

MEDICINAL HERBS

→

Infants and children:
Treating infants and children under
2 with any herbal preparation
is hazardous.

Others:
• None are expected if you are beyond
childhood, under 45, not pregnant,
basically healthy, take it for only a
short time and do not exceed
manufacturer's recommended dose.
• Frequent use is not recommended.
Less potent laxative herbs are
available.

Storage:
• Store in cool, dry area away from
direct light, but don't freeze.
• Store safely out of reach of children.
• Don't store in bathroom medicine
cabinet. Heat and moisture may
change the action of the herb.

Safe dosage:
Consult your doctor for the appropriate dose for your condition.

 Toxicity

Rated relatively safe when taken in
appropriate quantities for short
periods of time

For symptoms of toxicity: See
*Adverse Reactions, Side Effects or
Overdose Symptoms* section below.

 Adverse Reactions, Side Effects or Overdose Symptoms

Signs and symptoms	What to do
Cramping, abdominal pain	Discontinue. Call doctor immediately.
Diarrhea (explosive, watery)	Discontinue. Call doctor immediately.

Coconut

 Basic Information

Biological name (genus and species):
Cocus nucifera

Parts used for medicinal purposes:
Oil from seeds

Chemicals this herb contains:
• Fixed oil (see Glossary)
• Tannins (see Glossary)
• Trilaurin
• Trimyristin
• Triolein
• Tripalmatic acid
• Tripalmatin
• Tristearin

 Known Effects

• Prevents secretion of fluids
• Interferes with absorption of iron
and other minerals when
taken internally

Miscellaneous information:
• Coconut is used in making soaps,
scalp applications, hand creams and
some foodstuffs.
• Coconut-oil based soaps are useful
for marine purposes because they
are not easily separated by saltwater
or salty solutions.

Possible Additional Effects

No additional effects are known.

Warnings and Precautions

Don't take if you:

Have any chronic disease of the gastrointestinal tract, such as stomach or duodenal ulcers, reflux esophagitis, ulcerative colitis, spastic colitis, diverticulosis or diverticulitis.

Consult your doctor if you:

• Take this herb for any medical problem that doesn't improve in 2 weeks (There may be safer, more effective treatments.)
• Take any medicinal drugs or herbs including aspirin, laxatives, cold and cough remedies, antacids, vitamins, minerals, amino acids, supplements, other prescription or nonprescription drugs

Pregnancy:

Pregnant women should experience no problems taking usual amounts as part of a balanced diet. Other products extracted from this herb have not been proved to cause problems.

Breastfeeding:

Breastfed infants of lactating mothers should experience no problems when mother takes usual amounts as part of a balanced diet. Other products extracted from this herb have not been proved to cause problems.

Infants and children:

Treating infants and children under 2 with any herbal preparation is hazardous.

Others:

None are expected if you are beyond childhood, under 45, not pregnant, basically healthy, take it for only a short time and do not exceed manufacturer's recommended dose.

Storage:

• Store in cool, dry area away from direct light, but don't freeze.
• Store safely out of reach of children.
• Don't store in bathroom medicine cabinet. Heat and moisture may change the action of the herb.

Safe dosage:

Consult your doctor for the appropriate dose for your condition.

Toxicity

Comparative-toxicity rating is not available from standard references.

For symptoms of toxicity: See *Adverse Reactions, Side Effects or Overdose Symptoms* section below.

Adverse Reactions, Side Effects or Overdose Symptoms

Signs and symptoms	What to do
Diarrhea	Discontinue. Call doctor immediately.

MEDICINAL HERBS

Cohosh, Blue (Papoose Root, Squaw Root)

Basic Information

Biological name (genus and species):
Caulophyllum thalictroides

Parts used for medicinal purposes:
Roots

Chemicals this herb contains:
- Coulosaponin
- Leontin, a saponin (see Glossary)
- Methylcystine

Known Effects

- Stimulates contraction of smooth muscle (blood vessels and small muscles surrounding certain arteries and muscle fibers in the uterus)
- Raises blood pressure

Possible Additional Effects

- May treat menstrual problems
- May stimulate uterine contractions during labor

Warnings and Precautions

Don't take if you:
- Are pregnant, think you may be pregnant or plan pregnancy in the near future
- Have any chronic disease of the gastrointestinal tract, such as stomach or duodenal ulcers, reflux esophagitis, ulcerative colitis, spastic colitis, diverticulosis or diverticulitis

Consult your doctor if you:
- Take this herb for any medical problem that doesn't improve in 2 weeks (There may be safer, more effective treatments.)
- Take any medicinal drugs or herbs including aspirin, laxatives, cold and cough remedies, antacids, vitamins, minerals, amino acids, supplements, other prescription or nonprescription drugs

Pregnancy:
Dangers outweigh any possible benefits. Don't use.

Breastfeeding:
Dangers outweigh any possible benefits. Don't use.

Infants and children:
Treating infants and children under 2 with any herbal preparation is hazardous.

Others:
Don't self-medicate for any purpose. Cohosh may cause toxic symptoms.

Storage:
- Store in cool, dry area away from direct light, but don't freeze.
- Store safely out of reach of children.
- Don't store in bathroom medicine cabinet. Heat and moisture may change the action of the herb.

Safe dosage:
Consult your doctor for the appropriate dose for your condition.

Toxicity

Rated slightly dangerous, particularly in children, persons over 55 and those who take larger than appropriate quantities for extended periods of time

For symptoms of toxicity: See *Adverse Reactions, Side Effects or Overdose Symptoms* section below.

Adverse Reactions, Side Effects or Overdose Symptoms

Signs and symptoms	What to do
Chest pain	Seek emergency treatment.
Convulsions	Seek emergency treatment.
Dilated pupils	Discontinue. Call doctor immediately.
Headache	Discontinue. Call doctor immediately.
Nausea or vomiting	Discontinue. Call doctor immediately.
Stomach irritation, with possible bleeding	Discontinue. Call doctor immediately.
Thirst	Discontinue. Call doctor when convenient.
Weakness	Discontinue. Call doctor immediately.

Cohosh, White

Basic Information

Biological name (genus and species):
Actaea alba, A. arguta

Parts used for medicinal purposes:
Various parts of the entire plant, frequently differing by country and culture

Chemicals this herb contains:
• Glycosides (see Glossary)
• Protoanemonin
• Volatile oils (see Glossary)

Known Effects
Irritates mucous membranes

Possible Additional Effects
• Potential mild sedative to relieve anxiety
• May help bring on menstruation

Warnings and Precautions

Don't take if you:
• Are pregnant, think you may be pregnant or plan pregnancy in the near future
• Have any chronic disease of the gastrointestinal tract, such as stomach or duodenal ulcers, reflux esophagitis, ulcerative colitis, spastic colitis, diverticulosis or diverticulitis

Consult your doctor if you:
• Take this herb for any medical problem that doesn't improve in 2 weeks (There may be safer, more effective treatments.)
• Take any medicinal drugs or herbs including aspirin, laxatives, cold and cough remedies, antacids, vitamins, minerals, amino acids, supplements, other prescription or nonprescription drugs

Pregnancy:
Dangers outweigh any possible benefits. Don't use.

MEDICINAL HERBS

Breastfeeding:
Dangers outweigh any possible
benefits. Don't use.

Infants and children:
Treating infants and children under
2 with any herbal preparation
is hazardous.

Others:
This product will not help you and
may cause toxic symptoms.

Storage:
• Store in cool, dry area away from
  direct light, but don't freeze.
• Store safely out of reach of children.
• Don't store in bathroom medicine
  cabinet. Heat and moisture may
  change the action of the herb.

Safe dosage:
Consult your doctor for the appropriate dose for your condition.

Toxicity

Comparative-toxicity rating is not available from standard references.

For symptoms of toxicity: See
*Adverse Reactions, Side Effects or
Overdose Symptoms* section below.

Adverse Reactions, Side Effects or Overdose Symptoms

Signs and symptoms	What to do
Diarrhea (sometimes bloody)	Discontinue. Call doctor immediately.
Hallucinations	Seek emergency treatment.
Nausea or vomiting	Discontinue. Call doctor immediately.
Skin rashes or eye irritation, if used on skin or in eye	Discontinue. Call doctor immediately.

Coltsfoot (Coughwort, Horse-hoof)

Basic Information

Biological name (genus and species):
Tussilago farfara

Parts used for medicinal purposes:
• Berries/fruits
• Leaves

Chemicals this herb contains:
• Caoutchouc
• Pectin
• Resin (see Glossary)
• Tannins (see Glossary)
• Volatile oils (see Glossary)

Known Effects

No proven medicinal effects are known.

Miscellaneous information:
• Has been found to have carcinogenic
  properties
• Available as tincture, capsule, bulk

Possible Additional Effects

Internal use:
May treat persistent cough—bronchitis,
allergic, whooping

External use:
May soothe various skin disorders

 Warnings and Precautions

Don't take if you:
Are pregnant, think you may be pregnant or plan pregnancy in the near future.

Consult your doctor if you:
• Take this herb for any medical problem that doesn't improve in 2 weeks (There may be safer, more effective treatments.)
• Take any medicinal drugs or herbs including aspirin, laxatives, cold and cough remedies, antacids, vitamins, minerals, amino acids, supplements, other prescription or nonprescription drugs

Pregnancy:
Don't use unless prescribed by your doctor.

Breastfeeding:
Don't use unless prescribed by your doctor.

Infants and children:
Treating infants and children under 2 with any herbal preparation is hazardous.

Others:
None are expected if you are beyond childhood, under 45, not pregnant, basically healthy, take it for only a short time and do not exceed manufacturer's recommended dose.

Storage:
• Store in cool, dry area away from direct light, but don't freeze.
• Store safely out of reach of children.
• Don't store in bathroom medicine cabinet. Heat and moisture may change the action of the herb.

Safe dosage:
Consult your doctor for the appropriate dose for your condition.

 Toxicity

Coltsfoot is rated relatively safe when taken in small quantities for short periods of time; however, cumulative effects may produce malignant growths.

For symptoms of toxicity: See *Adverse Reactions, Side Effects or Overdose Symptoms* section below.

 Adverse Reactions, Side Effects or Overdose Symptoms

Signs and symptoms	What to do
Abdominal pain	Discontinue. Call doctor immediately.
Fever	Discontinue. Call doctor immediately.
Jaundice (yellow skin and eyes)	Discontinue. Call doctor immediately.
Nausea or vomiting	Discontinue. Call doctor immediately.

MEDICINAL HERBS

Cottonwood (Balm of Gilead)

Basic Information

Biological name (genus and species):
Populus deltoides, P. candicans

Parts used for medicinal purposes:
Roots

Chemicals this herb contains:
Salicin

Known Effects

- Anti-inflammatory
- Reduces pain
- Reduces fever

Miscellaneous information:
Used extensively by Native Americans
for many disorders.

Possible Additional Effects

- May relieve toothache
- May treat arthritis
- May treat heart diseases
- May treat any illness accompanied by
  fever, pain or inflammation

Warnings and Precautions

Don't take if you:
Are pregnant, think you may be
pregnant or plan pregnancy in the
near future.

Consult your doctor if you:
- Take this herb for any medical
  problem that doesn't improve in
  2 weeks (There may be safer, more
  effective treatments.)
- Take any medicinal drugs or
  herbs including aspirin, laxatives,
  cold and cough remedies, antacids,
  vitamins, minerals, amino acids,
  supplements, other prescription
  or nonprescription drugs

Pregnancy:
Don't use unless prescribed by
your doctor.

Breastfeeding:
Don't use unless prescribed by
your doctor.

Infants and children:
Treating infants and children under
2 with any herbal preparation
is hazardous.

Others:
None are expected if you are beyond
childhood, under 45, not pregnant,
basically healthy, take it for only a short
time and do not exceed manufacturer's
recommended dose.

Storage:
- Store in cool, dry area away from
  direct light, but don't freeze.
- Store safely out of reach of children.
- Don't store in bathroom medicine
  cabinet. Heat and moisture may
  change the action of the herb.

Safe dosage:
Consult your doctor for the appropriate dose for your condition.

Toxicity

Comparative-toxicity rating is not available from standard references.

For symptoms of toxicity: See
*Adverse Reactions, Side Effects or
Overdose Symptoms* section below.

Adverse Reactions, Side Effects or Overdose Symptoms

Signs and symptoms	What to do
Coma	Seek emergency treatment.
Confusion	Discontinue. Call doctor immediately.
Convulsions	Seek emergency treatment.

Couch Grass (Dog Grass, Triticum)

Basic Information

Biological name (genus and species):
Agropyrum repens

Parts used for medicinal purposes:
Roots

Chemicals this herb contains:
- Dextrose
- Gum (see Glossary)
- Inosite
- Lactic acid
- Levulose
- Mannite
- Silica
- Vannilin

Known Effects

- Helps body dispose of excess fluid by increasing amount of urine produced
- If contaminated with ergot, causes constriction of blood vessels and muscular spasm of uterus

Miscellaneous information:
Couch grass is frequently contaminated with a poisonous fungus containing ergot. Discard any grass that has a black coating.

Possible Additional Effects

- May protect scraped tissues
- Potential nutrient
- May treat bladder infections
- May treat arthritis

Warnings and Precautions

Don't take if you:
- Are pregnant, think you may be pregnant or plan pregnancy in the near future
- Have any chronic disease of the gastrointestinal tract, such as stomach or duodenal ulcers, reflux esophagitis, ulcerative colitis, spastic colitis, diverticulosis or diverticulitis

MEDICINAL HERBS

➡

Consult your doctor if you:

- Take this herb for any medical problem that doesn't improve in 2 weeks (There may be safer, more effective treatments.)
- Take any medicinal drugs or herbs including aspirin, laxatives, cold and cough remedies, antacids, vitamins, minerals, amino acids, supplements, other prescription or nonprescription drugs

Pregnancy:

Dangers outweigh any possible benefits. Don't use.

Breastfeeding:

Dangers outweigh any possible benefits. Don't use.

Infants and children:

Treating infants and children under 2 with any herbal preparation is hazardous.

Others:

None are expected if you are beyond childhood, under 45, not pregnant, basically healthy, take it for only a short time and do not exceed manufacturer's recommended dose.

Storage:

- Store in cool, dry area away from direct light, but don't freeze.
- Store safely out of reach of children.
- Don't store in bathroom medicine cabinet. Heat and moisture may change the action of the herb.

Safe dosage:

Consult your doctor for the appropriate dose for your condition.

 Toxicity

Comparative-toxicity rating is not available from standard references.

For symptoms of toxicity: See *Adverse Reactions, Side Effects or Overdose Symptoms* section below.

 Adverse Reactions, Side Effects or Overdose Symptoms

Signs and symptoms	What to do
Only if contaminated with ergot:	
Coma	Seek emergency treatment.
Diarrhea	Discontinue. Call doctor when convenient.
Rapid, weak pulse	Seek emergency treatment.
Tingling, itching	Discontinue. Call doctor when convenient.
Unquenchable thirst	Discontinue. Call doctor immediately.
Vomiting	Discontinue. Call doctor immediately.

Cow Parsnip (Hogweed, Keck)

 Basic Information

Biological name (genus and species):
Heracleum lanatum

Parts used for medicinal purposes:
- Fruit
- Leaves
- Roots
- Seeds

Chemicals this herb contains:
Volatile oils (see Glossary)

Known Effects

- Decreases thickness and increases fluidity of mucus in lungs and bronchial tubes
- Depresses central nervous system
- Decreases spasm of smooth muscle or skeletal muscle

Miscellaneous information:

Young plants may look like hemlock, which is poisonous.

Possible Additional Effects

Fruits and leaves are potential sedatives.

Warnings and Precautions

Don't take if you:

Are pregnant, think you may be pregnant or plan pregnancy in the near future.

Consult your doctor if you:

- Take this herb for any medical problem that doesn't improve in 2 weeks (There may be safer, more effective treatments.)
- Take any medicinal drugs or herbs including aspirin, laxatives, cold and cough remedies, antacids, vitamins, minerals, amino acids, supplements, other prescription or nonprescription drugs

Pregnancy:

Dangers outweigh any possible benefits. Don't use.

Breastfeeding:

Dangers outweigh any possible benefits. Don't use.

Infants and children:

Treating infants and children under 2 with any herbal preparation is hazardous.

Others:

None are expected if you are beyond childhood, under 45, not pregnant, basically healthy, take it for only a short time and do not exceed manufacturer's recommended dose.

Storage:

- Store in cool, dry area away from direct light, but don't freeze.
- Store safely out of reach of children.
- Don't store in bathroom medicine cabinet. Heat and moisture may change the action of the herb.

Safe dosage:

Consult your doctor for the appropriate dose for your condition.

Toxicity

Comparative-toxicity rating is not available from standard references.

Adverse Reactions, Side Effects or Overdose Symptoms

None are expected.

MEDICINAL HERBS

Cranesbill (Crowfoot)

Basic Information

Biological name (genus and species):
Geranium maculatum

Parts used for medicinal purposes:
- Leaves
- Roots

Chemicals this herb contains:
- Coloring materials
- Gallic acid
- Gum (see Glossary)
- Pectin
- Starch
- Sugar
- Tannins (see Glossary)

Known Effects

- Produces puckering
- Shrinks tissues
- Prevents secretion of fluids
- Interferes with absorption of iron and other minerals when taken internally

Miscellaneous information:
- Used as a mouthwash and a gargle for sore throat
- Used in traps to kill Japanese beetles which are attracted to it (They die when they eat cranesbill leaves.)
- Used as a poultice (see Glossary)
- Occasionally used as a means of applying medications

Possible Additional Effects

- May increase blood clotting
- Potential astringent
- May decrease nosebleeds
- May treat bleeding from stomach, mouth, intestines
- May treat diarrhea.

Warnings and Precautions

Don't take if you:
- Are pregnant, think you may be pregnant or plan pregnancy in the near future
- Have any chronic disease of the gastrointestinal tract, such as stomach or duodenal ulcers, reflux esophagitis, ulcerative colitis, spastic colitis, diverticulosis or diverticulitis

Consult your doctor if you:
- Take this herb for any medical problem that doesn't improve in 2 weeks (There may be safer, more effective treatments.)
- Take any medicinal drugs or herbs including aspirin, laxatives, cold and cough remedies, antacids, vitamins, minerals, amino acids, supplements, other prescription or nonprescription drugs

Pregnancy:
Don't use unless prescribed by your doctor.

Breastfeeding:
Don't use unless prescribed by your doctor.

Infants and children:
Treating infants and children under 2 with any herbal preparation is hazardous.

Others:
None are expected if you are beyond childhood, under 45, not pregnant, basically healthy, take it for only a short time and do not exceed manufacturer's recommended dose.

Storage:
- Store in cool, dry area away from direct light, but don't freeze.
- Store safely out of reach of children.
- Don't store in bathroom medicine cabinet. Heat and moisture may change the action of the herb.

Safe dosage:

Consult your doctor for the appropriate dose for your condition.

Toxicity

Comparative-toxicity rating is not available from standard references.

For symptoms of toxicity: See *Adverse Reactions, Side Effects or Overdose Symptom* section below.

Adverse Reactions, Side Effects or Overdose Symptoms

Signs and symptoms	What to do
Diarrhea	Discontinue. Call doctor immediately.
Kidney damage characterized by blood in urine, decreased urine flow, swelling of hands and feet	Seek emergency treatment.
Nausea or vomiting	Discontinue. Call doctor immediately.

Cubeb (Java Pepper, Tailed Pepper)

Basic Information

Biological name (genus and species): *Piper cubeba*

Parts used for medicinal purposes: Berries/fruits

Chemicals this herb contains:
- Cubebic acid
- Cubebin
- Fixed oil (see Glossary)
- Gum (see Glossary)
- Resin (see Glossary)
- Sesquiterpene alcohol
- Terpenes (see Glossary)
- Volatile oils (see Glossary)

Known Effects

Cubebic acid irritates the ureter, bladder and urethra.

Miscellaneous information:

Active chemicals are in fully grown, unripe fruit.

Possible Additional Effects

- May help body dispose of excess fluid by increasing amount of urine produced
- Potential urinary antiseptic
- May decrease thickness and increase fluidity of mucus in lungs and bronchial tubes
- May help expel gas from intestinal tract

MEDICINAL HERBS

→

Warnings and Precautions

Don't take if you:
- Are pregnant, think you may be pregnant or plan pregnancy in the near future
- Have any chronic disease of the gastrointestinal tract, such as stomach or duodenal ulcers, reflux esophagitis, ulcerative colitis, spastic colitis, diverticulosis or diverticulitis

Consult your doctor if you:
- Take this herb for any medical problem that doesn't improve in 2 weeks (There may be safer, more effective treatments.)
- Have chronic intestinal disease; cubeb may make it worse

Pregnancy:
Don't use unless prescribed by your doctor.

Breastfeeding:
Don't use unless prescribed by your doctor.

Infants and children:
Treating infants and children under 2 with any herbal preparation is hazardous.

Others:
None are expected if you are beyond childhood, under 45, not pregnant, basically healthy, take it for only a short time and do not exceed manufacturer's recommended dose.

Storage:
- Store in cool, dry area away from direct light, but don't freeze.
- Store safely out of reach of children.
- Don't store in bathroom medicine cabinet. Heat and moisture may change the action of the herb.

Safe dosage:
Consult your doctor for the appropriate dose for your condition.

 ## Toxicity

Comparative-toxicity rating is not available from standard references.

For symptoms of toxicity: See *Adverse Reactions, Side Effects or Overdose Symptoms* section below.

 ## Adverse Reactions, Side Effects or Overdose Symptoms

Signs and symptoms	What to do
Nausea or vomiting	Discontinue. Call doctor immediately.

Elderberry (Elder)

 ## Basic Information

Biological name (genus and species):
Sambucus nigra

Parts used for medicinal purposes:
- Bark
- Berries/fruits
- Inner bark
- Leaves

Chemicals this herb contains:
- Albumin
- Cyanide
- Hydrocyanic acid
- Resin (see Glossary)

- Rutin
- Sambucine
- Sambunigrin (found in stem; breaks down to cyanide)
- Tannic acid
- Tyrosine
- Viburnic acid
- Vitamin C
- Volatile oils (see Glossary)
- Wax (see Glossary)

Known Effects

- Irritates the gastrointestinal tract and acts as a laxative and purgative
- Causes vomiting (sometimes)

Miscellaneous information:
Stems contain cyanide and can be extremely toxic.

Possible Additional Effects

- May help treat headache
- May help treat arthritis
- May help treat gout
- May help treat the common cold
- May help treat fevers
- May help treat sore throat
- May ease discomfort of menstrual cramps
- May promote healing of bruises and sprains when used as a poultice (see Glossary)
- May help treat skin irritations

Warnings and Precautions

Don't take if you:
- Are pregnant, think you may be pregnant or plan pregnancy in the near future
- Have any chronic disease of the gastrointestinal tract, such as stomach or duodenal ulcers, reflux esophagitis, ulcerative colitis, spastic colitis, diverticulosis or diverticulitis

Consult your doctor if you:
- Take this herb for any medical problem that doesn't improve in 2 weeks (There may be safer, more effective treatments.)
- Take any medicinal drugs or herbs including aspirin, laxatives, cold and cough remedies, antacids, vitamins, minerals, amino acids, supplements, other prescription or nonprescription drugs

Pregnancy:
Dangers outweigh any possible benefits. Don't use.

Breastfeeding:
Dangers outweigh any possible benefits. Don't use.

Infants and children:
Treating infants and children under 2 with any herbal preparation is hazardous.

Others:
- Ripe berries are probably nontoxic. They should be eaten only after cooking.
- Beware of stems. Enough cyanide from them could be fatal.

Storage:
- Store in cool, dry area away from direct light, but don't freeze.
- Store safely out of reach of children.
- Don't store in bathroom medicine cabinet. Heat and moisture may change the action of the herb.

Safe dosage:
Consult your doctor for the appropriate dose for your condition.

Toxicity

- Elderberry is rated slightly dangerous, particularly in children, persons over 55 and those who take larger than appropriate quantities for extended periods of time.
- Raw seeds are toxic.

MEDICINAL HERBS

➜

- Roots, stems and leaves can cause cyanide poisoning.

For symptoms of toxicity: See *Adverse Reactions, Side Effects or Overdose Symptoms* section below.

 Adverse Reactions, Side Effects or Overdose Symptoms

Signs and symptoms	What to do
Abdominal pain	Discontinue. Call doctor immediately.
Diarrhea	Discontinue. Call doctor immediately.
Nausea or vomiting	Discontinue. Call doctor immediately.

Fennel (Finocchio)

 Basic Information

Biological name (genus and species): *Foeniculum vulgare*

Parts used for medicinal purposes:
- Berries/fruits
- Roots
- Stems

Chemicals this herb contains:
- Anethole
- Fixed oil (see Glossary)
- Volatile oils (see Glossary)

 Known Effects

- Helps expel gas from intestinal tract
- Stimulates respiration
- Increases stomach acidity
- Treats dyspepsia
- Helps treat common colds
- Treats coughs
- Treats colic

Miscellaneous information:
- Used as a flavoring
- Available in dry bulk, oil and tinctures

 Possible Additional Effects

May treat diarrhea

 Warnings and Precautions

Don't take if you:
- Are pregnant, think you may be pregnant or plan pregnancy in the near future
- Have any chronic disease of the gastrointestinal tract, such as stomach or duodenal ulcers, reflux esophagitis, ulcerative colitis, spastic colitis, diverticulosis or diverticulitis

Consult your doctor if you:
- Take this herb for any medical problem that doesn't improve in 2 weeks (There may be safer, more effective treatments.)
- Take any medicinal drugs or herbs including aspirin, laxatives, cold and cough remedies, antacids, vitamins, minerals, amino acids, supplements, other prescription or nonprescription drugs

Pregnancy:
Dangers outweigh any possible benefits. Don't use.

Breastfeeding:
Dangers outweigh any possible benefits. Don't use.

Infants and children:
Treating infants and children under 2 with any herbal preparation is hazardous.

Others:
None are expected if you are beyond childhood, under 45, not pregnant, basically healthy, take it for only a short time and do not exceed manufacturer's recommended dose.

Storage:
- Store in cool, dry area away from direct light, but don't freeze.
- Store safely out of reach of children.

- Don't store in bathroom medicine cabinet. Heat and moisture may change the action of the herb.

Safe dosage:
Consult your doctor for the appropriate dose for your condition.

 Toxicity

Generally regarded as safe when taken in appropriate quantities for short periods of time

For symptoms of toxicity: See *Adverse Reactions, Side Effects or Overdose Symptoms* section below.

 Adverse Reactions, Side Effects or Overdose Symptoms

Signs and symptoms	What to do
Oil extracted from fennel may cause	
Congestive heart failure	Seek emergency treatment.
Nausea or vomiting	Discontinue. Call doctor immediately.
Rash	Discontinue. Call doctor when convenient.
Seizures	Seek emergency treatment.

Fenugreek

 Basic Information

Biological name (genus and species): *Trigonella foenumgraecum*

Parts used for medicinal purposes: Seeds

Chemicals this herb contains:
- Choline
- Fixed oil (see Glossary)
- Iron
- Lecithin
- Mucilage (see Glossary)
- Phosphates (see Glossary)
- Protein

- Trigonelline
- Trimethylamine
- Volatile oils (see Glossary)

Known Effects

- Increases stomach acidity
- Reduces sore throat

Miscellaneous information:

- Fenugreek has a disagreeable odor and bitter taste.
- It is prescribed frequently by veterinarians, particularly for horses.
- Fenugreek is available in bulk seeds, capsules and tinctures.

Possible Additional Effects

- Potential bulk laxative (seeds)
- May protect scraped tissues
- May reduce arthritic pain
- May promote lactation

Warnings and Precautions

Don't take if you:

Are pregnant, think you may be pregnant or plan pregnancy in the near future.

Consult your doctor if you:

- Take this herb for any medical problem that doesn't improve in 2 weeks (There may be safer, more effective treatments.)
- Take any medicinal drugs or herbs including aspirin, laxatives, cold and cough remedies, antacids, vitamins, minerals, amino acids, supplements, other prescription or nonprescription drugs

Pregnancy:
Don't use unless prescribed by your doctor.

Breastfeeding:
Don't use unless prescribed by your doctor.

Infants and children:
Treating infants and children under 2 with any herbal preparation is hazardous.

Storage:

- Store in cool, dry area away from direct light, but don't freeze.
- Store safely out of reach of children.
- Don't store in bathroom medicine cabinet. Heat and moisture may change the action of the herb.

Safe dosage:
Consult your doctor for the appropriate dose for your condition.

Toxicity

Rated relatively safe when taken in appropriate quantities for short periods of time

Adverse Reactions, Side Effects or Overdose Symptoms

None are expected.

Fritillaria (Bei Mu, Snake's Head)

Basic Information

Biological name (genus and species):
Fritillaria verticillata, F. meleagris

Parts used for medicinal purposes:
Roots

Chemicals this herb contains:
- Fritimine
- Fritilline
- Peimine
- Peiminine
- Verticilline
- Verticine

(Peimine and peiminine may resemble steroid hormones.)

Known Effects

- May decrease blood pressure
- May increase blood sugar

Miscellaneous information:
Only roots have medicinal properties.

Possible Additional Effects

- May affect the electrical system of the heart (because of peimine and peiminine)
- May reduce fevers
- May decrease thickness and increase fluidity of mucus in lungs and bronchial tubes
- May increase flow of breast milk in lactating women

Warnings and Precautions

Don't take if you:
- Are pregnant, think you may be pregnant or plan pregnancy in the near future
- Have heart disease

Consult your doctor if you:
- Take this herb for any medical problem that doesn't improve in 2 weeks (There may be safer, more effective treatments.)
- Take any medicinal drugs or herbs including aspirin, laxatives, cold and cough remedies, antacids, vitamins, minerals, amino acids, supplements, other prescription or nonprescription drugs

Pregnancy:
Dangers outweigh any possible benefits. Don't use.

Breastfeeding:
Dangers outweigh any possible benefits. Don't use.

Infants and children:
Treating infants and children under 2 with any herbal preparation is hazardous.

Others:
None are expected if you are beyond childhood, under 45, not pregnant, basically healthy, take it for only a short time and do not exceed manufacturer's recommended dose.

Storage:
- Store in cool, dry area away from direct light, but don't freeze.
- Store safely out of reach of children.

MEDICINAL HERBS

- Don't store in bathroom medicine cabinet. Heat and moisture may change the action of the herb.

Safe dosage:

Consult your doctor for the appropriate dose for your condition.

 Toxicity

Comparative-toxicity rating is not available from standard references.

For symptoms of toxicity: See *Adverse Reactions, Side Effects or Overdose Symptoms* section below.

 Adverse Reactions, Side Effects or Overdose Symptoms

Signs and symptoms	What to do
Heart block characterized by slow heart rate (below 50)	Seek emergency treatment.
Heartbeat irregularity	Discontinue. Call doctor immediately.

Galanga Major & Minor (Chinese Ginger, India Root)

 Basic Information

Biological name (genus and species): *Alpinia galanga, A. officinarum*

Parts used for medicinal purposes: Various parts of the entire plant, frequently differing by country and culture

Chemicals this herb contains:

- Cineole
- Galangin
- Galangol
- Kaempferid
- Resin (see Glossary)
- Volatile oils (see Glossary)

 Known Effects

Antibacterial effect acts against bacterial germs, such as streptococci, staphylococci and coliform bacteria.

Miscellaneous information:

- Related botanically and pharmacologically to ginger
- Used by ancient Greeks and Arabs

 Possible Additional Effects

- May help expel gas from intestinal tract
- May treat impotence
- May reduce excess phlegm caused by allergies
- May treat painful teeth and gums
- May stimulate respiration

 Warnings and Precautions

Don't take if you:

- Are pregnant, think you may be pregnant or plan pregnancy in the near future
- Have any chronic disease of the gastrointestinal tract, such as stomach or duodenal ulcers, reflux

esophagitis, ulcerative colitis, spastic colitis, diverticulosis or diverticulitis

Consult your doctor if you:
- Take this herb for any medical problem that doesn't improve in 2 weeks (There may be safer, more effective treatments.)
- Take any medicinal drugs or herbs including aspirin, laxatives, cold and cough remedies, antacids, vitamins, minerals, amino acids, supplements, other prescription or nonprescription drugs

Pregnancy:
Don't use unless prescribed by your doctor.

Breastfeeding:
Don't use unless prescribed by your doctor.

Infants and children:
Treating infants and children under 2 with any herbal preparation is hazardous.

Others:
None are expected if you are beyond childhood, under 45, not pregnant, basically healthy, take it for only a short time and do not exceed manufacturer's recommended dose.

Storage:
- Store in cool, dry area away from direct light, but don't freeze.
- Store safely out of reach of children.
- Don't store in bathroom medicine cabinet. Heat and moisture may change the action of the herb.

Safe dosage:
Consult your doctor for the appropriate dose for your condition.

Toxicity

Comparative-toxicity rating is not available from standard references.

For symptoms of toxicity: See *Adverse Reactions, Side Effects or Overdose Symptoms* section below.

Adverse Reactions, Side Effects or Overdose Symptoms

Signs and symptoms	What to do
Diarrhea	Discontinue. Call doctor immediately.
Nausea or vomiting	Discontinue. Call doctor immediately.

Galega (European Goat Rue)

Basic Information

Biological name (genus and species):
Galega officinalis

Parts used for medicinal purposes:
Various parts of the entire plant, frequently differing by country and culture

Chemicals this herb contains:
- Bitters (see Glossary)
- Galegine
- Tannins (see Glossary)

Known Effects
- Reduces blood sugar
- Interferes with absorption of iron and other minerals when taken internally

MEDICINAL HERBS

➜

Miscellaneous information:
Plant smells bad when it is bruised.

Possible Additional Effects

- May treat diabetes
- Increases flow of breast milk in lactating women

Warnings and Precautions

Don't take if you:
Are pregnant, think you may be pregnant or plan pregnancy in the near future.

Consult your doctor if you:
- Take this herb for any medical problem that doesn't improve in 2 weeks (There may be safer, more effective treatments.)
- Take any medicinal drugs or herbs including aspirin, laxatives, cold and cough remedies, antacids, vitamins, minerals, amino acids, supplements, other prescription or nonprescription drugs

Pregnancy:
Don't use unless prescribed by your doctor.

Breastfeeding:
Don't use unless prescribed by your doctor.

Infants and children:
Treating infants and children under 2 with any herbal preparation is hazardous.

Others:
None are expected if you are beyond childhood, under 45, not pregnant, basically healthy, take it for only a short time and do not exceed manufacturer's recommended dose.

Storage:
- Store in cool, dry area away from direct light, but don't freeze.
- Store safely out of reach of children.
- Don't store in bathroom medicine cabinet. Heat and moisture may change the action of the herb.

Safe dosage:
Consult your doctor for the appropriate dose for your condition.

Toxicity

Comparative-toxicity rating is not available from standard references.

For symptoms of toxicity: See *Adverse Reactions, Side Effects or Overdose Symptoms* section below.

Adverse Reactions, Side Effects or Overdose Symptoms

Signs and symptoms	What to do
Headache	Discontinue. Call doctor when convenient.
Jitters	Discontinue. Call doctor when convenient.
Weakness	Discontinue. Call doctor immediately.

Gambier (Gambir, Pale Catechu)

Basic Information

Biological name (genus and species):
Uncaria gambir

Parts used for medicinal purposes:
- Leaves
- Twigs

Chemicals this herb contains:
- Catechin
- Catechu-tannic acid
- Tannins (see Glossary)

Known Effects

- Shrinks tissues
- Prevents secretion of fluids
- Interferes with absorption of iron and other minerals when taken internally

Possible Additional Effects

- May decrease unusual bleeding
- May treat chronic diarrhea
- May treat sore throats as a gargle

Warnings and Precautions

Don't take if you:

Have any chronic disease of the gastrointestinal tract, such as stomach or duodenal ulcers, reflux esophagitis, ulcerative colitis, spastic colitis, diverticulosis or diverticulitis.

Consult your doctor if you:

- Take this herb for any medical problem that doesn't improve in 2 weeks (There may be safer, more effective treatments.)
- Take any medicinal drugs or herbs including aspirin, laxatives, cold and cough remedies, antacids, vitamins, minerals, amino acids, supplements, other prescription or nonprescription drugs

Pregnancy:

Dangers outweigh any possible benefits. Don't use.

Breastfeeding:

Dangers outweigh any possible benefits. Don't use.

Infants and children:

Treating infants and children under 2 with any herbal preparation is hazardous.

Storage:

- Store in cool, dry area away from direct light, but don't freeze.
- Store safely out of reach of children.
- Don't store in bathroom medicine cabinet. Heat and moisture may change the action of the herb.

Safe dosage:

Consult your doctor for the appropriate dose for your condition.

Toxicity

Rated relatively safe when taken in appropriate quantities for short periods of time

For symptoms of toxicity: See *Adverse Reactions, Side Effects or Overdose Symptoms* section below.

MEDICINAL HERBS

→

Adverse Reactions, Side Effects or Overdose Symptoms

Signs and symptoms	What to do
Diarrhea	Discontinue. Call doctor immediately.
Kidney damage characterized by blood in urine, decreased urine flow, swelling of hands and feet	Seek emergency treatment.
Vomiting	Discontinue. Call doctor immediately.

Gentian (Yellow Gentian)

Basic Information

Biological name (genus and species):
Gentiana lutea

Parts used for medicinal purposes:
Roots

Chemicals this herb contains:
- Gentiamarin
- Gentiin
- Gentiopicrin
- Gentisin
- Sugar
- Xanthone pigment

Known Effects

- Irritates mucous membranes
- Kills plasmodium, which causes malaria

Miscellaneous information:
Used since ancient times in Greece.

Possible Additional Effects

- May increase contractions of stomach muscles
- May stimulate gastric secretions
- May stimulate appetite when used as a tonic
- May aid digestion

Warnings and Precautions

Don't take if you:
- Are pregnant, think you may be pregnant or plan pregnancy in the near future
- Have any chronic disease of the gastrointestinal tract, such as stomach or duodenal ulcers, reflux esophagitis, ulcerative colitis, spastic colitis, diverticulosis or diverticulitis

Consult your doctor if you:
- Take this herb for any medical problem that doesn't improve in 2 weeks (There may be safer, more

effective treatments.)

- Take any medicinal drugs or herbs including aspirin, laxatives, cold and cough remedies, antacids, vitamins, minerals, amino acids, supplements, other prescription or nonprescription drugs

Pregnancy:
Don't use unless prescribed by your doctor.

Breastfeeding:
Don't use unless prescribed by your doctor.

Infants and children:
Treating infants and children under 2 with any herbal preparation is hazardous.

Others:
None are expected if you are beyond childhood, under 45, not pregnant, basically healthy, take it for only a short time and do not exceed manufacturer's recommended dose.

Storage:
- Store in cool, dry area away from direct light, but don't freeze.
- Store safely out of reach of children.
- Don't store in bathroom medicine cabinet. Heat and moisture may change the action of the herb.

Safe dosage:
Consult your doctor for the appropriate dose for your condition.

 Toxicity

Rated relatively safe when taken in appropriate quantities for short periods of time.

For symptoms of toxicity: See *Adverse Reactions, Side Effects or Overdose Symptoms* section below.

 Adverse Reactions, Side Effects or Overdose Symptoms

Signs and symptoms	What to do
Nausea or vomiting	Discontinue. Call doctor immediately.

German Chamomile (Hungarian Chamomile, Matricaria)

 Basic Information

Biological name (genus and species): *Matricaria chamomilla*

Parts used for medicinal purposes: Petals/flower

Chemicals this herb contains:
- Alphabisabolol
- Azulene
- Fatty acid
- Furfural
- Paraffin hydrocarbons
- Sesquiterpene
- Sesquiterpene alcohol
- Tannins (see Glossary)

 Known Effects

- Anti-inflammatory
- Weakens muscles
- Interferes with absorption of iron and other minerals when taken internally

Miscellaneous information:
- Ice cream, candy and liqueur manufacturers use small, nontoxic amounts for flavoring.
- It is also used as a tonic.

➜

MEDICINAL HERBS

Possible Additional Effects

- Relieves spasms in skeletal or smooth muscle
- Is used as a tonic
- Potential sedative
- May help expel gas from intestinal tract

Warnings and Precautions

Don't take if you:

- Are pregnant, think you may be pregnant or plan pregnancy in the near future
- Have any chronic disease of the gastrointestinal tract, such as stomach or duodenal ulcers, reflux esophagitis, ulcerative colitis, spastic colitis, diverticulosis or diverticulitis

Consult your doctor if you:

- Take this herb for any medical problem that doesn't improve in 2 weeks (There may be safer, more effective treatments.)
- Take any medicinal drugs or herbs including aspirin, laxatives, cold and cough remedies, antacids, vitamins, minerals, amino acids, supplements, other prescription or nonprescription drugs

Pregnancy:

Don't use unless prescribed by your doctor.

Breastfeeding:

Don't use unless prescribed by your doctor.

Infants and children:

Treating infants and children under 2 with any herbal preparation is hazardous.

Others:

None are expected if you are beyond childhood, under 45, not pregnant, basically healthy, take it for only a short time and do not exceed manufacturer's recommended dose.

Storage:

- Store in cool, dry area away from direct light, but don't freeze.
- Store safely out of reach of children.
- Don't store in bathroom medicine cabinet. Heat and moisture may change the action of the herb.

Safe dosage:

Consult your doctor for the appropriate dose for your condition.

Toxicity

Generally regarded as safe when taken in appropriate quantities for short periods of time

For symptoms of toxicity: See *Adverse Reactions, Side Effects or Overdose Symptoms* section below.

Adverse Reactions, Side Effects or Overdose Symptoms

Signs and symptoms	What to do
Diarrhea	Discontinue. Call doctor immediately.
Excess sedation	Discontinue. Call doctor immediately.
Nausea or vomiting	Discontinue. Call doctor immediately.
Skin eruptions	Discontinue. Call doctor when convenient.

Grape Hyacinth

 Basic Information

Biological name (genus and species):
Muscari racemosum, M. comosum

Parts used for medicinal purposes:
Bulb

Chemicals this herb contains:
• Comisic acid
• Saponin (see Glossary)

 Known Effects

Irritates gastrointestinal tract

 Possible Additional Effects

• May treat constipation
• May stimulate central nervous system
• May help body dispose of excess fluid by increasing amount of urine produced

 Warnings and Precautions

Don't take if you:
• Are pregnant, think you may be pregnant or plan pregnancy in the near future
• Have any chronic disease of the gastrointestinal tract, such as stomach or duodenal ulcers, reflux esophagitis, ulcerative colitis, spastic colitis, diverticulosis or diverticulitis

Consult your doctor if you:
• Take this herb for any medical problem that doesn't improve in 2 weeks (There may be safer, more effective treatments.)

• Take any medicinal drugs or herbs including aspirin, laxatives, cold and cough remedies, antacids, vitamins, minerals, amino acids, supplements, other prescription or nonprescription drugs

Pregnancy:
Dangers outweigh any possible benefits. Don't use.

Breastfeeding:
Dangers outweigh any possible benefits. Don't use.

Infants and children:
Treating infants and children under 2 with any herbal preparation is hazardous.

Others:
No evidence of any useful therapeutic effect exists. Don't use.

Storage:
• Store in cool, dry area away from direct light, but don't freeze.
• Store safely out of reach of children.
• Don't store in bathroom medicine cabinet. Heat and moisture may change the action of the herb.

Safe dosage:
Consult your doctor for the appropriate dose for your condition.

 Toxicity

Comparative-toxicity rating is not available from standard references.

For symptoms of toxicity: See *Adverse Reactions, Side Effects or Overdose Symptoms* section below.

MEDICINAL HERBS

→

Adverse Reactions, Side Effects or Overdose Symptoms

Signs and symptoms	What to do
Diarrhea	Discontinue. Call doctor immediately.
Nausea or vomiting	Discontinue. Call doctor immediately.

Grindelia (Gumweed, Rosinweed)

Basic Information

Biological name (genus and species):
Grindelia camporum, G. squarrosa

Parts used for medicinal purposes:
Leaves

Chemicals this herb contains:
- Balsamic resin
- Grindelol
- Robustic acid
- Saponins (see Glossary)
- Tannins (see Glossary)
- Volatile oils (see Glossary)

Known Effects

- Depresses central nervous system (in high amounts)
- Dilates pupils of eyes
- Decreases heart rate
- Increases blood pressure
- Interferes with absorption of iron and other minerals when taken internally

Miscellaneous information:
Used in poultices (see Glossary) as a means of applying medications.

Possible Additional Effects

- May decrease thickness and increase fluidity of mucus in lungs and bronchial tubes
- Potential sedative
- May treat asthma
- May treat bronchitis
- May soothe and heal burns when applied topically
- May treat vaginitis

Warnings and Precautions

Don't take if you:
Are pregnant, think you may be pregnant or plan pregnancy in the near future.

Consult your doctor if you:
- Take this herb for any medical problem that doesn't improve in 2 weeks (There may be safer, more effective treatments.)
- Take any medicinal drugs or herbs including aspirin, laxatives, cold and cough remedies, antacids, vitamins, minerals, amino acids, supplements, other prescription or nonprescription drugs

Pregnancy:
Dangers outweigh any possible
benefits. Don't use.

Breastfeeding:
Dangers outweigh any possible
benefits. Don't use.

Infants and children:
Treating infants and children under
2 with any herbal preparation
is hazardous.

Storage:
- Store in cool, dry area away from
  direct light, but don't freeze.
- Store safely out of reach of children.
- Don't store in bathroom medicine
  cabinet. Heat and moisture may
  change the action of the herb.

Safe dosage:
Consult your doctor for the appropriate dose for your condition.

Toxicity

Rated slightly dangerous, particularly in
children, persons over 55 and those
who take larger than appropriate
quantities for extended periods of time

For symptoms of toxicity: See
*Adverse Reactions, Side Effects or
Overdose Symptoms* section below.

Adverse Reactions, Side Effects or Overdose Symptoms

Signs and symptoms	What to do
Kidney damage characterized by blood in urine, decreased urine flow, swelling of hands and feet	Seek emergency treatment.

Guaiac

Basic Information

Biological name (genus and species):
Guaiacum officinale, G. sanctum

Parts used for medicinal purposes:
Stems

Chemicals this herb contains:
- Guaiaconic acid
- Guaiaretic acid
- Resin (see Glossary)
- Saponin (see Glossary)
- Vanillin

Known Effects
- Irritates gastrointestinal tract
- Increases perspiration

- Tests for oxidizing enzymes to detect
  blood in stool or urine

Miscellaneous information:
When added to a stool specimen,
hydrogen peroxide and guaiac estab-
lish the presence or absence of blood.
This test is a useful screening proce-
dure to detect malignant and nonma-
lignant disorders of the intestinal tract.

Possible Additional Effects
- May treat arthritis
- May treat scrofula
- May treat constipation
- May reduce edema

MEDICINAL HERBS

Warnings and Precautions

Don't take if you:
- Are pregnant, think you may be pregnant or plan pregnancy in the near future
- Have any chronic disease of the gastrointestinal tract, such as stomach or duodenal ulcers, reflux esophagitis, ulcerative colitis, spastic colitis, diverticulosis or diverticulitis

Consult your doctor if you:
- Take this herb for any medical problem that doesn't improve in 2 weeks (There may be safer, more effective treatments.)
- Take any medicinal drugs or herbs including aspirin, laxatives, cold and cough remedies, antacids, vitamins, minerals, amino acids, supplements, other prescription or nonprescription drugs

Pregnancy:
Dangers outweigh any possible benefits. Don't use.

Breastfeeding:
Dangers outweigh any possible benefits. Don't use.

Infants and children:
Treating infants and children under 2 with any herbal preparation is hazardous.

Others:
None are expected if you are beyond childhood, under 45, not pregnant, basically healthy, take it for only a short time and do not exceed manufacturer's recommended dose.

Storage:
- Store in cool, dry area away from direct light, but don't freeze.
- Store safely out of reach of children.
- Don't store in bathroom medicine cabinet. Heat and moisture may change the action of the herb.

Safe dosage:
Consult your doctor for the appropriate dose for your condition.

 ## Toxicity

Comparative-toxicity rating is not available from standard references.

For symptoms of toxicity: See *Adverse Reactions, Side Effects or Overdose Symptoms* section below.

 ## Adverse Reactions, Side Effects or Overdose Symptoms

Signs and symptoms	What to do
Nausea or vomiting	Discontinue. Call doctor immediately.

Harmel (African Rue, Syrian Rue, Wild Rue)

 ## Basic Information

Biological name (genus and species):
Peganum harmala

Parts used for medicinal purposes:
Various parts of the entire plant, frequently differing by country and culture

Chemicals this herb contains:
- Harmaline
- Harmalol
- Harmine
- Peganine

Known Effects

- Causes hallucinations
- Destroys bacteria (germs) and suppresses their growth or reproduction

Miscellaneous information:
Wild rue is often abused where it grows in Arizona, New Mexico and Texas.

Possible Additional Effects

- May destroy intestinal worms
- May decrease pain

Warnings and Precautions

Don't take if you:
Are pregnant, think you may be pregnant or plan pregnancy in the near future.

Consult your doctor if you:
- Take this herb for any medical problem that doesn't improve in 2 weeks (There may be safer, more effective treatments.)
- Take any medicinal drugs or herbs including aspirin, laxatives, cold and cough remedies, antacids, vitamins, minerals, amino acids, supplements, other prescription or nonprescription drugs

Pregnancy:
Dangers outweigh any possible benefits. Don't use.

Breastfeeding:
Dangers outweigh any possible benefits. Don't use.

Infants and children:
Treating infants and children under 2 with any herbal preparation is hazardous.

Others:
Dangers outweigh any possible benefits. Do use.

Storage:
- Store in cool, dry area away from direct light, but don't freeze.
- Store safely out of reach of children.
- Don't store in bathroom medicine cabinet. Heat and moisture may change the action of the herb.

Safe dosage:
Consult your doctor for the appropriate dose for your condition.

Toxicity

Rated slightly dangerous, particularly in children, persons over 55 and those who take larger than appropriate quantities for extended periods of time

For symptoms of toxicity: See *Adverse Reactions, Side Effects or Overdose Symptoms* section below.

Adverse Reactions, Side Effects or Overdose Symptoms

Signs and symptoms	What to do
Hallucinations	Seek emergency treatment.
Muscle weakness	Discontinue. Call doctor immediately.

MEDICINAL HERBS

Heliotrope (Turnsole)

Basic Information

Biological name (genus and species):
Heliotropium europaeum

Parts used for medicinal purposes:
• Juice
• Leaves
• Seeds

Chemicals this herb contains:
• Heliotrine
• Lasiocarpine

Known Effects

• Kills liver cells
• Stimulates production of bile

Miscellaneous information:
Heliotrope is a common weed.

Possible Additional Effects

Leaves and juice may treat ulcers,
warts, polyps and tumors.

Warnings and Precautions

Don't take if you:
Are pregnant, think you may be
pregnant or plan pregnancy in the
near future.

Consult your doctor if you:
• Take this herb for any medical
  problem that doesn't improve in
  2 weeks (There may be safer, more
  effective treatments.)
• Take any medicinal drugs or
  herbs including aspirin, laxatives,
  cold and cough remedies, antacids,
  vitamins, minerals, amino acids,
  supplements, other prescription
  or nonprescription drugs

Pregnancy:
Dangers outweigh any possible
benefits. Don't use.

Breastfeeding:
Dangers outweigh any possible
benefits. Don't use.

Infants and children:
Treating infants and children under
2 with any herbal preparation
is hazardous.

Storage:
• Store in cool, dry area away from
  direct light, but don't freeze.
• Store safely out of reach of children.
• Don't store in bathroom medicine
  cabinet. Heat and moisture may
  change the action of the herb.

Safe dosage:
Consult your doctor for the appropriate dose for your condition.

Toxicity

Rated slightly dangerous, particularly in
children, persons over 55 and those
who take larger than appropriate
quantities for extended periods of time

For symptoms of toxicity: See
*Adverse Reactions, Side Effects or
Overdose Symptoms* section below.

Adverse Reactions, Side Effects or Overdose Symptoms

Signs and symptoms	What to do
Jaundice (yellow skin and eyes)	Discontinue. Call doctor immediately.

Hellebore (American Hellebore, Green Hellebore)

Basic Information

Biological name (genus and species):
Veratrum viride

Parts used for medicinal purposes:
- Rhizomes
- Root

Chemicals this herb contains:
- Germidine
- Germitrine
- Jervine
- Pseudojervine
- Rubijervine
- Veratrum alkaloids

Known Effects

- Decreases blood pressure
- Decreases heart rate
- Depresses central nervous system

Possible Additional Effects

- May treat hypertension
- May treat toxemia of pregnancy
- May irritate gastrointestinal system

Warnings and Precautions

Don't take if you:
- Are pregnant, think you may be pregnant or plan pregnancy in the near future
- Have any chronic disease of the gastrointestinal tract, such as stomach or duodenal ulcers, reflux esophagitis, ulcerative colitis, spastic colitis, diverticulosis or diverticulitis

Consult your doctor if you:
- Take this herb for any medical problem that doesn't improve in 2 weeks (There may be safer, more effective treatments.)
- Take any medicinal drugs or herbs including aspirin, laxatives, cold and cough remedies, antacids, vitamins, minerals, amino acids, supplements, other prescription or nonprescription drugs

Pregnancy:
Dangers outweigh any possible benefits. Don't use.

Breastfeeding:
Dangers outweigh any possible benefits. Don't use.

Infants and children:
Treating infants and children under 2 with any herbal preparation is hazardous.

Others:
All parts of the plant may be toxic.

Storage:
- Store in cool, dry area away from direct light, but don't freeze.
- Store safely out of reach of children.
- Don't store in bathroom medicine cabinet. Heat and moisture may change the action of the herb.

Safe dosage:
Consult your doctor for the appropriate dose for your condition.

Toxicity

Rated dangerous, particularly in children, persons over 55 and those who take larger than appropriate quantities for extended periods of time

MEDICINAL HERBS

→

For symptoms of toxicity: See *Adverse Reactions, Side Effects or Overdose Symptoms* section below.

Adverse Reactions, Side Effects or Overdose Symptoms

Signs and symptoms	What to do
Abdominal pain	Discontinue. Call doctor immediately.
Burning sensation in mouth	Discontinue. Call doctor when convenient.
Diarrhea	Discontinue. Call doctor immediately.
Headache	Discontinue. Call doctor when convenient.
Nausea or vomiting	Discontinue. Call doctor immediately.
Precipitous blood-pressure drop: symptoms include faintness, cold sweat, paleness, rapid pulse	Seek emergency treatment.

Helonias (Fairy Wand, False Unicorn Root)

Basic Information

Biological name (genus and species): *Chamaelirium luteum*

Parts used for medicinal purposes: Roots

Chemicals this herb contains:
• Chamaelirin
• Saponin (see Glossary)

Known Effects

• Irritates gastrointestinal system
• Helps body dispose of excess fluid by increasing amount of urine produced
• Produces puckering

Possible Additional Effects

• May prevent miscarriage
• May treat menopause symptoms
• May increase appetite
• Potential vigorous laxative

Warnings and Precautions

Don't take if you:
• Are pregnant, think you may be pregnant or plan pregnancy in the near future
• Have any chronic disease of the gastrointestinal tract, such as stomach or duodenal ulcers, reflux esophagitis, ulcerative colitis, spastic colitis, diverticulosis or diverticulitis

Consult your doctor if you:
• Take this herb for any medical problem that doesn't improve in 2 weeks (There may be safer, more effective treatments.)
• Take any medicinal drugs or herbs including aspirin, laxatives, cold and cough remedies, antacids, vitamins, minerals, amino acids, supplements, other prescription or nonprescription drugs

Pregnancy:
Dangers outweigh any possible benefits. Don't use.

Breastfeeding:
Dangers outweigh any possible benefits. Don't use.

Infants and children:
Treating infants and children under 2 with any herbal preparation is hazardous.

Others:
None are expected if you are beyond childhood, under 45, not pregnant, basically healthy, take it for only a short time and do not exceed manufacturer's recommended dose.

Storage:
- Store in cool, dry area away from direct light, but don't freeze.
- Store safely out of reach of children.
- Don't store in bathroom medicine cabinet. Heat and moisture may change the action of the herb.

Safe dosage:
Consult your doctor for the appropriate dose for your condition.

 Toxicity

Comparative-toxicity rating is not available from standard references.

For symptoms of toxicity: See *Adverse Reactions, Side Effects or Overdose Symptoms* section below.

 Adverse Reactions, Side Effects or Overdose Symptoms

Signs and symptoms	What to do
Diarrhea	Discontinue. Call doctor immediately.
Nausea	Discontinue. Call doctor immediately.

Henbane (Hyoscyamus)

 Basic Information

Biological name (genus and species):
Hyoscyamus niger

Parts used for medicinal purposes:
- Berries/fruits
- Leaves
- Roots

Chemicals this herb contains:
- Hyoscyamine
- Scopolamine

 Known Effects

Blocks effects of parasympathetic nervous system, causing increased heart rate, dilated pupils, dry mouth, hallucinations, urinary retention, reduced contractions of gastrointestinal tract

Miscellaneous information:
- Henbane is poisonous, especially to children!
- It's used as a mouthwash and painkiller.

 Possible Additional Effects

- May treat whooping cough
- May treat asthma
- Potential sedative

MEDICINAL HERBS

Warnings and Precautions

Don't take if you:

• Are pregnant, think you may be pregnant or plan pregnancy in the near future
• Have any chronic disease of the gastrointestinal tract, such as stomach or duodenal ulcers, reflux esophagitis, ulcerative colitis, spastic colitis, diverticulosis or diverticulitis

Consult your doctor if you:

• Take this herb for any medical problem that doesn't improve in 2 weeks (There may be safer, more effective treatments.)
• Take any medicinal drugs or herbs including aspirin, laxatives, cold and cough remedies, antacids, vitamins, minerals, amino acids, supplements, other prescription or nonprescription drugs

Pregnancy:

Dangers outweigh any possible benefits. Don't use.

Breastfeeding:

Dangers outweigh any possible benefits. Don't use.

Infants and children:

Treating infants and children under 2 with any herbal preparation is hazardous.

Others:

None are expected if you are beyond childhood, under 45, not pregnant, basically healthy, take it for only a short time and do not exceed manufacturer's recommended dose.

Storage:

• Store in cool, dry area away from direct light, but don't freeze.
• Store safely out of reach of children.
• Don't store in bathroom medicine cabinet. Heat and moisture may change the action of the herb.

Safe dosage:

Consult your doctor for the appropriate dose for your condition.

Toxicity

Comparative-toxicity rating is not available from standard references.

For symptoms of toxicity: See *Adverse Reactions, Side Effects or Overdose Symptoms* section below.

Adverse Reactions, Side Effects or Overdose Symptoms

Signs and symptoms	What to do
Delirium	Seek emergency treatment.
Hallucinations	Seek emergency treatment.
Rapid heartbeat	Seek emergency treatment.

Hop, Common

Basic Information

Biological name (genus and species):
Humulus lupulus

Parts used for medicinal purposes:
Berries/fruits

Chemicals this herb contains:

• Humulene
• Lupulinic acid
• Lupulone

Known Effects

Inhibits growth and development of germs

Miscellaneous information:
- If fruit is not fresh, it smells bad.
- Hops are used extensively in the brewing industry.
- It produces odors because it evaporates at room temperature.

 Possible Additional Effects

Potential tonic

 Warnings and Precautions

Don't take if you:
Are pregnant, think you may be pregnant or plan pregnancy in the near future.

Consult your doctor if you:
- Take this herb for any medical problem that doesn't improve in 2 weeks (There may be safer, more effective treatments.)
- Take any medicinal drugs or herbs including aspirin, laxatives, cold and cough remedies, antacids, vitamins, minerals, amino acids, supplements, other prescription or nonprescription drugs

Pregnancy:
Don't use unless prescribed by your doctor.

Breastfeeding:
Don't use unless prescribed by your doctor.

Infants and children:
Treating infants and children under 2 with any herbal preparation is hazardous.

Others:
None are expected if you are beyond childhood, under 45, not pregnant, basically healthy, take it for only a short time and do not exceed manufacturer's recommended dose.

Storage:
- Store in cool, dry area away from direct light, but don't freeze.
- Store safely out of reach of children.
- Don't store in bathroom medicine cabinet. Heat and moisture may change the action of the herb.

Safe dosage:
Consult your doctor for the appropriate dose for your condition.

 Toxicity

Rated relatively safe when taken in appropriate quantities for short periods of time

For symptoms of toxicity: See *Adverse Reactions, Side Effects or Overdose Symptoms* section below.

 Adverse Reactions, Side Effects or Overdose Symptoms

Signs and symptoms	What to do
Diarrhea	Discontinue. Call doctor immediately.
Upset stomach	Discontinue. Call doctor immediately.

MEDICINAL HERBS

Horehound

Basic Information

Biological name (genus and species):
Marrubium vulgare

Parts used for medicinal purposes:
- Flowers
- Leaves

Chemicals this herb contains:
- Marrubiin
- Resin (see Glossary)
- Tannins (see Glossary)
- Volatile oils (see Glossary)

Known Effects

- Helps expel gas from intestinal tract
- Decreases thickness and increases fluidity of mucus in lungs and bronchial tubes

Miscellaneous information:
- Leaves and flowers are used to make tincture.
- It's also available as tea and lozenges.

Possible Additional Effects

- Potential cough and cold remedy
- May treat whooping cough

Warnings and Precautions

Don't take if you:
- Are pregnant, think you may be pregnant or plan pregnancy in the near future
- Have any chronic disease of the gastrointestinal tract, such as stomach or duodenal ulcers, reflux esophagitis, ulcerative colitis, spastic colitis, diverticulosis or diverticulitis

Consult your doctor if you:
- Take this herb for any medical problem that doesn't improve in 2 weeks (There may be safer, more effective treatments.)
- Take any medicinal drugs or herbs including aspirin, laxatives, cold and cough remedies, antacids, vitamins, minerals, amino acids, supplements, other prescription or nonprescription drugs
- Have heart disease
- Are over 65

Pregnancy:
Don't use unless prescribed by your doctor.

Breastfeeding:
Don't use unless prescribed by your doctor.

Infants and children:
Treating infants and children under 2 with any herbal preparation is hazardous.

Others:
None are expected if you are beyond childhood, under 45, not pregnant, basically healthy, take it for only a short time and do not exceed manufacturer's recommended dose.

Storage:
- Store in cool, dry area away from direct light, but don't freeze.
- Store safely out of reach of children.
- Don't store in bathroom medicine cabinet. Heat and moisture may change the action of the herb.

Safe dosage:
Consult your doctor for the appropriate dose for your condition.

Toxicity

Comparative-toxicity rating is not available from standard references.

For symptoms of toxicity: See *Adverse Reactions, Side Effects or Overdose Symptoms* section below.

Adverse Reactions, Side Effects or Overdose Symptoms

Signs and symptoms	What to do
Diarrhea	Discontinue. Call doctor immediately.
Nausea or vomiting	Discontinue. Call doctor immediately.

Horse Chestnut

Basic Information

Biological name (genus and species):
Aesculus hippocastanum

Parts used for medicinal purposes:
• Bark
• Leaves
• Seeds/nuts

Chemicals this herb contains:
• Aescin
• Coumarins
• Flavonoids (quercetin, kaempferol)
• Saponin (see Glossary)

Known Effects

• Increases bleeding time (a laboratory test for blood clotting)
• Irritates mucous membrane
• Restricts edema
• Increases blood return to heart
• Diuretic

Miscellaneous information:
• There are more reliable, safer anticoagulants approved by the FDA. Eating even a few nuts can cause toxic symptoms.
• Superstitious adults carry seeds in their pockets to cure arthritis.

Possible Additional Effects

• Potential anticoagulant
• Potential sunscreen (4 percent solution)
• May help treat varicose veins

Warnings and Precautions

Don't take if you:
• Are pregnant, think you may be pregnant or plan pregnancy in the near future
• Have any chronic disease of the gastrointestinal tract, such as stomach or duodenal ulcers, reflux esophagitis, ulcerative colitis, spastic colitis, diverticulosis or diverticulitis

Consult your doctor if you:
• Take this herb for any medical problem that doesn't improve in 2 weeks (There may be safer, more effective treatments.)
• Take any medicinal drugs or herbs including aspirin, laxatives, cold and cough remedies, antacids, vitamins, minerals, amino acids, supplements, other prescription or nonprescription drugs

MEDICINAL HERBS

→

Pregnancy:
Dangers outweigh any possible benefits. Don't use.

Breastfeeding:
Dangers outweigh any possible benefits. Don't use.

Infants and children:
Treating infants and children under 2 with any herbal preparation is hazardous.

Storage:
- Store in cool, dry area away from direct light, but don't freeze.
- Store safely out of reach of children.
- Don't store in bathroom medicine cabinet. Heat and moisture may change the action of the herb.

Safe dosage:
Consult your doctor for the appropriate dose for your condition.

Toxicity

Rated slightly dangerous, particularly in children, persons over 55 and those who take larger than appropriate quantities for extended periods of time

For symptoms of toxicity: See *Adverse Reactions, Side Effects or Overdose Symptoms* section below.

Adverse Reactions, Side Effects or Overdose Symptoms

Signs and symptoms	What to do
Gastrointestinal upset	Discontinue. Call doctor immediately.
Lack of coordination	Discontinue. Call doctor immediately.
Nausea or vomiting	Discontinue. Call doctor immediately.
Unusual bleeding	Discontinue. Call doctor immediately.

Horsemint

Basic Information

Biological name (genus and species):
Monarda punctata

Parts used for medicinal purposes:
- Leaves
- Stems

Chemicals this herb contains:
- Carvacrol
- Cymene
- D-limonene
- Linalool
- Monarda oil
- Thymol

Known Effects

- Irritates tissues and mucous membranes
- Kills germs when used on the skin for external infections

Possible Additional Effects

Internal use:
- May kill intestinal parasites
- May help expel gas from intestinal tract

- May treat abdominal cramps
- May treat nausea

External use:
- May kill fungus infections on skin
- May kill bacterial infections on skin

 Warnings and Precautions

Don't take if you:
- Are pregnant, think you may be pregnant or plan pregnancy in the near future
- Have any chronic disease of the gastrointestinal tract, such as stomach or duodenal ulcers, reflux esophagitis, ulcerative colitis, spastic colitis, diverticulosis or diverticulitis

Consult your doctor if you:
- Take this herb for any medical problem that doesn't improve in 2 weeks (There may be safer, more effective treatments.)
- Take any medicinal drugs or herbs including aspirin, laxatives, cold and cough remedies, antacids, vitamins, minerals, amino acids, supplements, other prescription or nonprescription drugs

Pregnancy:
Don't use unless prescribed by your doctor.

Breastfeeding:
Don't use unless prescribed by your doctor.

Infants and children:
Treating infants and children under 2 with any herbal preparation is hazardous.

Others:
None are expected if you are beyond childhood, under 45, not pregnant, basically healthy, take it for only a short time and do not exceed manufacturer's recommended dose.

Storage:
- Store in cool, dry area away from direct light, but don't freeze.
- Store safely out of reach of children.
- Don't store in bathroom medicine cabinet. Heat and moisture may change the action of the herb.

Safe dosage:
Consult your doctor for the appropriate dose for your condition.

 Toxicity

Comparative-toxicity rating is not available from standard references.

For symptoms of toxicity: See *Adverse Reactions, Side Effects or Overdose Symptoms* section below.

 Adverse Reactions, Side Effects or Overdose Symptoms

Signs and symptoms	What to do
Diarrhea	Discontinue. Call doctor immediately.
Nausea or vomiting	Discontinue. Call doctor immediately.
Skin rash when used on skin	Discontinue. Call doctor when convenient.

MEDICINAL HERBS

Horseradish

Basic Information

Biological name (genus and species):
Armoracia lapathifolia, Cochlearia armoracia

Parts used for medicinal purposes:
Roots

Chemicals this herb contains:
- Allyl isothiocyanate
- Sinigrin

Known Effects

External use:
- Irritates skin
- Helps clear sinuses

Internal use:
Irritates gastrointestinal tract

Miscellaneous information:
- Horseradish is used to add flavor to foods.
- No effects are expected on the body, either good or bad, when this herb is used in very small amounts to enhance the flavor of food.

Possible Additional Effects

No additional effects are known.

Warnings and Precautions

Don't take if you:
- Are pregnant, think you may be pregnant or plan pregnancy in the near future
- Have any chronic disease of the gastrointestinal tract, such as stomach or duodenal ulcers, reflux esophagitis, ulcerative colitis, spastic colitis, diverticulosis or diverticulitis

Consult your doctor if you:
- Take this herb for any medical problem that doesn't improve in 2 weeks (There may be safer, more effective treatments.)
- Take any medicinal drugs or herbs including aspirin, laxatives, cold and cough remedies, antacids, vitamins, minerals, amino acids, supplements, other prescription or nonprescription drugs

Pregnancy:
Don't use unless prescribed by your doctor.

Breastfeeding:
Don't use unless prescribed by your doctor.

Infants and children:
Treating infants and children under 2 with any herbal preparation is hazardous.

Others:
Eating large amounts of raw root can be toxic.

Storage:
- Store in cool, dry area away from direct light, but don't freeze.
- Store safely out of reach of children.
- Don't store in bathroom medicine cabinet. Heat and moisture may change the action of the herb.

Safe dosage:
Consult your doctor for the appropriate dose for your condition.

Toxicity

Comparative-toxicity rating is not available from standard references.

For symptoms of toxicity: See *Adverse Reactions, Side Effects or Overdose Symptoms* section below.

 Adverse Reactions, Side Effects or Overdose Symptoms

Signs and symptoms	What to do
Diarrhea, with blood	Discontinue. Call doctor immediately.
Nausea or vomiting	Discontinue. Call doctor immediately.
Vomiting, with blood	Seek emergency treatment.

Horsetails (Bottle Brush, Field Horsetail, Shave Grass)

 Basic Information

Biological name (genus and species): *Equisetum arvense*

Parts used for medicinal purposes: Stems

Chemicals this herb contains:
• Alkaloids
• Flavonoids
• Phenolic acids
• Silicic acid
• Silicates
• Sterols

 Known Effects

No proven medicinal effects are known.

 Possible Additional Effects

• May treat bladder infections
• May treat prostatitis
• May help body dispose of excess fluid by increasing amount of urine produced
• May help heal sores on skin

 Warnings and Precautions

Don't take if you:
• Are pregnant, think you may be pregnant or plan pregnancy in the near future
• Have heart disease or high blood pressure—use only under doctor's care

Consult your doctor if you:
• Take this herb for any medical problem that doesn't improve in 2 weeks (There may be safer, more effective treatments.)
• Take any medicinal drugs or herbs including aspirin, laxatives, cold and cough remedies, antacids, vitamins, minerals, amino acids, supplements, other prescription or nonprescription drugs

Pregnancy:
Dangerous. Don't use.

Breastfeeding:
Dangerous. Don't use.

Infants and children:
Treating infants and children under 2 with any herbal preparation is hazardous.

MEDICINAL HERBS

→

Others:

None are expected if you are beyond childhood, under 45, not pregnant, basically healthy, take it for only a short time and do not exceed manufacturer's recommended dose.

Storage:

- Store in cool, dry area away from direct light, but don't freeze.
- Store safely out of reach of children.
- Don't store in bathroom medicine cabinet. Heat and moisture may change the action of the herb.

Safe dosage:

Consult your doctor for the appropriate dose for your condition.

 Toxicity

Rated slightly dangerous, particularly in children, persons over 55 and those who take larger than appropriate quantities for extended periods of time

For symptoms of toxicity: See *Adverse Reactions, Side Effects or Overdose Symptoms* section below.

 Adverse Reactions, Side Effects or Overdose Symptoms

Signs and symptoms	What to do
Cold hands and feet	Discontinue. Call doctor when convenient.
Fever	Discontinue. Call doctor immediately.
Heartbeat irregularities	Seek emergency treatment.
Muscle weakness	Discontinue. Call doctor immediately.
Trouble walking	Discontinue. Call doctor immediately.
Weight loss	Discontinue. Call doctor when convenient.

Houseleek (Jupiter's Eye, Thor's Beard)

 Basic Information

Biological name (genus and species): *Sempervivum tectorum*

Parts used for medicinal purposes: Leaves

Chemicals this herb contains: Malic acid

 Known Effects

- Shrinks tissues
- Prevents secretion of fluids

 Possible Additional Effects

- May help body dispose of excess fluid by increasing amount of urine produced
- May treat insect bites, burns, bruises, skin disease when used as a poultice (see Glossary)

 Warnings and Precautions

Don't take if you:

- Are pregnant, think you may be pregnant or plan pregnancy in the near future

- Have any chronic disease of the gastrointestinal tract, such as stomach or duodenal ulcers, reflux esophagitis, ulcerative colitis, spastic colitis, diverticulosis or diverticulitis

Consult your doctor if you:
- Take this herb for any medical problem that doesn't improve in 2 weeks (There may be safer, more effective treatments.)
- Take any medicinal drugs or herbs including aspirin, laxatives, cold and cough remedies, antacids, vitamins, minerals, amino acids, supplements, other prescription or nonprescription drugs

Pregnancy:
Don't use unless prescribed by your doctor.

Breastfeeding:
Don't use unless prescribed by your doctor.

Infants and children:
Treating infants and children under 2 with any herbal preparation is hazardous.

Others:
None are expected if you are beyond childhood, under 45, not pregnant, basically healthy, take it for only a short time and do not exceed manufacturer's recommended dose.

Storage:
- Store in cool, dry area away from direct light, but don't freeze.
- Store safely out of reach of children.
- Don't store in bathroom medicine cabinet. Heat and moisture may change the action of the herb.

Safe dosage:
Consult your doctor for the appropriate dose for your condition.

 Toxicity

Comparative-toxicity rating is not available from standard references.

For symptoms of toxicity: See *Adverse Reactions, Side Effects or Overdose Symptoms* section below.

 Adverse Reactions, Side Effects or Overdose Symptoms

Signs and symptoms	What to do
Diarrhea, watery, explosive	Discontinue. Call doctor immediately.
Vomiting	Discontinue. Call doctor immediately.

Huckleberry

 Basic Information

Biological name (genus and species):
Gaylussacia baccata

Parts used for medicinal purposes:
Entire plant

Chemicals this herb contains:
- Fatty acids
- Hydroquinone
- Loeanolic acid
- Neomyrtillin
- Tannins (see Glossary)
- Ursolic acid

MEDICINAL HERBS

Known Effects

- Decreases blood sugar
- Helps body dispose of excess fluid by increasing amount of urine produced
- Interferes with absorption of iron and other minerals when taken internally

Possible Additional Effects

- May treat diarrhea
- May treat gastroenteritis
- May treat and prevent scurvy

Warnings and Precautions

Don't take if you:
Are allergic to blueberries or huckleberries.

Consult your doctor if you:
- Take this herb for any medical problem that doesn't improve in 2 weeks (There may be safer, more effective treatments.)
- Take any medicinal drugs or herbs including aspirin, laxatives, cold and cough remedies, antacids, vitamins, minerals, amino acids, supplements, other prescription or nonprescription drugs

Pregnancy:
Pregnant women should experience no problems taking usual amounts as part of a balanced diet. Other products extracted from this herb have not been proved to cause problems.

Breastfeeding:
Breastfed infants of lactating mothers should experience no problems when mother takes usual amounts as part of a balanced diet. Other products extracted from this herb have not been proved to cause problems.

Infants and children:
Treating infants and children under 2 with any herbal preparation is hazardous.

Others:
None are expected if you are beyond childhood, under 45, not pregnant, basically healthy, take it for only a short time and do not exceed manufacturer's recommended dose.

Storage:
- Store in cool, dry area away from direct light, but don't freeze.
- Store safely out of reach of children.
- Don't store in bathroom medicine cabinet. Heat and moisture may change the action of the herb.

Safe dosage:
Consult your doctor for the appropriate dose for your condition.

Toxicity

Generally regarded as safe when taken in appropriate quantities for short periods of time

Adverse Reactions, Side Effects or Overdose Symptoms

None are expected.

Hydrangea (Peegee, Seven Barks)

Basic Information

Biological name (genus and species):
Hydrangea paniculata

Parts used for medicinal purposes:
Roots

Chemicals this herb contains:
- Hydrangin (can change to cyanide)
- Resin (see Glossary)
- Saponin (see Glossary)
- Volatile oils (see Glossary)

Known Effects

- Helps expel gas from intestinal tract
- Shrinks tissues
- Prevents secretion of fluids

Miscellaneous information:
- Leaves contain cyanide.
- Smoking this herb can cause mind-altering effects and toxicity.

Possible Additional Effects

- May treat cystitis
- May treat bladder stones
- May treat dyspepsia

Warnings and Precautions

Don't take if you:
- Are pregnant, think you may be pregnant or plan pregnancy in the near future
- Have any chronic disease of the gastrointestinal tract, such as stomach or duodenal ulcers, reflux esophagitis, ulcerative colitis, spastic colitis, diverticulosis or diverticulitis

Consult your doctor if you:
- Take this herb for any medical problem that doesn't improve in 2 weeks (There may be safer, more effective treatments.)
- Take any medicinal drugs or herbs including aspirin, laxatives, cold and cough remedies, antacids, vitamins, minerals, amino acids, supplements, other prescription or nonprescription drugs

Pregnancy:
Dangers outweigh any possible benefits. Don't use.

Breastfeeding:
Dangers outweigh any possible benefits. Don't use.

Infants and children:
Treating infants and children under 2 with any herbal preparation is hazardous.

Storage:
- Store in cool, dry area away from direct light, but don't freeze.
- Store safely out of reach of children.
- Don't store in bathroom medicine cabinet. Heat and moisture may change the action of the herb.

Safe dosage:
Consult your doctor for the appropriate dose for your condition.

Toxicity

Rated relatively safe when taken in appropriate quantities for short periods of time

For symptoms of toxicity: See *Adverse Reactions, Side Effects or Overdose Symptoms* section below.

MEDICINAL HERBS

➔

Adverse Reactions, Side Effects or Overdose Symptoms

Signs and symptoms	What to do
Dizziness	Discontinue. Call doctor immediately.
Heavy feeling in chest	Discontinue. Call doctor immediately.
Nausea or vomiting	Discontinue. Call doctor immediately.

Indian Nettle

Basic Information

Indian nettle is also called kuppi, mercury weed, Indian acalypha and hierba del cancer.

Biological name (genus and species): *Acalypha indica, A. virginica*

Parts used for medicinal purposes: Leaves

Chemicals this herb contains:
- Acalyphine
- Cyanogenic glycoside (see Glossary)
- Inositol methylether
- Resin (see Glossary)
- Triacetomamine
- Volatile oils (see Glossary)

Known Effects

- Irritates stomach lining
- Decreases thickness and increases fluidity of mucus in lungs and bronchial tubes
- Causes vomiting

Miscellaneous information:
- Basic ingredients are similar to ipecac
- Used as a mouthwash and a poultice (see Glossary)

Possible Additional Effects

May stimulate bowel movements

Warnings and Precautions

Don't take if you:
Are pregnant, think you may be pregnant or plan pregnancy in the near future.

Consult your doctor if you:
- Take this herb for any medical problem that doesn't improve in 2 weeks (There may be safer, more effective treatments.)
- Take any medicinal drugs or herbs including aspirin, laxatives, cold and cough remedies, antacids, vitamins, minerals, amino acids, supplements, other prescription or nonprescription drugs

Pregnancy:
Dangers outweigh any possible benefits. Don't use.

Breastfeeding:
Dangers outweigh any possible benefits. Don't use.

Infants and children:
Treating infants and children under 2 with any herbal preparation is hazardous.

Others:
None are expected if you are beyond childhood, under 45, not pregnant, basically healthy, take it for only a short time and do not exceed manufacturer's recommended dose.

Storage:
- Store in cool, dry area away from direct light, but don't freeze.
- Store safely out of reach of children.
- Don't store in bathroom medicine cabinet. Heat and moisture may change the action of the herb.

Safe dosage:
Consult your doctor for the appropriate dose for your condition.

Toxicity

Rated relatively safe when taken in appropriate quantities for short periods of time

For symptoms of toxicity: See *Adverse Reactions, Side Effects or Overdose Symptoms* section below.

Adverse Reactions, Side Effects or Overdose Symptoms

Signs and symptoms	What to do
Diarrhea	Discontinue. Call doctor immediately.
Nausea or vomiting	Discontinue. Call doctor immediately.

Indian Tobacco (Asthma Weed, Lobelia)

Basic Information

Biological name (genus and species):
Lobelia inflata

Parts used for medicinal purposes:
- Leaves
- Seeds

Chemicals this herb contains:
- Isolobinine
- Lobelanidine
- Lobelanine
- Lobeline
- Norlobelidione
- Norlobelol

Known Effects

- Large amounts stimulate central nervous system
- Small amounts depress central nervous system as blood level drops
- Activates vomiting center in people not accustomed to lobelia
- Effective expectorant

Miscellaneous information:
- Indian tobacco is sometimes advertised as "legal grass." Do not be misled! Toxic effects can be dangerous.
- It is not recommended for medicinal use.

MEDICINAL HERBS

→

Possible Additional Effects

No additional effects are known.

 ## Warnings and Precautions

Don't take if you:

- Are pregnant, think you may be pregnant or plan pregnancy in the near future
- Have any chronic disease of the gastrointestinal tract, such as stomach or duodenal ulcers, reflux esophagitis, ulcerative colitis, spastic colitis, diverticulosis or diverticulitis

Consult your doctor if you:

- Take this herb for any medical problem that doesn't improve in 2 weeks (There may be safer, more effective treatments.)
- Take any medicinal drugs or herbs including aspirin, laxatives, cold and cough remedies, antacids, vitamins, minerals, amino acids, supplements, other prescription or nonprescription drugs

Pregnancy:

Dangers outweigh any possible benefits. Don't use.

Breastfeeding:

Dangers outweigh any possible benefits. Don't use.

Infants and children:

Treating infants and children under 2 with any herbal preparation is hazardous.

Others:

Dangers outweigh any possible benefits. Don't use.

Storage:

- Store in cool, dry area away from direct light, but don't freeze.
- Store safely out of reach of children.
- Don't store in bathroom medicine cabinet. Heat and moisture may change the action of the herb.

Safe dosage:

Consult your doctor for the appropriate dose for your condition.

 ## Toxicity

Rated slightly dangerous, particularly in children, persons over 55 and those who take larger than appropriate quantities for extended periods of time.

For symptoms of toxicity: See *Adverse Reactions, Side Effects or Overdose Symptoms* section below.

 ## Adverse Reactions, Side Effects or Overdose Symptoms

Signs and symptoms	What to do
Coma	Seek emergency treatment.
Diarrhea	Discontinue. Call doctor immediately.
Excess salivation	Discontinue. Call doctor when convenient.
Excess tear formation	Discontinue. Call doctor when convenient.
Giddiness	Discontinue. Call doctor when convenient.
Headache	Discontinue. Call doctor when convenient.
Nausea or vomiting	Discontinue. Call doctor immediately.
Stupor	Seek emergency treatment.
Tremors	Discontinue. Call doctor immediately.

Indigo, Wild

 Basic Information

Biological name (genus and species):
Baptisia tinctoria

Parts used for medicinal purposes:
Roots

Chemicals this herb contains:
- Baptisine
- Baptisol
- Cytisine
- Quinolizidine

 Known Effects

- Irritates gastrointestinal lining
- Causes watery, explosive bowel movements
- Causes vomiting

Miscellaneous information:
Blue dye in wild indigo is inferior to domestically grown indigo.

 Possible Additional Effects

- May treat typhoid fever
- May treat amebiasis

 Warnings and Precautions

Don't take if you:
- Are pregnant, think you may be pregnant or plan pregnancy in the near future
- Have any chronic disease of the gastrointestinal tract, such as stomach or duodenal ulcers, reflux esophagitis, ulcerative colitis, spastic colitis, diverticulosis or diverticulitis

Consult your doctor if you:
- Take this herb for any medical problem that doesn't improve in 2 weeks (There may be safer, more effective treatments.)
- Take any medicinal drugs or herbs including aspirin, laxatives, cold and cough remedies, antacids, vitamins, minerals, amino acids, supplements, other prescription or nonprescription drugs

Pregnancy:
Dangers outweigh any possible benefits. Don't use.

Breastfeeding:
Dangers outweigh any possible benefits. Don't use.

Infants and children:
Treating infants and children under 2 with any herbal preparation is hazardous.

Others:
None are expected if you are beyond childhood, under 45, not pregnant, basically healthy, take it for only a short time and do not exceed manufacturer's recommended dose.

Storage:
- Store in cool, dry area away from direct light, but don't freeze.
- Store safely out of reach of children.
- Don't store in bathroom medicine cabinet. Heat and moisture may change the action of the herb.

Safe dosage:
At present no "safe" dosage has been established.

MEDICINAL HERBS

Toxicity

Comparative-toxicity rating is not available from standard references.

For symptoms of toxicity: See *Adverse Reactions, Side Effects or Overdose Symptoms* section below.

Adverse Reactions, Side Effects or Overdose Symptoms

Signs and symptoms	What to do
Diarrhea	Discontinue. Call doctor immediately.
Nausea or vomiting	Discontinue. Call doctor immediately.

Irish Moss

Basic Information

Biological name (genus and species): *Chondrus crispus, Gigartina mamillosa*

Parts used for medicinal purposes: Entire plant

Chemicals this herb contains:
- Bromine
- Calcium
- Carrageenan
- Chlorine
- Protein
- Sodium

Known Effects

- Protects scraped tissues
- Interferes with blood-clotting mechanism

Miscellaneous information:
- Used for hand lotions and as substitute for gelatin in jellies
- Chemically similar to agar, a substance used in laboratories as a base for growing germ cultures

Possible Additional Effects

- May help form bulky stools
- May treat coughs
- May treat diarrhea

Warnings and Precautions

Don't take if you:
- Are pregnant, think you may be pregnant or plan pregnancy in the near future
- Have any chronic disease of the gastrointestinal tract, such as stomach or duodenal ulcers, reflux esophagitis, ulcerative colitis, spastic colitis, diverticulosis or diverticulitis
- Take anticoagulants

Consult your doctor if you:
- Take this herb for any medical problem that doesn't improve in 2 weeks (There may be safer, more effective treatments.)
- Take any medicinal drugs or herbs including aspirin, laxatives, cold and cough remedies, antacids, vitamins, minerals, amino acids, supplements, other prescription or nonprescription drugs

Pregnancy:
Don't use unless prescribed by your doctor.

Breastfeeding:
Don't use unless prescribed by your doctor.

Infants and children:
Treating infants and children under 2 with any herbal preparation is hazardous.

Others:
None are expected if you are beyond childhood, under 45, not pregnant, basically healthy, take it for only a short time and do not exceed manufacturer's recommended dose.

Storage:
• Store in cool, dry area away from direct light, but don't freeze.
• Store safely out of reach of children.
• Don't store in bathroom medicine cabinet. Heat and moisture may change the action of the herb.

Safe dosage:
Consult your doctor for the appropriate dose for your condition.

Toxicity

Comparative-toxicity rating is not available from standard references.

For symptoms of toxicity: See *Adverse Reactions, Side Effects or Overdose Symptoms* section below.

Adverse Reactions, Side Effects or Overdose Symptoms

Signs and symptoms	What to do
May interact with other anticoagulants to increase anticoagulant effect	Discontinue. Call doctor immediately.
Nausea	Discontinue. Call doctor immediately.

Jalap Root

Basic Information

Jalap root is also known as conqueror root, high john root, ipomoea and turpeth.

Biological name (genus and species): *Exagonium purga*

Parts used for medicinal purposes: Roots

Chemicals this herb contains:
• Convolvulin
• Gum (see Glossary)
• Jalapin
• Jalapinolic acid
• Starch
• Sugar
• Volatile oils (see Glossary)

Known Effects
• Irritates the gastrointestinal system
• Laxative

Possible Additonal Benefits
No additional benefits are known.

➔

Warnings and Precautions

Don't take if you:

- Are pregnant, think you may be pregnant or plan pregnancy in the near future
- Have any chronic disease of the gastrointestinal tract, such as stomach or duodenal ulcers, reflux esophagitis, ulcerative colitis, spastic colitis, diverticulosis or diverticulitis

Consult your doctor if you:

- Take this herb for any medical problem that doesn't improve in 2 weeks (There may be safer, more effective treatments.)
- Take any medicinal drugs or herbs including aspirin, laxatives, cold and cough remedies, antacids, vitamins, minerals, amino acids, supplements, other prescription or nonprescription drugs

Pregnancy:

Dangers outweigh any possible benefits. Don't use.

Breastfeeding:

Dangers outweigh any possible benefits. Don't use.

Infants and children:

Treating infants and children under 2 with any herbal preparation is hazardous.

Others:

None are expected if you are beyond childhood, under 45, not pregnant, basically healthy, take it for only a short time and do not exceed manufacturer's recommended dose.

Storage:

- Store in cool, dry area away from direct light, but don't freeze.
- Store safely out of reach of children.
- Don't store in bathroom medicine cabinet. Heat and moisture may change the action of the herb.

Safe dosage:

Consult your doctor for the appropriate dose for your condition.

 # Toxicity

Comparative-toxicity rating is not available from standard references.

For symptoms of toxicity: See *Adverse Reactions, Side Effects or Overdose Symptoms* section below.

 # Adverse Reactions, Side Effects or Overdose Symptoms

Signs and symptoms	What to do
Diarrhea, explosive, watery, with possible fluid and electrolyte depletion, leading to weakness and possible heartbeat irregularities	Discontinue. Call doctor immediately.

Jamaican Dogwood (Fish-poison Tree)

Basic Information

Biological name (genus and species):
Piscidia piscipula

Parts used for medicinal purposes:
Bark

Chemicals this herb contains:
- Piscidin
- Rotenone

Known Effects

- Causes hallucinations
- Treats painful conditions
- Depresses uterine contractions

Miscellaneous information:
- Poisonous to fish
- Active chemicals in bark have odor similar to opium

Possible Additional Effects

- May produce euphoria
- May treat dysmenorrhea (painful menstruation)

Warnings and Precautions

Don't take if you:
Are pregnant, think you may be pregnant or plan pregnancy in the near future.

Consult your doctor if you:
- Take this herb for any medical problem that doesn't improve in 2 weeks (There may be safer, more effective treatments.)

- Take any medicinal drugs or herbs including aspirin, laxatives, cold and cough remedies, antacids, vitamins, minerals, amino acids, supplements, other prescription or nonprescription drugs

Pregnancy:
Don't use unless prescribed by your doctor.

Breastfeeding:
Don't use unless prescribed by your doctor.

Infants and children:
Treating infants and children under 2 with any herbal preparation is hazardous.

Others:
None are expected if you are beyond childhood, under 45, not pregnant, basically healthy, take it for only a short time and do not exceed manufacturer's recommended dose.

Storage:
- Store in cool, dry area away from direct light, but don't freeze.
- Store safely out of reach of children.
- Don't store in bathroom medicine cabinet. Heat and moisture may change the action of the herb.

Safe dosage:
Consult your doctor for the appropriate dose for your condition.

Toxicity

Rated slightly dangerous, particularly in children, persons over 55 and those who take larger than appropriate quantities for extended periods of time

MEDICINAL HERBS

→

For symptoms of toxicity: See *Adverse Reactions, Side Effects or Overdose Symptoms* section below.

Adverse Reactions, Side Effects or Overdose Symptoms

Signs and symptoms	What to do
Hallucinations	Seek emergency treatment.

Jequirity Bean (Crab's Eyes, Indian Licorice, Rosary Pea)

Basic Information

Biological name (genus and species): *Abrus precatorius*

Parts used for medicinal purposes: Seeds/beans

Chemicals this herb contains:
• Abrin
• Anthocyanins
• Indole alkaloids

Known Effects

Abrin in the seed causes cell destruction.

Miscellaneous information:
• No longer used therapeutically
• Causes toxic reactions with ingestion
• Common weed in Florida, Central America and South America

Possible Additional Effects

Used as drops to potentially treat eye problems

Warnings and Precautions

Don't take if you:
• Are pregnant, think you may be pregnant or plan pregnancy in the near future
• Have any chronic disease of the gastrointestinal tract, such as stomach or duodenal ulcers, reflux esophagitis, ulcerative colitis, spastic colitis, diverticulosis or diverticulitis

Consult your doctor if you:
• Take this herb for any medical problem that doesn't improve in 2 weeks (There may be safer, more effective treatments.)
• Take any medicinal drugs or herbs including aspirin, laxatives, cold and cough remedies, antacids, vitamins, minerals, amino acids, supplements, other prescription or nonprescription drugs

Pregnancy:
Dangers outweigh any possible benefits. Don't use.

Breastfeeding:
Dangers outweigh any possible benefits. Don't use.

Infants and children:
Treating infants and children under 2 with any herbal preparation is hazardous.

Others:

Dangers outweigh any possible benefits for anyone. Don't use. Swallowing even one bean can cause toxic symptoms hours or even days after eating.

Storage:

- Store in cool, dry area away from direct light, but don't freeze.
- Store safely out of reach of children.
- Don't store in bathroom medicine cabinet. Heat and moisture may change the action of the herb.

Safe dosage:

Consult your doctor for the appropriate dose for your condition.

 Toxicity

Rated dangerous, particularly in children, persons over 55 and those who take larger than appropriate quantities for extended periods of time

For symptoms of toxicity: See *Adverse Reactions, Side Effects or Overdose Symptoms* section below.

 Adverse Reactions, Side Effects or Overdose Symptoms

Signs and symptoms	What to do
Convulsions	Seek emergency treatment.
Diarrhea	Discontinue. Call doctor immediately.
Increased heart rate	Discontinue. Call doctor immediately.
Kidney damage characterized by blood in urine, decreased urine flow, swelling of hands and feet	Seek emergency treatment.
Nausea or vomiting	Discontinue. Call doctor immediately.

Jersey Tea (Red Root)

 Basic Information

Biological name (genus and species): *Ceanothus americanus*

Parts used for medicinal purposes: Roots

Chemicals this herb contains:

- Ceanothic acid
- Malonic acid
- Orthophosphoric acid
- Oxalic acid
- Pyrophosphoric acid
- Resin (see Glossary)
- Succinic acid
- Tannins (see Glossary)

 Known Effects

- Shrinks tissues
- Prevents secretion of fluids
- Increases blood clotting
- Interferes with absorption of iron and other minerals when taken internally

 Possible Additional Effects

- May treat syphilis (archaic)
- May treat "spleen" problems
- May stop mild bleeding from broken capillaries in skin
- May decrease thickness and increase fluidity of mucus in lungs and bronchial tubes

→

- Potential sedative
- May relieve spasm in skeletal muscle or smooth muscle
- May treat depression

 Warnings and Precautions

Don't take if you:
Are pregnant, think you may be pregnant or plan pregnancy in the near future.

Consult your doctor if you:
- Take this herb for any medical problem that doesn't improve in 2 weeks (There may be safer, more effective treatments.)
- Take any medicinal drugs or herbs including aspirin, laxatives, cold and cough remedies, antacids, vitamins, minerals, amino acids, supplements, other prescription or nonprescription drugs

Pregnancy:
Problems in pregnant women taking small or usual amounts have not been proved, but the chance of problems does exist. Don't use unless prescribed by your doctor.

Breastfeeding:
Don't use unless prescribed by your doctor.

Infants and children:
Treating infants and children under 2 with any herbal preparation is hazardous.

Others:
None are expected if you are beyond childhood, under 45, not pregnant, basically healthy, take it for only a short time and do not exceed manufacturer's recommended dose.

Storage:
- Store in cool, dry area away from direct light, but don't freeze.
- Store safely out of reach of children.
- Don't store in bathroom medicine cabinet. Heat and moisture may change the action of the herb.

Safe dosage:
Consult your doctor for the appropriate dose for your condition.

 Toxicity

Comparative-toxicity rating is not available from standard references.

For symptoms of toxicity: See *Adverse Reactions, Side Effects or Overdose Symptoms* section below.

 Adverse Reactions, Side Effects or Overdose Symptoms

Signs and symptoms	What to do
Prolonged minor bleeding	Discontinue. Call doctor immediately.

Jimson Weed (Sacred Datura, Stramonium, Thorn Apple)

 Basic Information

Biological name (genus and species):
Datura stramonium

Parts used for medicinal purposes:
• Leaves
• Seeds

Chemicals this herb contains:
• Atropine
• Hyoscyamine
• Scopolamine

 Known Effects

Negates normal activity of acetyl-choline, an important chemical at the synapses (connections between nerve cells) of heart, brain, smooth muscles and glands

Miscellaneous information:
• There are more refined, predictable sources for the active chemicals in jimson weed.
• The highest concentration of toxins are in seeds but toxins may be in all parts of the plant.

 Possible Additional Effects

• May treat asthma
• May treat gastrointestinal problems
• May produce hallucinations
• Potential sedative

 Warnings and Precautions

Don't take if you:
• Are pregnant, think you may be pregnant or plan pregnancy in the near future
• Have heart disease

Consult your doctor if you:
• Take this herb for any medical problem that doesn't improve in 2 weeks (There may be safer, more effective treatments.)
• Take any medicinal drugs or herbs including aspirin, laxatives, cold and cough remedies, antacids, vitamins, minerals, amino acids, supplements, other prescription or nonprescription drugs

Pregnancy:
Dangers outweigh any possible benefits. Don't use.

Breastfeeding:
Dangers outweigh any possible benefits. Don't use.

Infants and children:
Treating infants and children under 2 with any herbal preparation is hazardous.

Others:
Dangers outweigh any possible benefits. Don't use.

Storage:
• Store in cool, dry area away from direct light, but don't freeze.
• Store safely out of reach of children.
• Don't store in bathroom medicine cabinet. Heat and moisture may change the action of the herb.

MEDICINAL HERBS

Safe dosage:
Consult your doctor for the appropriate dose for your condition.

Toxicity

Rated dangerous, particularly in children, persons over 55 and those who take larger than appropriate quantities for extended periods of time

For symptoms of toxicity: See *Adverse Reactions, Side Effects or Overdose Symptoms* section below.

Adverse Reactions, Side Effects or Overdose Symptoms

Signs and symptoms	What to do
Convulsions	Seek emergency treatment.
Dilated pupils	Discontinue. Call doctor immediately.
Dry mouth	Discontinue. Call doctor when convenient.
Extremely fast heart rate	Seek emergency treatment.
Flushing	Discontinue. Call doctor when convenient.
Hallucinations	Seek emergency treatment.
Increased blood pressure	Discontinue. Call doctor immediately.
Unconsciousness	Seek emergency treatment.

Juniper, Common

Basic Information

Biological name (genus and species):
Juniperus communis

Parts used for medicinal purposes:
Berries/fruits

Chemicals this herb contains:
- Alcohols
- Alpha-pinene
- Cadinene
- Camphene
- Flavone
- Resin (see Glossary)
- Sabinene
- Sugar
- Tannins (see Glossary)
- Terpinene
- Volatile oils (see Glossary)

Known Effects

- Irritates kidneys
- Diuretic
- Can cause uterine contractions

Miscellaneous information:
Provides flavor in gin.

Possible Additional Effects

- May treat chronic kidney disorders
- May help body dispose of excess fluid by increasing amount of urine produced
- May treat digestive problems
- May help reduce high blood pressure by decreasing fluid retention
- Potential anti-inflammatory

Warnings and Precautions

Don't take if you:

- Are pregnant, think you may be pregnant or plan pregnancy in the near future
- Have any chronic disease of the gastrointestinal tract, such as stomach or duodenal ulcers, reflux esophagitis, ulcerative colitis, spastic colitis, diverticulosis or diverticulitis
- Have kidney disease or infection or a history of kidney problems

Consult your doctor if you:

- Take this herb for any medical problem that doesn't improve in 2 weeks (There may be safer, more effective treatments.)
- Take any medicinal drugs or herbs including aspirin, laxatives, cold and cough remedies, antacids, vitamins, minerals, amino acids, supplements, other prescription or nonprescription drugs

Pregnancy:

Juniper can cause uterine contractions. Don't use.

Breastfeeding:

Dangers outweigh any possible benefits. Don't use.

Infants and children:

Treating infants and children under 2 with any herbal preparation is hazardous.

Others:

- None expected if you are beyond childhood, under 45, not pregnant, basically healthy, take it for only a short time and do not exceed manufacturer's recommended dose
- For short-term use only

Storage:

- Store in cool, dry area away from direct light, but don't freeze.
- Store safely out of reach of children.
- Don't store in bathroom medicine cabinet. Heat and moisture may change the action of the herb.

Safe dosage:

Consult your doctor for the appropriate dose for your condition.

 ## Toxicity

Rated slightly dangerous, particularly in children, persons over 55 and those who take larger than appropriate quantities for extended periods of time

For symptoms of toxicity: See *Adverse Reactions, Side Effects or Overdose Symptoms* section below.

 ## Adverse Reactions, Side Effects or Overdose Symptoms

Signs and symptoms	What to do
Single dose:	
Allergy symptoms	Discontinue. Call doctor immediately.
Diarrhea, watery, explosive	Discontinue. Call doctor immediately.
Increased heart rate	Discontinue. Call doctor immediately.
Small, repeated doses:	
Convulsions	Seek emergency treatment.
Hallucinations	Seek emergency treatment.
Kidney damage characterized by blood in urine, decreased urine flow, swelling of hands and feet	Discontinue. Call doctor immediately.
Personality changes	Discontinue. Call doctor immediately.

MEDICINAL HERBS

Kelp

Basic Information

Biological name (genus and species):
Laminaria, Fucus, Sargassum

Parts used for medicinal purposes:
Leaves

Chemicals this herb contains:
• Alginic acid
• Bromine
• Iodine
• Potassium
• Sodium

Known Effects

Provides bulk for bowel movements

Miscellaneous information:
• Iodine can interfere with normal thyroid function.
• Iodine is used as a substitute for table salt.

Possible Additional Effects

• May treat chronic constipation without catharsis
• May soften stools
• May treat ulcers
• May control obesity

Warnings and Precautions

Don't take if you:
• Are pregnant, think you may be pregnant or plan pregnancy in the near future

• Are allergic to iodine in any form, particularly if you have had an allergic reaction to injected dye used for X-ray studies of the kidney or other organs

Consult your doctor if you:
• Take this herb for any medical problem that doesn't improve in 2 weeks (There may be safer, more effective treatments.)
• Take any medicinal drugs or herbs including aspirin, laxatives, cold and cough remedies, antacids, vitamins, minerals, amino acids, supplements, other prescription or nonprescription drugs

Pregnancy:
Don't use unless prescribed by your doctor.

Breastfeeding:
Don't use unless prescribed by your doctor.

Infants and children:
Treating infants and children under 2 with any herbal preparation is hazardous.

Others:
None are expected if you are beyond childhood, under 45, not pregnant, basically healthy, take it for only a short time and do not exceed manufacturer's recommended dose.

Storage:
• Store in cool, dry area away from direct light, but don't freeze.
• Store safely out of reach of children.
• Don't store in bathroom medicine cabinet. Heat and moisture may change the action of the herb.

Safe dosage:
Consult your doctor for the appropriate dose for your condition.

Toxicity

Comparative-toxicity rating is not available from standard references.

Adverse Reactions, Side Effects or Overdose Symptoms

None are expected.

Lemongrass

Basic Information

Biological name (genus and species):
Cymbopogon citratus

Parts used for medicinal purposes:
Various parts of the entire plant, frequently differing by country and culture

Chemicals this herb contains:
- Citronellal
- Methylneptenone
- Myrcene
- Terpene (see Glossary)
- Terpene alcohol

Known Effects

Kills insects, but less efficiently than malathion or parathione

Miscellaneous information:
Lemongrass is used in perfumes and sometimes as an insect repellent.

Possible Additional Effects

- May treat constipation
- May treat fever
- Potential pain reducer
- Potential sedative

Warnings and Precautions

Don't take if you:
- Are pregnant, think you may be pregnant or plan pregnancy in the near future
- Have any chronic disease of the gastrointestinal tract, such as stomach or duodenal ulcers, reflux esophagitis, ulcerative colitis, spastic colitis, diverticulosis or diverticulitis

Consult your doctor if you:
- Take this herb for any medical problem that doesn't improve in 2 weeks (There may be safer, more effective treatments.)
- Take any medicinal drugs or herbs including aspirin, laxatives, cold and cough remedies, antacids, vitamins, minerals, amino acids, supplements, other prescription or nonprescription drugs

Pregnancy:
Don't use unless prescribed by your doctor.

Breastfeeding:
Don't use unless prescribed by your doctor.

Infants and children:
Treating infants and children under 2 with any herbal preparation is hazardous.

MEDICINAL HERBS

→

Others:

None are expected if you are beyond childhood, under 45, not pregnant, basically healthy, take it for only a short time and do not exceed manufacturer's recommended dose.

Storage:

- Store in cool, dry area away from direct light, but don't freeze.
- Store safely out of reach of children.
- Don't store in bathroom medicine cabinet. Heat and moisture may change the action of the herb.

Safe dosage:

Consult your doctor for the appropriate dose for your condition.

 Toxicity

Comparative-toxicity rating is not available from standard references.

For symptoms of toxicity: See *Adverse Reactions, Side Effects or Overdose Symptoms* section below.

 Adverse Reactions, Side Effects or Overdose Symptoms

Signs and symptoms	What to do
Diarrhea	Discontinue. Call doctor immediately.
Nausea or vomiting	Discontinue. Call doctor immediately.

Licorice, Common (Licorice Root, Spanish Licorice Root)

 Basic Information

Biological name (genus and species):
Glycyrrhiza glabra

Parts used for medicinal purposes:
- Rhizomes
- Roots

Chemicals this herb contains:
- Asparagine
- Fat
- Glycyrrhizin
- Gum (see Glossary)
- Pentacyclic terpenes
- Protein
- Sugar
- Yellow dye

 Known Effects

- Decreases inflammation
- Provides estrogen-like hormone effects
- Decreases spasm of smooth muscle or skeletal muscle (asthma, allergic reactions)
- Decreases thickness and increases fluidity of mucus in lungs and bronchial tubes
- Cough suppressant
- Treats constipation, heartburn, ulcers

Miscellaneous information:

- Warning: Consuming large amounts of licorice may lead to high blood pressure.
- Licorice is available as liquid extract and capsules.
- Most licorice in the United States is anise-flavored candy, not true licorice.

Possible Additional Effects

- May protect scraped tissues (external use)
- May improve liver function

Warnings and Precautions

Don't take if you:
- Are pregnant, think you may be pregnant or plan pregnancy in the near future
- Have heart disease
- Take diuretics

Consult your doctor if you:
- Take this herb for any medical problem that doesn't improve in 2 weeks (There may be safer, more effective treatments.)
- Take any medicinal drugs or herbs including aspirin, laxatives, cold and cough remedies, antacids, vitamins, minerals, amino acids, supplements, other prescription or nonprescription drugs
- Have a history of heart disease
- Are over age 55

Pregnancy:
Dangers outweigh any possible benefits. Don't use.

Breastfeeding:
Dangers outweigh any possible benefits. Don't use.

Infants and children:
Treating infants and children under 2 with any herbal preparation is hazardous.

Others:
None are expected if you are beyond childhood, under 45, not pregnant, basically healthy, take it for only a short time and do not exceed manufacturer's recommended dose.

Storage:
- Store in cool, dry area away from direct light, but don't freeze.
- Store safely out of reach of children.
- Don't store in bathroom medicine cabinet. Heat and moisture may change the action of the herb.

Safe dosage:
Consult your doctor for the appropriate dose for your condition.

Toxicity

Rated slightly dangerous, particularly in children, persons over 55 and those who take larger than appropriate quantities for extended periods of time

For symptoms of toxicity: See *Adverse Reactions, Side Effects or Overdose Symptoms* section below.

Adverse Reactions, Side Effects or Overdose Symptoms

Signs and symptoms	What to do
High blood pressure	Discontinue. Call doctor immediately.
Effects of sodium retention:	
Edema	Discontinue. Call doctor immediately.
Lung congestion	Discontinue. Call doctor immediately.
Effects of sodium depletion:	
Heartbeat irregularities	Discontinue. Call doctor immediately.
Nausea	Discontinue. Call doctor immediately.
Weakness	Discontinue. Call doctor immediately.

MEDICINAL HERBS

Liferoot (Golden Groundsel, Squaw Weed)

Basic Information

Biological name (genus and species):
Senecio vulgaris, S. aureus

Parts used for medicinal purposes:
Roots

Chemicals this herb contains:
Pyrrolizidine

Known Effects

- Increases blood pressure
- Stimulates uterine contractions

Miscellaneous information:
Pyrrolizidine has a high potential for causing liver disorders, including cancer.

Possible Additional Effects

- May treat menstrual irregularities
- May treat dysmenorrhea (painful menstruation)
- May treat excessive menstrual bleeding (menorrhagia)
- May help relieve vaginal discharge
- May cause overdue labor to begin

Warnings and Precautions

Don't take if you:
Are pregnant, think you may be pregnant or plan pregnancy in the near future.

Consult your doctor if you:
- Take this herb for any medical problem that doesn't improve in 2 weeks (There may be safer, more effective treatments.)
- Take any medicinal drugs or herbs including aspirin, laxatives, cold and cough remedies, antacids, vitamins, minerals, amino acids, supplements, other prescription or nonprescription drugs

Pregnancy:
Dangers outweigh any possible benefits. Don't use.

Breastfeeding:
Dangers outweigh any possible benefits. Don't use.

Infants and children:
Treating infants and children under 2 with any herbal preparation is hazardous.

Others:
None are expected if you are beyond childhood, under 45, not pregnant, basically healthy, take it for only a short time and do not exceed manufacturer's recommended dose.

Storage:
- Store in cool, dry area away from direct light, but don't freeze.
- Store safely out of reach of children.
- Don't store in bathroom medicine cabinet. Heat and moisture may change the action of the herb.

Safe dosage:
Consult your doctor for the appropriate dose for your condition.

Toxicity

Rated slightly dangerous, particularly in children, persons over 55 and those who take larger than appropriate quantities for extended periods of time

For symptoms of toxicity: See *Adverse Reactions, Side Effects or Overdose Symptoms* section below.

Adverse Reactions, Side Effects or Overdose Symptoms

Signs and symptoms	What to do
Abnormal liver-function tests	Discontinue. Call doctor immediately.
Jaundice (yellow skin and eyes)	Discontinue. Call doctor immediately.

Lily-of-the-Valley

Basic Information

Biological name (genus and species): *Convallaria majalis*

Parts used for medicinal purposes:
- Berries/fruits
- Petals/flower
- Roots

Chemicals this herb contains:
- Convallamarin
- Convallarin
- Convallatoxin (highly toxic)

Known Effects

- Increases efficiency of heart-muscle contraction
- Helps body dispose of excess fluid by increasing amount of urine produced

Miscellaneous information:

Although lily-of-the-valley has similar action to digitalis, there are safer, less expensive, more reliable products to use.

Possible Additional Effects

- May treat congestive heart failure
- May treat heartbeat irregularities
- May improve circulation

Warnings and Precautions

Don't take if you:
- Are pregnant, think you may be pregnant or plan pregnancy in the near future
- Have any chronic disease of the gastrointestinal tract, such as stomach or duodenal ulcers, reflux esophagitis, ulcerative colitis, spastic colitis, diverticulosis or diverticulitis

Consult your doctor if you:
- Take this herb for any medical problem that doesn't improve in 2 weeks (There may be safer, more effective treatments.)
- Take any medicinal drugs or herbs including aspirin, laxatives, cold and cough remedies, antacids, vitamins, minerals, amino acids, supplements, other prescription or nonprescription drugs

MEDICINAL HERBS

→

Pregnancy:
Dangers outweigh any possible
benefits. Don't use.

Breastfeeding:
Dangers outweigh any possible
benefits. Don't use.

Infants and children:
Treating infants and children under
2 with any herbal preparation
is hazardous.

Others:
Dangers outweigh any possible
benefits. Don't use.

Storage:
• Store in cool, dry area away from
  direct light, but don't freeze.
• Store safely out of reach of children.
• Don't store in bathroom medicine
  cabinet. Heat and moisture may
  change the action of the herb.

Safe dosage:
Consult your doctor for the appropriate dose for your condition.

Toxicity

Rated dangerous, particularly in
children, persons over 55 and those
who take larger than appropriate
quantities for extended periods of time

For symptoms of toxicity: See
*Adverse Reactions, Side Effects or
Overdose Symptoms* section below.

Adverse Reactions, Side Effects or Overdose Symptoms

Signs and symptoms	What to do
Heartbeat irregularities	Seek emergency treatment.
Nausea or vomiting	Discontinue. Call doctor immediately.

Linden Tree

Basic Information

The linden tree is called a lime tree in
Europe.

Biological name (genus and species):
Tilia europaea

Parts used for medicinal purposes:
Petals/flower

Chemicals this herb contains:
• Tannins (see Glossary)
• Volatile oils (see Glossary)

Known Effects

• Decreases spasm of smooth or
  skeletal muscle
• Increases perspiration
• Clears excess mucous from lungs
• Promotes digestion

Possible Additional Effects

• May treat coughs
• May decrease thickness and increase
  fluidity of mucus in lungs and
  bronchial tubes
• May reduce fever

• May have relaxing effect to help treat insomnia, nervous tension

Warnings and Precautions

Don't take if you:
Are pregnant, think you may be pregnant or plan pregnancy in the near future.

Consult your doctor if you:
• Take this herb for any medical problem that doesn't improve in 2 weeks (There may be safer, more effective treatments.)
• Take any medicinal drugs or herbs including aspirin, laxatives, cold and cough remedies, antacids, vitamins, minerals, amino acids, supplements, other prescription or nonprescription drugs
• Have a history of heart disease

Pregnancy:
Don't use unless prescribed by your doctor.

Breastfeeding:
Don't use unless prescribed by your doctor.

Infants and children:
Treating infants and children under 2 with any herbal preparation is hazardous.

Others:
None are expected if you are beyond childhood, under 45, not pregnant, basically healthy, take it for only a short time and do not exceed manufacturer's recommended dose.

Storage:
• Store in cool, dry area away from direct light, but don't freeze.
• Store safely out of reach of children.
• Don't store in bathroom medicine cabinet. Heat and moisture may change the action of the herb.

Safe dosage:
Consult your doctor for the appropriate dose for your condition.

Toxicity

Rated relatively safe when taken in appropriate quantities for short periods of time

For symptoms of toxicity: See *Adverse Reactions, Side Effects or Overdose Symptoms* section below.

Adverse Reactions, Side Effects or Overdose Symptoms

Signs and symptoms	What to do
Drowsiness	Discontinue. Call doctor when convenient.

MEDICINAL HERBS

Mace (Nutmeg)

 Basic Information

Biological name (genus and species):
Myristica fragrans

Parts used for medicinal purposes:
- Fibrous covering
- Seeds

Chemicals this herb contains:
- Elemicin
- Eugenol
- Fixed oil (see Glossary)
- Isoeugenol
- Isomethyleugenol
- Methoxyeugenol
- Methyleugenol
- Myristicin
- Protein
- Starch

 Known Effects

- Stimulates muscular movement of intestinal tract
- Stimulates central nervous system
- Helps treat diarrhea and indigestion
- Removes excess gas from gastrointestinal tract

Miscellaneous information:
- No effects are expected on the body, either good or bad, when the herb is used in very small amounts to enhance the flavor of food.
- Nutmeg is the seed. Mace is the fibrous covering.
- It is available as a powder and tincture.

 Possible Additional Effects

- May produce hallucinations
- May alter mood
- May treat digestive disorders
- May treat cholera

 Warnings and Precautions

Don't take if you:
- Are pregnant, think you may be pregnant or plan pregnancy in the near future
- Have any chronic disease of the gastrointestinal tract, such as stomach or duodenal ulcers, reflux esophagitis, ulcerative colitis, spastic colitis, diverticulosis or diverticulitis

Consult your doctor if you:
- Take any medicinal drugs or herbs including aspirin, laxatives, cold and cough remedies, antacids, vitamins, minerals, amino acids, supplements, other prescription or nonprescription drugs
- Are over age 60

Pregnancy:
Dangers outweigh any possible benefits. Don't use.

Breastfeeding:
Dangers outweigh any possible benefits. Don't use.

Infants and children:
Treating infants and children under 2 with any herbal preparation is hazardous.

Others:
Mind-altering and hallucinogenic effects are unpleasant. Do not use nutmeg for these purposes.

Storage:
- Store in cool, dry area away from direct light, but don't freeze.
- Store safely out of reach of children.
- Don't store in bathroom medicine cabinet. Heat and moisture may change the action of the herb.

Safe dosage:
Consult your doctor for the appropriate dose for your condition.

 Toxicity

- Mace is rated slightly dangerous, particularly in children, persons over 55 and those who take larger than appropriate quantities for extended periods of time.
- Narcotic properties—known to be toxic in humans—can cause delirium, disorientation and drunkenness.

For symptoms of toxicity: See *Adverse Reactions, Side Effects or Overdose Symptoms* section below.

 Adverse Reactions, Side Effects or Overdose Symptoms

Signs and symptoms	What to do
Diarrhea	Discontinue. Call doctor immediately.
Drowsiness	Discontinue. Call doctor when convenient.
Hallucinations	Seek emergency treatment.
Nausea or vomiting	Discontinue. Call doctor immediately.
Reduced body temperature	Discontinue. Call doctor immediately.
Weak, thready, rapid pulse	Seek emergency treatment.

Malabar Nut (Vasaka)

 Basic Information

Biological name (genus and species):
Adhatoda vasica

Parts used for medicinal purposes:
Leaves

Chemicals this herb contains:
- Adhatodic acid
- Peganine
- Vasicine

 Known Effects

- Dilates bronchial tubes
- Decreases thickness and increases fluidity of mucus in lungs and bronchial tubes

 Possible Additional Effects

- May treat coughs and colds
- May treat bronchitis
- May treat asthma

 Warnings and Precautions

Don't take if you:
- Are pregnant, think you may be pregnant or plan pregnancy in the near future
- Have any chronic disease of the gastrointestinal tract, such as stomach or duodenal ulcers, reflux esophagitis, ulcerative colitis, spastic colitis, diverticulosis or diverticulitis

MEDICINAL HERBS

→

Consult your doctor if you:
- Take this herb for any medical problem that doesn't improve in 2 weeks (There may be safer, more effective treatments.)
- Take any medicinal drugs or herbs including aspirin, laxatives, cold and cough remedies, antacids, vitamins, minerals, amino acids, supplements, other prescription or nonprescription drugs

Pregnancy:
Don't use unless prescribed by your doctor.

Breastfeeding:
Don't use unless prescribed by your doctor.

Infants and children:
Treating infants and children under 2 with any herbal preparation is hazardous.

Others:
None are expected if you are beyond childhood, under 45, not pregnant, basically healthy, take it for only a short time and do not exceed manufacturer's recommended dose.

Storage:
- Store in cool, dry area away from direct light, but don't freeze.
- Store safely out of reach of children.
- Don't store in bathroom medicine cabinet. Heat and moisture may change the action of the herb.

Safe dosage:
Consult your doctor for the appropriate dose for your condition.

 Toxicity

Rated slightly dangerous, particularly in children, persons over 55 and those who take larger than appropriate quantities for extended periods of time

For symptoms of toxicity: See *Adverse Reactions, Side Effects or Overdose Symptoms* section below.

 Adverse Reactions, Side Effects or Overdose Symptoms

Signs and symptoms	What to do
Diarrhea	Discontinue. Call doctor immediately.
Nausea or vomiting	Discontinue. Call doctor immediately.

Male Fern (Aspidium)

 Basic Information

Biological name (genus and species):
Dryopteris filix-mas

Parts used for medicinal purposes:
- Leaves
- Roots

Chemicals this herb contains:
- Alkanes
- Oleo resin
- Resins
- Triterpenes
- Volatile oils (see Glossary)

Known Effects

- Destroys intestinal worms
- Decreases normal muscle function
- Interferes with absorption of iron and other minerals when taken internally

Possible Additional Effects

No additional effects are known.

Warnings and Precautions

Don't take if you:

- Are pregnant, think you may be pregnant or plan pregnancy in the near future
- Have any chronic disease of the gastrointestinal tract, such as stomach or duodenal ulcers, reflux esophagitis, ulcerative colitis, spastic colitis, diverticulosis or diverticulitis
- Are over age 55
- Have heart disease
- Have kidney disease

Consult your doctor if you:

- Take this herb for any medical problem that doesn't improve in 2 weeks (There may be safer, more effective treatments.)
- Take any medicinal drugs or herbs including aspirin, laxatives, cold and cough remedies, antacids, vitamins, minerals, amino acids, supplements, other prescription or nonprescription drugs

Pregnancy:

Dangers outweigh any possible benefits. Don't use.

Breastfeeding:

Dangers outweigh any possible benefits. Don't use.

Infants and children:

Treating infants and children under 2 with any herbal preparation is hazardous.

Others:

Dangers outweigh any possible benefits. Don't use.

Storage:

- Store in cool, dry area away from direct light, but don't freeze.
- Store safely out of reach of children.
- Don't store in bathroom medicine cabinet. Heat and moisture may change the action of the herb.

Safe dosage:

Consult your doctor for the appropriate dose for your condition.

Toxicity

Rated dangerous, particularly in children, persons over 55 and those who take larger than appropriate quantities for extended periods of time

For symptoms of toxicity: See *Adverse Reactions, Side Effects or Overdose Symptoms* section below.

Adverse Reactions, Side Effects or Overdose Symptoms

Signs and symptoms	What to do
Abdominal cramping	Discontinue. Call doctor when convenient.
Breathing difficulty	Seek emergency treatment.
Coma	Seek emergency treatment.
Convulsions	Seek emergency treatment.
Diarrhea	Discontinue. Call doctor immediately.
Headache	Discontinue. Call doctor when convenient.
Heartbeat irregularities	Seek emergency treatment.
Nausea or vomiting	Discontinue. Call doctor immediately.
Vision impairment	Discontinue. Call doctor when convenient.

Mandrake (Love Apple, Satan's Apple)

Basic Information

Biological name (genus and species):
Mandragora officinarum

Parts used for medicinal purposes:
Roots

Chemicals this herb contains:
- Hyoscyamine
- Mandragorin
- Scopolamine

Known Effects

- Increases heart rate
- Dilates pupils
- Causes dry mouth
- Causes urinary retention
- Causes hallucinations
- Reduces muscular movements of intestinal tract

Possible Additional Effects

- May relieve pain
- Potential sedative
- Potential aphrodisiac
- May treat ulcers
- May treat skin diseases
- May treat hemorrhoids
- May cause explosive, watery diarrhea
- Potential anesthetic

Warnings and Precautions

Don't take if you:
- Are pregnant, think you may be pregnant or plan pregnancy in the near future
- Have heart disease

Consult your doctor if you:
- Take this herb for any medical problem that doesn't improve in 2 weeks (There may be safer, more effective treatments.)
- Take any medicinal drugs or herbs including aspirin, laxatives, cold and cough remedies, antacids, vitamins, minerals, amino acids, supplements, other prescription or nonprescription drugs

Pregnancy:
Dangers outweigh any possible benefits. Don't use.

Breastfeeding:
Dangers outweigh any possible benefits. Don't use.

Infants and children:
Treating infants and children under 2 with any herbal preparation is hazardous.

Others:
None are expected if you are beyond childhood, under 45, not pregnant, basically healthy, take it for only a short time and do not exceed manufacturer's recommended dose.

Storage:
- Store in cool, dry area away from direct light, but don't freeze.
- Store safely out of reach of children.
- Don't store in bathroom medicine cabinet. Heat and moisture may change the action of the herb.

Safe dosage:
Consult your doctor for the appropriate dose for your condition.

Toxicity

Rated dangerous, particularly in children, persons over 55 and those who take larger than appropriate quantities for extended periods of time

For symptoms of toxicity: See *Adverse Reactions, Side Effects or Overdose Symptoms* section below.

 Adverse Reactions, Side Effects or Overdose Symptoms

Signs and symptoms	What to do
Coma	Seek emergency treatment.
Confusion	Discontinue. Call doctor immediately.
Irregular heartbeat	Seek emergency treatment.

Marshmallow Plant

 Basic Information

Biological name (genus and species): *Althaea officinalis*

Parts used for medicinal purposes:
• Leaves
• Roots

Chemicals this herb contains:
• Asparagine
• Fat
• Mucilage (see Glossary)
• Pectin
• Starch
• Sugar

 Known Effects

• Softens or soothes skin
• Helps treat sore throat, cough, colds, sinusitis

Miscellaneous information:
• Marshmallow plant is used as a "filler" in a variety of pills.
• It is available in dried bulk, capsules, tincture and is used as a poultice (see Glossary) for applying medications.

 Possible Additional Effects

• May protect injured or scraped skin
• May treat kidney stones
• May treat indigestion

 Warnings and Precautions

Don't take if you:
• Are pregnant, think you may be pregnant or plan pregnancy in the near future
• Have any chronic disease of the gastrointestinal tract, such as stomach or duodenal ulcers, reflux esophagitis, ulcerative colitis, spastic colitis, diverticulosis or diverticulitis

Consult your doctor if you:
• Take this herb for any medical problem that doesn't improve in 2 weeks (There may be safer, more effective treatments.)
• Take any medicinal drugs or herbs including aspirin, laxatives, cold and cough remedies, antacids, vitamins, minerals, amino acids, supplements, other prescription or nonprescription drugs

MEDICINAL HERBS

➜

Pregnancy:
Don't use unless prescribed by your doctor.

Breastfeeding:
Don't use unless prescribed by your doctor.

Infants and children:
Treating infants and children under 2 with any herbal preparation is hazardous.

Others:
None are expected if you are beyond childhood, under 45, not pregnant, basically healthy, take it for only a short time and do not exceed manufacturer's recommended dose.

Storage:
• Store in cool, dry area away from direct light, but don't freeze.

• Store safely out of reach of children.
• Don't store in bathroom medicine cabinet. Heat and moisture may change the action of the herb.

Safe dosage:
Consult your doctor for the appropriate dose for your condition.

 Toxicity

Comparative-toxicity rating is not available from standard references.

 Adverse Reactions, Side Effects or Overdose Symptoms

None are expected.

Mayapple (American Mandrake, Podophyllum)

 Basic Information

Biological name (genus and species):
Podophyllum peltatum

Parts used for medicinal purposes:
Roots

Chemicals this herb contains:
• Alpha-peltatin
• Beta-peltatin
• Podophyllotoxin

 Known Effects

• Inhibits or prevents cell division
• Stimulates gastrointestinal tract
• Induces vomiting

 Possible Additional Effects

• May treat constipation and recurrent fecal impactions
• May cause testicular cancer (Certain components are under study.)

 Warnings and Precautions

Don't take if you:
• Are pregnant, think you may be pregnant or plan pregnancy in the near future
• Have any chronic disease of the gastrointestinal tract, such as stomach or duodenal ulcers, reflux esophagitis, ulcerative colitis, spastic colitis, diverticulosis or diverticulitis

Consult your doctor if you:
- Take this herb for any medical problem that doesn't improve in 2 weeks (There may be safer, more effective treatments.)
- Take any medicinal drugs or herbs including aspirin, laxatives, cold and cough remedies, antacids, vitamins, minerals, amino acids, supplements, other prescription or nonprescription drugs

Pregnancy:
Don't use unless prescribed by your doctor.

Breastfeeding:
Don't use unless prescribed by your doctor.

Infants and children:
Treating infants and children under 2 with any herbal preparation is hazardous.

Others:
None are expected if you are beyond childhood, under 45, not pregnant, basically healthy, take it for only a short time and do not exceed manufacturer's recommended dose.

Storage:
- Store in cool, dry area away from direct light, but don't freeze.
- Store safely out of reach of children.

- Don't store in bathroom medicine cabinet. Heat and moisture may change the action of the herb.

Safe dosage:
Consult your doctor for the appropriate dose for your condition.

Toxicity

Rated slightly dangerous, particularly in children, persons over 55 and those who take larger than appropriate quantities for extended periods of time

For symptoms of toxicity: See *Adverse Reactions, Side Effects or Overdose Symptoms* section below.

Adverse Reactions, Side Effects or Overdose Symptoms

Signs and symptoms	What to do
Diarrhea	Discontinue. Call doctor immediately.
Drowsiness	Discontinue. Call doctor when convenient.
Lethargy	Discontinue. Call doctor when convenient.
Nausea or vomiting	Discontinue. Call doctor immediately.
Unconsciousness	Seek emergency treatment.

Meadowsweet (Queen-of-the-Meadow, Spirea)

Basic Information

Biological name (genus and species):
Filipendula ulmaria

Parts used for medicinal purposes:
- Petals/flower
- Roots

Chemicals this herb contains:
- Gallic acid
- Methyl salicylate
- Salicylic acid
- Salicylic aldehyde
- Tannic acid
- Volatile oils (see Glossary)

➜

MEDICINAL HERBS

Known Effects

- Helps treat gastrointestinal upset
- Helps treat headaches

Possible Additional Effects

- May help body dispose of excess fluid by increasing amount of urine produced
- May treat diarrhea
- May reduce pain
- May relieve menstrual cramps

Warnings and Precautions

Don't take if you:

- Are pregnant, think you may be pregnant or plan pregnancy in the near future
- Have chronic kidney problems

Consult your doctor if you:

- Take this herb for any medical problem that doesn't improve in 2 weeks (There may be safer, more effective treatments.)
- Take any medicinal drugs or herbs including aspirin, laxatives, cold and cough remedies, antacids, vitamins, minerals, amino acids, supplements, other prescription or nonprescription drugs

Pregnancy:

Don't use unless prescribed by your doctor—contains salicylates.

Breastfeeding:

Don't use unless prescribed by your doctor—contains salicylates.

Infants and children:

Treating infants and children under 2 with any herbal preparation is hazardous.

Others:

None are expected if you are beyond childhood, under 45, not pregnant, basically healthy, take it for only a short time and do not exceed manufacturer's recommended dose.

Storage:

- Store in cool, dry area away from direct light, but don't freeze.
- Store safely out of reach of children.
- Don't store in bathroom medicine cabinet. Heat and moisture may change the action of the herb.

Safe dosage:

Consult your doctor for the appropriate dose for your condition.

Toxicity

Generally regarded as safe when taken in appropriate quantities for short periods of time

For symptoms of toxicity: See *Adverse Reactions, Side Effects or Overdose Symptoms* section below.

Adverse Reactions, Side Effects or Overdose Symptoms

Signs and symptoms	What to do
Coma	Seek emergency treatment.
Kidney damage characterized by blood in urine, decreased urine flow, swelling of hands and feet	Seek emergency treatment.
Lethargy	Discontinue. Call doctor when convenient.
Unconsciousness	Seek emergency treatment.
Upset stomach	Discontinue. Call doctor when convenient.

Mexican Sarsaparilla

Basic Information

Biological name (genus and species):
Smilax aristolochiaefolia, S. regelii, S. febrifuga, S. ornata

Parts used for medicinal purposes:
• Bark
• Berries
• Roots

Chemicals this herb contains:
• Resin (see Glossary)
• Sarsasapogenin
• Smilagenin
• Starch
• Stigmasterol
• Volatile oils (see Glossary)

Known Effects

• Irritates mucous membranes
• Irritates gastrointestinal tract

Miscellaneous information:
• Berries are edible.
• Berries, bark and other parts of plant are used to make the soft drink of the same name.

Possible Additional Effects

• May relieve toothache
• May temporarily relieve constipation

Warnings and Precautions

Don't take if you:
Are pregnant, think you may be pregnant or plan pregnancy in the near future.

Consult your doctor if you:
• Take this herb for any medical problem that doesn't improve in 2 weeks (There may be safer, more effective treatments.)
• Take any medicinal drugs or herbs including aspirin, laxatives, cold and cough remedies, antacids, vitamins, minerals, amino acids, supplements, other prescription or nonprescription drugs

Pregnancy:
Don't use unless prescribed by your doctor.

Breastfeeding:
Don't use unless prescribed by your doctor.

Infants and children:
Treating infants and children under 2 with any herbal preparation is hazardous.

Others:
None are expected if you are beyond childhood, under 45, not pregnant, basically healthy, take it for only a short time and do not exceed manufacturer's recommended dose.

Storage:
• Store in cool, dry area away from direct light, but don't freeze.
• Store safely out of reach of children.
• Don't store in bathroom medicine cabinet. Heat and moisture may change the action of the herb.

MEDICINAL HERBS

Safe dosage:
Consult your doctor for the appropriate dose for your condition.

Toxicity

Rated relatively safe when taken in appropriate quantities for short periods of time

Adverse Reactions, Side Effects or Overdose Symptoms

None are expected.

Milkweed, Common (Blood-flower)

Basic Information

Biological name (genus and species):
Asclepias syriaca

Parts used for medicinal purposes:
Roots

Chemicals this herb contains:
• Asclepiadin
• Asclepione (a bitter)
• Galitoxin

Known Effects

• Irritates and stimulates gastrointestinal tract
• Decreases thickness and increases fluidity of mucus in lungs and bronchial tubes
• Increases perspiration

Miscellaneous information:
All parts of milkweed may be toxic.

Possible Additional Effects

• May treat bronchitis
• May treat arthritis

Warnings and Precautions

Don't take if you:
• Are pregnant, think you may be pregnant or plan pregnancy in the near future
• Have any chronic disease of the gastrointestinal tract, such as stomach or duodenal ulcers, reflux esophagitis, ulcerative colitis, spastic colitis, diverticulosis or diverticulitis

Consult your doctor if you:
• Take this herb for any medical problem that doesn't improve in 2 weeks (There may be safer, more effective treatments.)
• Take any medicinal drugs or herbs including aspirin, laxatives, cold and cough remedies, antacids, vitamins, minerals, amino acids, supplements, other prescription or nonprescription drugs

Pregnancy:
Dangers outweigh any possible benefits. Don't use.

Breastfeeding:
Dangers outweigh any possible benefits. Don't use.

Infants and children:
Treating infants and children under 2 with any herbal preparation is hazardous.

Others:
Dangers outweigh any possible benefits. Don't use.

Storage:
• Store in cool, dry area away from direct light, but don't freeze.
• Store safely out of reach of children.
• Don't store in bathroom medicine cabinet. Heat and moisture may change the action of the herb.

Safe dosage:
Consult your doctor for the appropriate dose for your condition.

 Toxicity

Rated slightly dangerous, particularly in children, persons over 55 and those who take larger than appropriate quantities for extended periods of time

For symptoms of toxicity: See *Adverse Reactions, Side Effects or Overdose Symptoms* section below.

Adverse Reactions, Side Effects or Overdose Symptoms

Signs and symptoms	What to do
Coma	Seek emergency treatment.
Diarrhea	Discontinue. Call doctor immediately.
Drowsiness	Discontinue. Call doctor when convenient.
Jaundice (yellow skin and eyes)	Discontinue. Call doctor immediately.
Kidney damage characterized by blood in urine, decreased urine flow, swelling of hands and feet	Seek emergency treatment.
Lethargy	Discontinue. Call doctor when convenient.
Loss of appetite	Discontinue. Call doctor when convenient.
Nausea or vomiting	Discontinue. Call doctor immediately.
Seizures	Seek emergency treatment.
Unsteady walk	Discontinue. Call doctor immediately.

MEDICINAL HERBS

→

Milkwort

 ## Basic Information

Biological name (genus and species):
Polygala vulgaris, P. senega

Parts used for medicinal purposes:
Roots

Chemicals this herb contains:
Saponins (see Glossary)

 ## Known Effects

- Increases secretions from bronchial tubes
- Irritates intestinal tract
- Decreases thickness and increases fluidity of mucus in lungs and bronchial tubes
- Helps body dispose of excess fluid by increasing amount of urine produced
- Increases perspiration

 ## Possible Additional Effects

- May treat croup
- May treat arthritis
- May treat hives
- May treat gout
- May treat pleurisy
- May treat constipation
- May increase milk production in lactating women

 ## Warnings and Precautions

Don't take if you:
- Are pregnant, think you may be pregnant or plan pregnancy in the near future
- Have any chronic disease of the gastrointestinal tract, such as stomach or duodenal ulcers, reflux esophagitis, ulcerative colitis, spastic colitis, diverticulosis or diverticulitis

Consult your doctor if you:
- Take this herb for any medical problem that doesn't improve in 2 weeks (There may be safer, more effective treatments.)
- Take any medicinal drugs or herbs including aspirin, laxatives, cold and cough remedies, antacids, vitamins, minerals, amino acids, supplements, other prescription or nonprescription drugs

Pregnancy:
Dangers outweigh any possible benefits. Don't use.

Breastfeeding:
Dangers outweigh any possible benefits. Don't use.

Infants and children:
Treating infants and children under 2 with any herbal preparation is hazardous.

Others:
None are expected if you are beyond childhood, under 45, not pregnant, basically healthy, take it for only a short time and do not exceed manufacturer's recommended dose.

Storage:

- Store in cool, dry area away from direct light, but don't freeze.
- Store safely out of reach of children.
- Don't store in bathroom medicine cabinet. Heat and moisture may change the action of the herb.

Safe dosage:

Consult your doctor for the appropriate dose for your condition.

 Toxicity

Comparative-toxicity rating is not available from standard references.

For symptoms of toxicity: See *Adverse Reactions, Side Effects or Overdose Symptoms* section below.

 Adverse Reactions, Side Effects or Overdose Symptoms

Signs and symptoms	What to do
Coma	Seek emergency treatment.
Diarrhea	Discontinue. Call doctor immediately.
Drowsiness	Discontinue. Call doctor when convenient.
Lethargy	Discontinue. Call doctor when convenient.
Nausea, violent	Discontinue. Call doctor immediately.
Vomiting	Discontinue. Call doctor immediately.

Mistletoe

 Basic Information

Biological name (genus and species): *Phoradendron serotinum, Viscum album*

Parts used for medicinal purposes:
- Berries/fruits
- Leaves
- Stems

Chemicals this herb contains:
- Beta-phenylethylamine
- Tyramine
- Viscotoxins

 Known Effects

- Stimulates central nervous system
- Causes contraction of smooth muscle

Miscellaneous information:

Mistletoe is particularly dangerous for people taking monoamine-oxidase medications to treat high blood pressure.

 Possible Additional Effects

- May relieve nervousness
- May reduce high blood pressure

MEDICINAL HERBS

→

Warnings and Precautions

Don't take if you:

- Are pregnant, think you may be pregnant or plan pregnancy in the near future
- Have any chronic disease of the gastrointestinal tract, such as stomach or duodenal ulcers, reflux esophagitis, ulcerative colitis, spastic colitis, diverticulosis or diverticulitis

Consult your doctor if you:

- Take this herb for any medical problem that doesn't improve in 2 weeks (There may be safer, more effective treatments.)
- Take any medicinal drugs or herbs including aspirin, laxatives, cold and cough remedies, antacids, vitamins, minerals, amino acids, supplements, other prescription or nonprescription drugs
- Wish to use this herb—it is considered poisonous

Pregnancy:
Dangers outweigh any possible benefits. Don't use.

Breastfeeding:
Dangers outweigh any possible benefits. Don't use.

Infants and children:
Treating infants and children under 2 with any herbal preparation is hazardous.

Others:
Do not allow children to eat the berries of this popular Christmas plant. As few as one or two berries may cause toxic symptoms.

Storage:

- Store in cool, dry area away from direct light, but don't freeze.
- Store safely out of reach of children.
- Don't store in bathroom medicine cabinet. Heat and moisture may change the action of the herb.

Safe dosage:
Consult your doctor for the appropriate dose for your condition.

 ## Toxicity

Rated slightly dangerous, particularly in children, persons over 55 and those who take larger than appropriate quantities for extended periods of time

For symptoms of toxicity: See *Adverse Reactions, Side Effects or Overdose Symptoms* section below.

 ## Adverse Reactions, Side Effects or Overdose Symptoms

Signs and symptoms	What to do
Convulsions	Seek emergency treatment.
Diarrhea	Discontinue. Call doctor immediately.
Hallucinations	Seek emergency treatment.
Headache	Discontinue. Call doctor immediately.
Increased blood pressure	Discontinue. Call doctor immediately.
Muscle spasms	Discontinue. Call doctor immediately.
Nausea or vomiting	Discontinue. Call doctor immediately.
Slow heartbeat	Seek emergency treatment.

Mormon Tea (Brigham Tea, Nevada Jointfir)

Basic Information

Biological name (genus and species):
Ephedra nevadensis, E. trifurca

Parts used for medicinal purposes:
Stems

Chemicals this herb contains:
Ephedrine

Known Effects

- Stimulates central nervous system
- Increases blood pressure
- Increases heart rate

Miscellaneous information:
Mormon tea has no value in treating bronchial asthma.

Possible Additional Effects

vate mood
- May reduce symptoms of congestive heart failure, kidney failure, liver failure
- May decrease appetite
- May stimulate energy
- May reduce symptoms of fatigue

STOP Warnings and Precautions

Don't take if you:
- Are pregnant, think you may be pregnant or plan pregnancy in the near future
- Have diabetes mellitus, because it impedes control with diet and insulin
- Have heart disease

Consult your doctor if you:
- Take this herb for any medical problem that doesn't improve in 2 weeks (There may be safer, more effective treatments.)
- Take any medicinal drugs or herbs including aspirin, laxatives, cold and cough remedies, antacids, vitamins, minerals, amino acids, supplements, other prescription or nonprescription drugs

Pregnancy:
Dangers outweigh any possible benefits. Don't use.

Breastfeeding:
Dangers outweigh any possible benefits. Don't use.

Infants and children:
Treating infants and children under 2 with any herbal preparation is hazardous.

Others:
None are expected if you are beyond childhood, under 45, not pregnant, basically healthy, take it for only a short time and do not exceed manufacturer's recommended dose.

MEDICINAL HERBS

→

Storage:
- Store in cool, dry area away from direct light, but don't freeze.
- Store safely out of reach of children.
- Don't store in bathroom medicine cabinet. Heat and moisture may change the action of the herb.

Safe dosage:

Consult your doctor for the appropriate dose for your condition.

 Toxicity

Rated slightly dangerous, particularly in children, persons over 55 and those who take larger than appropriate quantities for extended periods of time

For symptoms of toxicity: See *Adverse Reactions, Side Effects or Overdose Symptoms* section below.

 Adverse Reactions, Side Effects or Overdose Symptoms

Signs and symptoms	What to do
Excessively high blood pressure	Seek emergency treatment.
Irregular heartbeat	Seek emergency treatment.
Rapid heartbeat	Discontinue. Call doctor immediately.

Morning Glory

 Basic Information

Biological name (genus and species):
Ipomoea purpurea

Parts used for medicinal purposes:
Seeds

Chemicals this herb contains:
- Cetyl alcohol
- Dihydroxycinnamic acid
- Lysergic acid
- Scopoletin

 Known Effects

- Stimulates central nervous system
- Stimulates gastrointestinal tract

 Possible Additional Effects

- May cause hallucinations
- Potential purgative for constipation
- May elevate mood

Warnings and Precautions

Don't take if you:

- Are pregnant, think you may be pregnant or plan pregnancy in the near future
- Have any chronic disease of the gastrointestinal tract, such as stomach or duodenal ulcers, reflux esophagitis, ulcerative colitis, spastic colitis, diverticulosis or diverticulitis

Consult your doctor if you:

- Take this herb for any medical problem that doesn't improve in 2 weeks (There may be safer, more effective treatments.)
- Take any medicinal drugs or herbs including aspirin, laxatives, cold and cough remedies, antacids, vitamins, minerals, amino acids, supplements, other prescription or nonprescription drugs

Pregnancy:

Don't use unless prescribed by your doctor.

Breast-feeding:

Don't use unless prescribed by your doctor.

Infants and children:

Treating infants and children under 2 with any herbal preparation is hazardous.

Others:

None are expected if you are beyond childhood, under 45, not pregnant, basically healthy, take it for only a short time and do not exceed manufacturer's recommended dose.

Storage:

- Store in cool, dry area away from direct light, but don't freeze.
- Store safely out of reach of children.
- Don't store in bathroom medicine cabinet. Heat and moisture may change the action of the herb.

Safe dosage:

Consult your doctor for the appropriate dose for your condition.

 ## Toxicity

Rated slightly dangerous, particularly in children, persons over 55 and those who take larger than appropriate quantities for extended periods of time

For symptoms of toxicity: See *Adverse Reactions, Side Effects or Overdose Symptoms* section below.

 ## Adverse Reactions, Side Effects or Overdose Symptoms

Signs and symptoms	What to do
Confusion	Discontinue. Call doctor immediately.
Diarrhea, explosive and watery	Discontinue. Call doctor immediately.
Disturbed vision	Discontinue. Call doctor immediately.
Hallucinations	Seek emergency treatment.
Nausea or vomiting	Discontinue. Call doctor immediately.

MEDICINAL HERBS

Mountain Ash (Rowan Tree)

Basic Information

Biological name (genus and species):
Sorbus aucuparia

Parts used for medicinal purposes:
• Berries/fruits
• Seeds

Chemicals this herb contains:
• Fixed oil (see Glossary)
• Malic acid
• Sorbic acid
• Sorbitol
• Sorbose

Known Effects

• Irritates and stimulates
gastrointestinal tract
• Helps body dispose of excess fluid
by increasing amount of
urine produced

Miscellaneous information:
Used as a sweetener.

Possible Additional Effects

• May prevent scurvy
• May treat hemorrhoids
• May treat stomach and
duodenal ulcers

Warnings and Precautions

Don't take if you:
Are pregnant, think you may be
pregnant or plan pregnancy in the
near future.

Consult your doctor if you:
• Take this herb for any medical
problem that doesn't improve in
2 weeks (There may be safer, more
effective treatments.)
• Take any medicinal drugs or
herbs including aspirin, laxatives,
cold and cough remedies, antacids,
vitamins, minerals, amino acids,
supplements, other prescription
or nonprescription drugs

Pregnancy:
Don't use unless prescribed by
your doctor.

Breastfeeding:
Problems in breastfed infants of
lactating mothers taking small or usual
amounts have not been proved, but the
chance of problems does exist. Don't
use unless prescribed by your doctor.

Infants and children:
Treating infants and children under
2 with any herbal preparation
is hazardous.

Others:
None are expected if you are beyond
childhood, under 45, not pregnant,
basically healthy, take it for only a short
time and do not exceed manufacturer's
recommended dose.

Storage:
• Store in cool, dry area away from
direct light, but don't freeze.
• Store safely out of reach of children.
• Don't store in bathroom medicine
cabinet. Heat and moisture may
change the action of the herb.

Safe dosage:
Consult your doctor for the appropriate dose for your condition.

Toxicity

Comparative-toxicity rating is not available from standard references.

For symptoms of toxicity: See *Adverse Reactions, Side Effects or Overdose Symptoms* section below.

Adverse Reactions, Side Effects or Overdose Symptoms

Signs and symptoms	What to do
Diarrhea	Discontinue. Call doctor immediately.

Mountain Tobacco (Leopard's Bane, Wolf's Bane)

Basic Information

Biological name (genus and species):
Arnica montana

Parts used for medicinal purposes:
Petals/flower

Chemicals this herb contains:
- Angelic acid
- Arnidiol
- Choline
- Fatty acids
- Formic acid
- Thymohydroquinone

Known Effects

- Provides counterirritation (see Glossary) when applied to skin overlying an inflamed or irritated joint
- Depresses central nervous system
- Irritates gastrointestinal tract

Possible Additional Effects

May relieve discomfort of sprains, strains, bruises when applied to skin over injury

Warnings and Precautions

Don't take if you:
- Are pregnant, think you may be pregnant or plan pregnancy in the near future
- Have any chronic disease of the gastrointestinal tract, such as stomach or duodenal ulcers, reflux esophagitis, ulcerative colitis, spastic colitis, diverticulosis or diverticulitis

Consult your doctor if you:
- Take this herb for any medical problem that doesn't improve in 2 weeks (There may be safer, more effective treatments.)
- Take any medicinal drugs or herbs including aspirin, laxatives, cold and cough remedies, antacids, vitamins, minerals, amino acids, supplements, other prescription or nonprescription drugs

Pregnancy:
Dangers outweigh any possible benefits. Don't use.

Breastfeeding:
Dangers outweigh any possible benefits. Don't use.

MEDICINAL HERBS

→

Infants and children:
Treating infants and children under 2 with any herbal preparation is hazardous.

Others:
Don't take internally. Probably safe for application to skin.

Storage:
• Store in cool, dry area away from direct light, but don't freeze.
• Store safely out of reach of children.
• Don't store in bathroom medicine cabinet. Heat and moisture may change the action of the herb.

Safe dosage:
Consult your doctor for the appropriate dose for your condition.

 Toxicity

Rated slightly dangerous, particularly in children, persons over 55 and those who take larger than appropriate quantities for extended periods of time

For symptoms of toxicity: See *Adverse Reactions, Side Effects or Overdose Symptoms* section below.

 Adverse Reactions, Side Effects or Overdose Symptoms

Signs and symptoms	What to do
Diarrhea, explosive, watery	Discontinue. Call doctor immediately.
Heartbeat irregularities	Seek emergency treatment.
Muscle weakness	Discontinue. Call doctor immediately.
Nausea or vomiting	Discontinue. Call doctor immediately.
Precipitous blood-pressure drop: symptoms include faintness, cold sweat, paleness, rapid pulse	Seek emergency treatment.

Mulberry

 Basic Information

Biological name (genus and species):
Morus rubra

Parts used for medicinal purposes:
• Bark
• Berries/fruits

Chemicals this herb contains:
Unidentified

 Known Effects
• Stimulates gastrointestinal tract
• Depresses central nervous system

 Possible Additional Effects
• May reduce fever
• May induce drowsiness
• Potential mild laxative

Warnings and Precautions

Don't take if you:
- Are pregnant, think you may be pregnant or plan pregnancy in the near future
- Have any chronic disease of the gastrointestinal tract, such as stomach or duodenal ulcers, reflux esophagitis, ulcerative colitis, spastic colitis, diverticulosis or diverticulitis

Consult your doctor if you:
- Take this herb for any medical problem that doesn't improve in 2 weeks (There may be safer, more effective treatments.)
- Take any medicinal drugs or herbs including aspirin, laxatives, cold and cough remedies, antacids, vitamins, minerals, amino acids, supplements, other prescription or nonprescription drugs

Pregnancy:
Dangers outweigh any possible benefits. Don't use.

Breastfeeding:
Dangers outweigh any possible benefits. Don't use.

Infants and children:
Treating infants and children under 2 with any herbal preparation is hazardous.

Others:
This product will not help you and may cause toxic symptoms.

Storage:
- Store in cool, dry area away from direct light, but don't freeze.
- Store safely out of reach of children.
- Don't store in bathroom medicine cabinet. Heat and moisture may change the action of the herb.

Safe dosage:
Consult your doctor for the appropriate dose for your condition.

 ## Toxicity

Comparative-toxicity rating is not available from standard references.

For symptoms of toxicity: See *Adverse Reactions, Side Effects or Overdose Symptoms* section below.

 ## Adverse Reactions, Side Effects or Overdose Symptoms

Signs and symptoms	What to do
Diarrhea	Discontinue. Call doctor immediately.
Hallucinations	Seek emergency treatment.
Nausea or vomiting	Discontinue. Call doctor immediately.

MEDICINAL HERBS

Myrtle

Basic Information

Biological name (genus and species):
Myrtus communis

Parts used for medicinal purposes:
Leaves

Chemicals this herb contains:
• D-pinene
• Eucalyptol
• Myrtenol

Known Effects

• Myrtle irritates mucous membranes.
• Large amounts may depress central nervous system.

Miscellaneous information:
Myrtle is used as a condiment, flavoring, perfume essence and gargle.

Possible Additional Effects

• May treat stomach irritations
• May treat bronchitis
• May treat cystitis

Warnings and Precautions

Don't take if you:
• Are pregnant, think you may be pregnant or plan pregnancy in the near future
• Have chronic kidney disease

Consult your doctor if you:
• Take this herb for any medical problem that doesn't improve in 2 weeks (There may be safer, more effective treatments.)

• Take any medicinal drugs or herbs including aspirin, laxatives, cold and cough remedies, antacids, vitamins, minerals, amino acids, supplements, other prescription or nonprescription drugs

Pregnancy:
Don't use unless prescribed by your doctor.

Breastfeeding:
Don't use unless prescribed by your doctor.

Infants and children:
Treating infants and children under 2 with any herbal preparation is hazardous.

Others:
None are expected if you are beyond childhood, under 45, not pregnant, basically healthy, take it for only a short time and do not exceed manufacturer's recommended dose.

Storage:
• Store in cool, dry area away from direct light, but don't freeze.
• Store safely out of reach of children.
• Don't store in bathroom medicine cabinet. Heat and moisture may change the action of the herb.

Safe dosage:
Consult your doctor for the appropriate dose for your condition.

Toxicity

Comparative-toxicity rating is not available from standard references.

For symptoms of toxicity: See *Adverse Reactions, Side Effects or Overdose Symptoms* section below.

Adverse Reactions, Side Effects or Overdose Symptoms

Signs and symptoms	What to do
Coma	Seek emergency treatment.
Convulsions	Seek emergency treatment.
Kidney damage characterized by blood in urine, decreased urine flow, swelling of hands and feet	Seek emergency treatment.

Oak Bark

Basic Information

Biological name (genus and species):
Quercus

Parts used for medicinal purposes:
• Bark
• Seeds

Chemicals this herb contains:
Quercitannic acid

Known Effects

• Anti-inflammatory
• Relieves sore throats when used as a gargle
• Helps treat strains

Possible Additional Effects

• May treat hemorrhoids
• May treat diarrhea
• Potential mouthwash for inflammation

Warnings and Precautions

Don't take if you:
• Are pregnant, think you may be pregnant or plan pregnancy in the near future
• Have any chronic disease of the gastrointestinal tract, such as stomach or duodenal ulcers, reflux esophagitis, ulcerative colitis, spastic colitis, diverticulosis or diverticulitis

Consult your doctor if you:
• Take this herb for any medical problem that doesn't improve in 2 weeks (There may be safer, more effective treatments.)
• Take any medicinal drugs or herbs including aspirin, laxatives, cold and cough remedies, antacids, vitamins, minerals, amino acids, supplements, other prescription or nonprescription drugs

Pregnancy:
Dangers outweigh any possible benefits. Don't use.

MEDICINAL HERBS

➜

Breastfeeding:
Dangers outweigh any possible benefits. Don't use.

Infants and children:
Treating infants and children under 2 with any herbal preparation is hazardous.

Others:
None are expected if you are beyond childhood, under 45, not pregnant, basically healthy, take it for only a short time and do not exceed manufacturer's recommended dose.

Storage:
• Store in cool, dry area away from direct light, but don't freeze.
• Store safely out of reach of children.
• Don't store in bathroom medicine cabinet. Heat and moisture may change the action of the herb.

Safe dosage:
Consult your doctor for the appropriate dose for your condition.

 Toxicity

Comparative-toxicity rating is not available from standard references.

For symptoms of toxicity: See *Adverse Reactions, Side Effects or Overdose Symptoms* section below.

 Adverse Reactions, Side Effects or Overdose Symptoms

Signs and symptoms	What to do
Constipation	Discontinue. Call doctor when convenient.
Dry mouth	Discontinue. Call doctor when convenient.
Increased urination	Discontinue. Call doctor when convenient.
Jaundice (yellow skin and eyes)	Discontinue. Call doctor immediately.
Kidney damage characterized by blood in urine, decreased urine flow, swelling of hands and feet	Seek emergency treatment.
Skin eruptions	Discontinue. Call doctor when convenient.
Thirst	Discontinue. Call doctor when convenient.

Orris Root (Black Flag)

 Basic Information

Biological name (genus and species):
Iris versicolor

Parts used for medicinal purposes:
Roots

Chemicals this herb contains:
• Gum (see Glossary)
• Oleoresin (see Glossary)
• Tannins (see Glossary)

 Known Effects

• Depresses central nervous system
• Causes vomiting
• Interferes with absorption of iron and other minerals when taken internally

Possible Additional Effects

- May treat skin disorders
- May treat arthritis
- May treat tumors

Warnings and Precautions

Don't take if you:

- Are pregnant, think you may be pregnant or plan pregnancy in the near future
- Have any chronic disease of the gastrointestinal tract, such as stomach or duodenal ulcers, reflux esophagitis, ulcerative colitis, spastic colitis, diverticulosis or diverticulitis

Consult your doctor if you:

- Take this herb for any medical problem that doesn't improve in 2 weeks (There may be safer, more effective treatments.)
- Take any medicinal drugs or herbs including aspirin, laxatives, cold and cough remedies, antacids, vitamins, minerals, amino acids, supplements, other prescription or nonprescription drugs

Pregnancy:

Problems in pregnant women taking small or usual amounts have not been proved, but the chance of problems does exist. Don't use unless prescribed by your doctor.

Breastfeeding:

Problems in breastfed infants of lactating mothers taking small or usual amounts have not been proved, but the chance of problems does exist. Don't use unless prescribed by your doctor.

Infants and children:

Treating infants and children under 2 with any herbal preparation is hazardous.

Others:

Don't use. This product will not help you and may cause toxic symptoms.

Storage:

- Store in cool, dry area away from direct light, but don't freeze.
- Store safely out of reach of children.
- Don't store in bathroom medicine cabinet. Heat and moisture may change the action of the herb.

Safe dosage:

Consult your doctor for the appropriate dose for your condition.

Toxicity

Rated relatively safe when taken in appropriate quantities for short periods of time

For symptoms of toxicity: See *Adverse Reactions, Side Effects or Overdose Symptoms* section below.

Adverse Reactions, Side Effects or Overdose Symptoms

Signs and symptoms	What to do
Burning sensation in throat and mouth	Discontinue. Call doctor when convenient.
Cramping, abdominal pain	Discontinue. Call doctor when convenient.
Diarrhea, watery	Discontinue. Call doctor immediately.
Nausea or vomiting	Discontinue. Call doctor immediately.

Papaya

Basic Information

Biological name (genus and species):
Carica papaya

Parts used for medicinal purposes:
- Berries/fruits
- Inner bark
- Stems

Chemicals this herb contains:
- Amylolytic enzyme
- Caricin
- Myrosin
- Peptidase
- Vitamins C and E

Known Effects

- Stimulates stomach to increase secretions
- Releases histamine from body tissues
- Depresses central nervous system
- Kills some intestinal parasites

Miscellaneous information:
- No problems expected when eaten as a common food
- Used as a meat tenderizer

Possible Additional Effects

- May aid digestion
- May liquify excessive mucus in mouth and stomach
- May treat sore teeth (inner bark)

Warnings and Precautions

Don't take if you:
- Are pregnant, think you may be pregnant or plan pregnancy in the near future
- Have any chronic disease of the gastrointestinal tract, such as stomach or duodenal ulcers, reflux esophagitis, ulcerative colitis, spastic colitis, diverticulosis or diverticulitis

Consult your doctor if you:
- Take this herb for any medical problem that doesn't improve in 2 weeks (There may be safer, more effective treatments.)
- Take any medicinal drugs or herbs including aspirin, laxatives, cold and cough remedies, antacids, vitamins, minerals, amino acids, supplements, other prescription or nonprescription drugs

Pregnancy:
Pregnant women should experience no problems taking usual amounts as part of a balanced diet. Other products extracted from this herb have not been proved to cause problems.

Breastfeeding:
Breastfed infants of lactating mothers should experience no problems when mother takes usual amounts as part of a balanced diet. Other products extracted from this herb have not been proved to cause problems.

Infants and children:
Treating infants and children under 2 with any herbal preparation is hazardous.

Others:

None are expected if you are beyond childhood, under 45, not pregnant, basically healthy, take it for only a short time and do not exceed manufacturer's recommended dose.

Storage:

- Store in cool, dry area away from direct light, but don't freeze.
- Store safely out of reach of children.
- Don't store in bathroom medicine cabinet. Heat and moisture may change the action of the herb.

Safe dosage:

Consult your doctor for the appropriate dose for your condition.

 Toxicity

Generally regarded as safe when taken in appropriate quantities for short periods of time

For symptoms of toxicity: See *Adverse Reactions, Side Effects or Overdose Symptoms* section below.

 Adverse Reactions, Side Effects or Overdose Symptoms

Signs and symptoms	What to do
Heartburn caused by irritation of lower part of esophagus	Discontinue. Call doctor when convenient.

Partridgeberry (Squawvine)

 Basic Information

Biological name (genus and species): *Mitchella repens*

Parts used for medicinal purposes: Stems

Chemicals this herb contains:
- Dextrin
- Mucilage (see Glossary)
- Saponins (see Glossary)
- Wax (see Glossary)

 Known Effects

- Helps body dispose of excess fluid by increasing amount of urine produced
- Shrinks tissues
- Prevents secretion of fluids

 Possible Additional Effects

- May make labor less difficult
- May help flow of milk in lactating women
- May treat insomnia
- May decrease diarrhea
- May treat congestive heart failure, kidney failure, liver failure

MEDICINAL HERBS

➔

Warnings and Precautions

Don't take if you:
Are pregnant, think you may be pregnant or plan pregnancy in the near future.

Consult your doctor if you:
• Take this herb for any medical problem that doesn't improve in 2 weeks (There may be safer, more effective treatments.)
• Take any medicinal drugs or herbs including aspirin, laxatives, cold and cough remedies, antacids, vitamins, minerals, amino acids, supplements, other prescription or nonprescription drugs

Pregnancy:
Don't use unless prescribed by your doctor.

Breastfeeding:
Don't use unless prescribed by your doctor.

Infants and children:
Treating infants and children under 2 with any herbal preparation is hazardous.

Others:
None are expected if you are beyond childhood, under 45, not pregnant, basically healthy, take it for only a short time and do not exceed manufacturer's recommended dose.

Storage:
• Store in cool, dry area away from direct light, but don't freeze.
• Store safely out of reach of children.
• Don't store in bathroom medicine cabinet. Heat and moisture may change the action of the herb.

Safe dosage:
Consult your doctor for the appropriate dose for your condition.

 Toxicity

Rated relatively safe when taken in appropriate quantities for short periods of time

 Adverse Reactions, Side Effects or Overdose Symptoms

None are expected.

Pasque Flower (May Flower, Pulsatilla)

 Basic Information

Biological name (genus and species):
Anemone pulsatilla

Parts used for medicinal purposes:
• Petals/flower
• Roots

Chemicals this herb contains:
• Anemone camphor
• Ranunculin
• Tannins (see Glossary)
• Volatile oils (see Glossary)

 Known Effects

• Irritates mucous membranes
• Shrinks tissues
• Prevents secretion of fluids
• Decreases thickness and increases fluidity of mucus in lungs and bronchial tubes
• Interferes with absorption of iron and other minerals when taken internally

Possible Additional Effects

- May treat menstrual disorders
- May depress sexual excitement
- May increase sexual strength

Warnings and Precautions

Don't take if you:

- Are pregnant, think you may be pregnant or plan pregnancy in the near future
- Have any chronic disease of the gastrointestinal tract, such as stomach or duodenal ulcers, reflux esophagitis, ulcerative colitis, spastic colitis, diverticulosis or diverticulitis

Consult your doctor if you:

- Take this herb for any medical problem that doesn't improve in 2 weeks (There may be safer, more effective treatments.)
- Take any medicinal drugs or herbs including aspirin, laxatives, cold and cough remedies, antacids, vitamins, minerals, amino acids, supplements, other prescription or nonprescription drugs

Pregnancy:

Dangers outweigh any possible benefits. Don't use.

Breastfeeding:

Dangers outweigh any possible benefits. Don't use.

Infants and children:

Treating infants and children under 2 with any herbal preparation is hazardous.

Others:

None are expected if you are beyond childhood, under 45, not pregnant, basically healthy, take it for only a short time and do not exceed manufacturer's recommended dose.

Storage:

- Store in cool, dry area away from direct light, but don't freeze.
- Store safely out of reach of children.
- Don't store in bathroom medicine cabinet. Heat and moisture may change the action of the herb.

Safe dosage:

Consult your doctor for the appropriate dose for your condition.

Toxicity

Rated slightly dangerous, particularly in children, persons over 55 and those who take larger than appropriate quantities for extended periods of time

For symptoms of toxicity: See *Adverse Reactions, Side Effects or Overdose Symptoms* section below.

Adverse Reactions, Side Effects or Overdose Symptoms

Signs and symptoms	What to do
Abdominal pain	Discontinue. Call doctor when convenient.
Diarrhea	Discontinue. Call doctor immediately.
Kidney damage characterized by blood in urine, decreased urine flow, swelling of hands and feet	Seek emergency treatment.
Nausea or vomiting	Discontinue. Call doctor immediately.

Passion Flower (Maypop)

 Basic Information

Biological name (genus and species):
Passiflora incarnata

Parts used for medicinal purposes:
• Flowers
• Fruit

Chemicals this herb contains:
• Cyanogenic glycosides (see Glossary)
• Harmaline
• Harman
• Harmine
• Harmol

 Known Effects

• Depresses nerve transfer in spinal cord and brain
• Increases respiratory rate
• Slightly depresses central nervous system
• Causes hallucinations

Miscellaneous information:
• Smoking passion flower reportedly causes mental changes similar to marijuana.
• It's available in capsules, herbal remedies or tinctures.
• No good human studies of clinical effectiveness exist.

 Possible Additional Effects

• May reduce headaches
• May aid against convulsions
• May help treat insomnia
• Potential "nerve tonic" for Parkinson's

 Warnings and Precautions

Don't take if you:
Are pregnant, think you may be pregnant or plan pregnancy in the near future.

Consult your doctor if you:
• Take this herb for any medical problem that doesn't improve in 2 weeks (There may be safer, more effective treatments.)
• Take any medicinal drugs or herbs including aspirin, laxatives, cold and cough remedies, antacids, vitamins, minerals, amino acids, supplements, other prescription or nonprescription drugs
• Are using other sleeping pills

Pregnancy:
Dangers outweigh any possible benefits. Don't use.

Breastfeeding:
Dangers outweigh any possible benefits. Don't use.

Infants and children:
Treating infants and children under 2 with any herbal preparation is hazardous.

Others:
This product will not help you. It may cause toxic symptoms.

Storage:
• Store in cool, dry area away from direct light, but don't freeze.
• Store safely out of reach of children.
• Don't store in bathroom medicine cabinet. Heat and moisture may change the action of the herb.

Safe dosage:
Consult your doctor for the appropriate dose for your condition.

Toxicity

Rated relatively safe when taken in appropriate quantities for short periods of time

For symptoms of toxicity: See *Adverse Reactions, Side Effects or Overdose Symptoms* section below.

Adverse Reactions, Side Effects or Overdose Symptoms

Signs and symptoms	What to do
Convulsions	Seek emergency treatment.
Decreased body temperature	Discontinue. Call doctor immediately.
Diarrhea	Discontinue. Call doctor immediately.
Hallucinations	Seek emergency treatment.
Muscle paralysis, including muscles used in breathing	Seek emergency treatment.
Nausea, vomiting, upset stomach	Discontinue. Call doctor immediately.
Sleepiness	Do not operate machinery or drive.

Peach

Basic Information

Biological name (genus and species): *Prunus persica* or other *Prunus* species

Parts used for medicinal purposes:
• Bark
• Leaves
• Roots
• Seeds

Chemicals this herb contains:
• Cyanide, especially in kernels
• Phloretin
• Volatile oils (see Glossary)

Known Effects

Irritates and stimulates gastrointestinal tract

Miscellaneous information:
• North American Indians made tea from the bark.
• The fruit, except for the peach pit, is safe.

Possible Additional Effects

• May treat constipation (leaves)
• May treat systemic infections (bark and roots)

Warnings and Precautions

Don't take if you:
• Are pregnant, think you may be pregnant or plan pregnancy in the near future
• Have any chronic disease of the gastrointestinal tract, such as stomach or duodenal ulcers, reflux

MEDICINAL HERBS

→

esophagitis, ulcerative colitis, spastic colitis, diverticulosis or diverticulitis

Consult your doctor if you:
- Take this herb for any medical problem that doesn't improve in 2 weeks (There may be safer, more effective treatments.)
- Take any medicinal drugs or herbs including aspirin, laxatives, cold and cough remedies, antacids, vitamins, minerals, amino acids, supplements, other prescription or nonprescription drugs

Pregnancy:
The dangers of taking this as a medicinal herb outweigh any possible benefits. Avoid pits! There should be no problems with the fruit.

Breastfeeding:
The dangers of taking this as a medicinal herb outweigh any possible benefits. Avoid pits! There should be no problems with the fruit.

Infants and children:
Treating infants and children under 2 with any herbal preparation is hazardous.

Others:
Pits will not help you and may cause toxic symptoms.

Storage:
- Store in cool, dry area away from direct light, but don't freeze.
- Store safely out of reach of children.
- Don't store in bathroom medicine cabinet. Heat and moisture may change the action of the herb.

Safe dosage:
Consult your doctor for the appropriate dose for your condition.

 Toxicity

Comparative-toxicity rating is not available from standard references.

For symptoms of toxicity: See *Adverse Reactions, Side Effects or Overdose Symptoms* section below.

 Adverse Reactions, Side Effects or Overdose Symptoms

Signs and symptoms	What to do
Diarrhea	Discontinue. Call doctor immediately.
Nausea or vomiting	Discontinue. Call doctor immediately.

Pellitory

 Basic Information

Biological name (genus and species):
Anacyclus pyrethrum

Parts used for medicinal purposes:
Various parts of the entire plant, frequently differing by country and culture

Chemicals this herb contains:
Pellitorine

 Known Effects

Kills insects

Miscellaneous information:
Tastes bitter.

Possible Additional Effects

- May relieve pain from toothache or gum infections
- May relieve facial pain
- May increase saliva flow

Warnings and Precautions

Don't take if you:

- Are pregnant, think you may be pregnant or plan pregnancy in the near future
- Have any chronic disease of the gastrointestinal tract, such as stomach or duodenal ulcers, reflux esophagitis, ulcerative colitis, spastic colitis, diverticulosis or diverticulitis

Consult your doctor if you:

- Take this herb for any medical problem that doesn't improve in 2 weeks (There may be safer, more effective treatments.)
- Take any medicinal drugs or herbs including aspirin, laxatives, cold and cough remedies, antacids, vitamins, minerals, amino acids, supplements, other prescription or nonprescription drugs

Pregnancy:

Don't use unless prescribed by your doctor.

Breastfeeding:

Don't use unless prescribed by your doctor.

Infants and children:

Treating infants and children under 2 with any herbal preparation is hazardous.

Others:

None are expected if you are beyond childhood, under 45, not pregnant, basically healthy, take it for only a short time and do not exceed manufacturer's recommended dose.

Storage:

- Store in cool, dry area away from direct light, but don't freeze.
- Store safely out of reach of children.
- Don't store in bathroom medicine cabinet. Heat and moisture may change the action of the herb.

Safe dosage:

Consult your doctor for the appropriate dose for your condition.

Toxicity

Comparative-toxicity rating is not available from standard references.

For symptoms of toxicity: See *Adverse Reactions, Side Effects or Overdose Symptoms* section below.

Adverse Reactions, Side Effects or Overdose Symptoms

Signs and symptoms	What to do
Diarrhea	Discontinue. Call doctor immediately.
Nausea or vomiting	Discontinue. Call doctor immediately.

MEDICINAL HERBS

Pennyroyal

Basic Information

Biological name (genus and species):
Mentha pulegium, Hedeoma pulegioides

Parts used for medicinal purposes:
Entire plant

Chemicals this herb contains:
Pulegone (yellow or green-yellow oil)

Known Effects

• Stimulates uterine contractions
• Depresses central nervous system
• Irritates mucous membranes
• Reddens skin by increasing blood supply to it
• Decongestant
• Can cause severe liver and kidney damage

Miscellaneous information:

• Pennyroyal is used as a flavoring agent.
• As little as 2 ounces of the essential oil can cause severe liver and kidney damage.
• It's also available as tinctures, dried leaves and flowers.
• The oil is toxic. Do not ingest.

Possible Additional Effects

• May decrease intestinal cramps and flatulence
• May help treat colds, coughs
• May regulate menstruation
• May reduce gas, indigestion

Warnings and Precautions

Don't take if you:

Are pregnant, think you may be pregnant or plan pregnancy in the near future.

Consult your doctor if you:

• Take this herb for any medical problem that doesn't improve in 2 weeks (There may be safer, more effective treatments.)
• Take any medicinal drugs or herbs including aspirin, laxatives, cold and cough remedies, antacids, vitamins, minerals, amino acids, supplements, other prescription or nonprescription drugs

Pregnancy:

Dangers outweigh any possible benefits. Don't use.

Breastfeeding:

Dangers outweigh any possible benefits. Don't use.

Infants and children:

Treating infants and children under 2 with any herbal preparation is hazardous.

Others:

Don't use in an attempt to induce abortion. Pennyroyal can be deadly.

Storage:

• Store in cool, dry area away from direct light, but don't freeze.
• Store safely out of reach of children.
• Don't store in bathroom medicine cabinet. Heat and moisture may change the action of the herb.

Safe dosage:
Consult your doctor for the appropriate dose for your condition.

 Toxicity

Rated relatively safe when taken in appropriate quantities for short periods of time

For symptoms of toxicity: See *Adverse Reactions, Side Effects or Overdose Symptoms* section below.

 Adverse Reactions, Side Effects or Overdose Symptoms

Signs and symptoms	What to do
Bleeding from gastrointestinal tract	Seek emergency treatment.
Blood in urine	Seek emergency treatment.
Jaundice (yellow skin and eyes)	Discontinue. Call doctor immediately.
Seizures	Seek emergency treatment.
Unusual vaginal bleeding	Seek emergency treatment.

Periwinkle (Madagascar or Cape Periwinkle, Old Maid)

 Basic Information

Biological name (genus and species):
Catharanthus roseus, Vinca rosea

Parts used for medicinal purposes:
Leaves

Chemicals this herb contains:
• Vinblastine
• Vincristine
• Vinleurosine
• Vinrosidine

 Known Effects

• Inhibits growth and development of germs
• Depresses bone-marrow production, damaging body's blood cell-manufacturing processes
• Effective in treatment of several different types of malignant tumors
• Reduces granulocytes (white blood cells) in body

Miscellaneous information:
When purified, derivatives of *Vinca* (vincristine sulfate, vinblastine sulfate) are used to treat cancer under rigidly controlled supervision.

 Possible Additional Effects

• May decrease inflammation when used as ointment
• May treat sore throats and inflamed tonsils
• May treat diabetes mellitus
• May cause hallucinations when smoked

 Warnings and Precautions

Don't take if you:
• Are pregnant, think you may be pregnant or plan pregnancy in the near future
• Have any chronic disease of the gastrointestinal tract, such as stomach or duodenal ulcers, reflux esophagitis, ulcerative colitis, spastic colitis, diverticulosis or diverticulitis

➜

Consult your doctor if you:
• Take this herb for any medical problem that doesn't improve in 2 weeks (There may be safer, more effective treatments.)
• Take any medicinal drugs or herbs including aspirin, laxatives, cold and cough remedies, antacids, vitamins, minerals, amino acids, supplements, other prescription or nonprescription drugs

Pregnancy:
Dangers outweigh any possible benefits. Don't use.

Breastfeeding:
Dangers outweigh any possible benefits. Don't use.

Infants and children:
Treating infants and children under 2 with any herbal preparation is hazardous.

Others:
This product will not help you and may cause toxic symptoms.

Storage:
• Store in cool, dry area away from direct light, but don't freeze.
• Store safely out of reach of children.
• Don't store in bathroom medicine cabinet. Heat and moisture may change the action of the herb.

Safe dosage:
Consult your doctor for the appropriate dose for your condition.

 Toxicity

Rated slightly dangerous, particularly in children, persons over 55 and those who take larger than appropriate quantities for extended periods of time

For symptoms of toxicity: See *Adverse Reactions, Side Effects or Overdose Symptoms* section below.

 Adverse Reactions, Side Effects or Overdose Symptoms

Signs and symptoms	What to do
Drowsiness	Discontinue. Call doctor when convenient.
Hair loss	Discontinue. Call doctor when convenient.
Nausea	Discontinue. Call doctor immediately.
Seizures	Seek emergency treatment.
Yellow eyes, dark urine and yellow skin resulting from destruction of some liver cells	Seek emergency treatment.

Pipsissewa

 Basic Information

Biological name (genus and species): *Chimaphila umbellata*

Parts used for medicinal purposes: Leaves

Chemicals this herb contains:
• Arbutin
• Chimaphilin
• Chlorophyll
• Ericolin
• Minerals
• Pectic acid
• Tannins (see Glossary)
• Ursolic acid

Known Effects

- Helps body dispose of excess fluid by increasing amount of urine produced
- Interferes with absorption of iron and other minerals when taken internally

Possible Additional Effects

- May treat indigestion or mild stomach upsets
- May treat irritations of urinary tract (kidney, bladder, urethra)

Warnings and Precautions

Don't take if you:
- Are pregnant, think you may be pregnant or plan pregnancy in the near future
- Have any chronic disease of the gastrointestinal tract, such as stomach or duodenal ulcers, reflux esophagitis, ulcerative colitis, spastic colitis, diverticulosis or diverticulitis

Consult your doctor if you:
- Take this herb for any medical problem that doesn't improve in 2 weeks (There may be safer, more effective treatments.)
- Take any medicinal drugs or herbs including aspirin, laxatives, cold and cough remedies, antacids, vitamins, minerals, amino acids, supplements, other prescription or nonprescription drugs

Pregnancy:
Dangers outweigh any possible benefits. Don't use.

Breastfeeding:
Dangers outweigh any possible benefits. Don't use.

Infants and children:
Treating infants and children under 2 with any herbal preparation is hazardous.

Others:
None are expected if you are beyond childhood, under 45, not pregnant, basically healthy, take it for only a short time and do not exceed manufacturer's recommended dose.

Storage:
- Store in cool, dry area away from direct light, but don't freeze.
- Store safely out of reach of children.
- Don't store in bathroom medicine cabinet. Heat and moisture may change the action of the herb.

Safe dosage:
Consult your doctor for the appropriate dose for your condition.

Toxicity

Comparative-toxicity rating is not available from standard references.

For symptoms of toxicity: See *Adverse Reactions, Side Effects or Overdose Symptoms* section below.

Adverse Reactions, Side Effects or Overdose Symptoms

Signs and symptoms	What to do
Diarrhea	Discontinue. Call doctor immediately.
Nausea or vomiting	Discontinue. Call doctor immediately.
Skin eruptions	Discontinue. Call doctor when convenient.

MEDICINAL HERBS

Pitcher Plant

 Basic Information

Biological name (genus and species):
Sarracenia

Parts used for medicinal purposes:
Roots

Chemicals this herb contains:
• Resin (see Glossary)
• Yellow dye

 Known Effects

• Irritates gastrointestinal tract
• Has diuretic properties

 Possible Additional Effects

• May treat constipation
• May treat indigestion

 Warnings and Precautions

Don't take if you:
Are pregnant, think you may be pregnant or plan pregnancy in the near future.

Consult your doctor if you:
• Take this herb for any medical problem that doesn't improve in 2 weeks (There may be safer, more effective treatments.)
• Take any medicinal drugs or herbs including aspirin, laxatives, cold and cough remedies, antacids, vitamins, minerals, amino acids, supplements, other prescription or nonprescription drugs

Pregnancy:
Don't use unless prescribed by your doctor.

Breastfeeding:
Don't use unless prescribed by your doctor.

Infants and children:
Treating infants and children under 2 with any herbal preparation is hazardous.

Others:
None are expected if you are beyond childhood, under 45, not pregnant, basically healthy, take it for only a short time and do not exceed manufacturer's recommended dose.

Storage:
• Store in cool, dry area away from direct light, but don't freeze.
• Store safely out of reach of children.
• Don't store in bathroom medicine cabinet. Heat and moisture may change the action of the herb.

Safe dosage:
Consult your doctor for the appropriate dose for your condition.

 Toxicity

Comparative-toxicity rating is not available from standard references.

 Adverse Reactions, Side Effects or Overdose Symptoms

None are expected.

Pleurisy Root (Butterfly Weed)

Basic Information

Biological name (genus and species):
Asclepias tuberosa

Parts used for medicinal purposes:
Roots

Chemicals this herb contains:
- Asclepiadin
- Asclepione
- Galitoxin
- Volatile oils (see Glossary)

Known Effects

- Decreases thickness and increases fluidity of mucus in lungs and bronchial tubes
- Irritates mucous membranes
- Stimulates and irritates gastrointestinal tract

Possible Additional Effects

- Potential mild laxative to cause watery, explosive bowel movements
- May increase perspiration
- May help treat pleurisy

Warnings and Precautions

Don't take if you:
- Are pregnant, think you may be pregnant or plan pregnancy in the near future
- Have any chronic disease of the gastrointestinal tract, such as stomach or duodenal ulcers, reflux esophagitis, ulcerative colitis, spastic colitis, diverticulosis or diverticulitis

Consult your doctor if you:
- Take this herb for any medical problem that doesn't improve in 2 weeks (There may be safer, more effective treatments.)
- Take any medicinal drugs or herbs including aspirin, laxatives, cold and cough remedies, antacids, vitamins, minerals, amino acids, supplements, other prescription or nonprescription drugs

Pregnancy:
Dangers outweigh any possible benefits. Don't use.

Breastfeeding:
Dangers outweigh any possible benefits. Don't use.

Infants and children:
Treating infants and children under 2 with any herbal preparation is hazardous.

Others:
Dangers outweigh any possible benefits. Don't use.

Storage:
- Store in cool, dry area away from direct light, but don't freeze.
- Store safely out of reach of children.
- Don't store in bathroom medicine cabinet. Heat and moisture may change the action of the herb.

Safe dosage:
Consult your doctor for the appropriate dose for your condition.

MEDICINAL HERBS

Toxicity

Comparative-toxicity rating is not available from standard references.

For symptoms of toxicity: See *Adverse Reactions, Side Effects or Overdose Symptoms* section below.

Adverse Reactions, Side Effects or Overdose Symptoms

Signs and symptoms	What to do
Appetite loss	Discontinue. Call doctor when convenient.
Coma	Seek emergency treatment.
Diarrhea	Discontinue. Call doctor immediately.
Lethargy	Discontinue. Call doctor when convenient.
Muscle weakness	Discontinue. Call doctor immediately.
Nausea or vomiting	Discontinue. Call doctor immediately.

Poke (Pokeweed, Skoke)

Basic Information

Biological name (genus and species):
Phytolacca americana

Parts used for medicinal purposes:
• Leaves
• Roots
• Seeds

Chemicals this herb contains:
• Asparagine
• Mitogen
• Phytolaccagenin
• Resin (see Glossary)
• Saponins (see Glossary)

Known Effects

Stimulates and irritates gastrointestinal tract

Miscellaneous information:
• All parts of native plants are poisonous. Don't take it. Children are especially vulnerable to toxic effects.

• Leaves are boiled and eaten as flavoring in some areas, particularly the southern United States. Used this way, pokeweed may be toxic. Don't use!

Possible Additional Effects

• May treat chronic arthritis
• May treat constipation

Warnings and Precautions

Don't take if you:
• Are pregnant, think you may be pregnant or plan pregnancy in the near future
• Have any chronic disease of the gastrointestinal tract, such as stomach or duodenal ulcers, reflux esophagitis, ulcerative colitis, spastic colitis, diverticulosis or diverticulitis

Consult your doctor if you:
- Take this herb for any medical problem that doesn't improve in 2 weeks (There may be safer, more effective treatments.)
- Take any medicinal drugs or herbs including aspirin, laxatives, cold and cough remedies, antacids, vitamins, minerals, amino acids, supplements, other prescription or nonprescription drugs

Pregnancy:
Dangers outweigh any possible benefits. Don't use.

Breastfeeding:
Dangers outweigh any possible benefits. Don't use.

Infants and children:
Treating infants and children under 2 with any herbal preparation is hazardous.

Others:
Handling roots may cause skin abrasions.

Storage:
- Store in cool, dry area away from direct light, but don't freeze.
- Store safely out of reach of children.

- Don't store in bathroom medicine cabinet. Heat and moisture may change the action of the herb.

Safe dosage:
Consult your doctor for the appropriate dose for your condition.

Toxicity

Comparative-toxicity rating is not available from standard references.

For symptoms of toxicity: See *Adverse Reactions, Side Effects or Overdose Symptoms* section below.

Adverse Reactions, Side Effects or Overdose Symptoms

Signs and symptoms	What to do
Decreased heart rate	Seek emergency treatment.
Diarrhea	Discontinue. Call doctor immediately.
Nausea or vomiting	Discontinue. Call doctor immediately.
Skin eruptions	Discontinue. Call doctor when convenient.

Pomegranate

Basic Information

Biological name (genus and species):
Punica granatum

Parts used for medicinal purposes:
- Bark
- Berries/fruits, including rind

Chemicals this herb contains:
- Isopelletierine
- Methyl-isopelletierine
- Pelletierine
- Pseudo-pelletierine
- Tannins (see Glossary)

Known Effects

Rind and bark:
- Shrinks tissues
- Prevents secretion of fluids
- Destroys intestinal worms
- Interferes with absorption of iron and other minerals when taken internally

➜

MEDICINAL HERBS

Miscellaneous information:
• Fruits are edible and nontoxic.
• Bark and rind contain herbal-medicinal properties.

 ## Possible Additional Effects

May treat stasis ulcers and bed sores

 ## Warnings and Precautions

Don't take if you:
• Are pregnant, think you may be pregnant or plan pregnancy in the near future
• Have any chronic disease of the gastrointestinal tract, such as stomach or duodenal ulcers, reflux esophagitis, ulcerative colitis, spastic colitis, diverticulosis or diverticulitis

Consult your doctor if you:
• Take this herb for any medical problem that doesn't improve in 2 weeks (There may be safer, more effective treatments.)
• Take any medicinal drugs or herbs including aspirin, laxatives, cold and cough remedies, antacids, vitamins, minerals, amino acids, supplements, other prescription or nonprescription drugs

Pregnancy:
Taken internally as a medicinal herb, dangers outweigh any possible benefits. Don't use. Eating fruit as part of your diet will not cause problems.

Breastfeeding:
Taken internally as a medicinal herb, dangers outweigh any possible benefits. Don't use. Eating fruit as part of your diet will not cause problems.

Infants and children:
Treating infants and children under 2 with any herbal preparation is hazardous.

Others:
Taken internally, dangers outweigh any possible benefits. Don't use.

Storage:
• Store in cool, dry area away from direct light, but don't freeze.
• Store safely out of reach of children.
• Don't store in bathroom medicine cabinet. Heat and moisture may change the action of the herb.

Safe dosage:
Consult your doctor for the appropriate dose for your condition.

 ## Toxicity

Comparative-toxicity rating is not available from standard references.

For symptoms of toxicity: See *Adverse Reactions, Side Effects or Overdose Symptoms* section below.

 ## Adverse Reactions, Side Effects or Overdose Symptoms

Signs and symptoms	What to do
Diarrhea	Discontinue. Call doctor immediately.
Dilated pupils	Seek emergency treatment.
Dizziness	Discontinue. Call doctor immediately.
Double vision	Seek emergency treatment.
Nausea or vomiting	Discontinue. Call doctor immediately.
Weakness	Discontinue. Call doctor immediately.

Poplar Bud

Basic Information

Biological name (genus and species):
Populus candicans

Parts used for medicinal purposes:
• Leaf bud

Chemicals this herb contains:
• Chrysin
• Gallic acid
• Humulene
• Malic acid
• Mannite
• Populin
• Resin (see Glossary)
• Salicin
• Tectochrysin

Known Effects

• Blocks pain impulses to brain
• Changes fever-control "thermostat" in brain
• Antioxidant

Miscellaneous information:
• Antioxidant effect helps prevent rancidity in ointments.
• Poplar bud is used as an additive in several pharmaceutical preparations.

Possible Additional Effects

• May reduce pain of sprains and bruises when applied to skin
• May treat coughs and colds when taken internally
• May reduce fever

STOP Warnings and Precautions

Don't take if you:
• Are pregnant, think you may be pregnant or plan pregnancy in the near future
• Have any chronic disease of the gastrointestinal tract, such as stomach or duodenal ulcers, reflux esophagitis, ulcerative colitis, spastic colitis, diverticulosis or diverticulitis

Consult your doctor if you:
• Take this herb for any medical problem that doesn't improve in 2 weeks (There may be safer, more effective treatments.)
• Take any medicinal drugs or herbs including aspirin, laxatives, cold and cough remedies, antacids, vitamins, minerals, amino acids, supplements, other prescription or nonprescription drugs

Pregnancy:
Don't use unless prescribed by your doctor.

Breastfeeding:
Don't use unless prescribed by your doctor.

Infants and children:
Treating infants and children under 2 with any herbal preparation is hazardous.

Others:
None are expected if you are beyond childhood, under 45, not pregnant, basically healthy, take it for only a short time and do not exceed manufacturer's recommended dose.

MEDICINAL HERBS

➜

Storage:
- Store in cool, dry area away from direct light, but don't freeze.
- Store safely out of reach of children.
- Don't store in bathroom medicine cabinet. Heat and moisture may change the action of the herb.

Safe dosage:
Consult your doctor for the appropriate dose for your condition.

 Toxicity

Comparative-toxicity rating is not available from standard references.

For symptoms of toxicity: See *Adverse Reactions, Side Effects or Overdose Symptoms* section below.

 Adverse Reactions, Side Effects or Overdose Symptoms

Signs and symptoms	What to do
Itching and redness of skin	Apply hydrocortisone ointment, available without prescription.
Skin rash	Apply hydrocortisone ointment, available without prescription.

Prickly Ash

 Basic Information

Biological name (genus and species): *Zanthoxylum americanum* (northern), *Zanthoxylum clavaherculus* (southern)

Parts used for medicinal purposes:
- Bark
- Berries/fruits

Chemicals this herb contains:
- Acid amide
- Asarinin
- Berberine
- Herculin
- Xanthoxyletin
- Xanthyletin

 Known Effects

- Stimulates and irritates gastrointestinal tract
- Increases perspiration

 Possible Additional Effects

- May stimulate appetite
- May treat arthritis
- May decrease flatulence

 Warnings and Precautions

Don't take if you:
- Are pregnant, think you may be pregnant or plan pregnancy in the near future
- Have any chronic disease of the gastrointestinal tract, such as stomach or duodenal ulcers, reflux esophagitis, ulcerative colitis, spastic colitis, diverticulosis or diverticulitis

Consult your doctor if you:
- Take this herb for any medical problem that doesn't improve in 2 weeks (There may be safer, more effective treatments.)

- Take any medicinal drugs or herbs including aspirin, laxatives, cold and cough remedies, antacids, vitamins, minerals, amino acids, supplements, other prescription or nonprescription drugs

Pregnancy:
Don't use unless prescribed by your doctor.

Breastfeeding:
Don't use unless prescribed by your doctor.

Infants and children:
Treating infants and children under 2 with any herbal preparation is hazardous.

Others:
None are expected if you are beyond childhood, under 45, not pregnant, basically healthy, take it for only a short time and do not exceed manufacturer's recommended dose.

Storage:
- Store in cool, dry area away from direct light, but don't freeze.
- Store safely out of reach of children.

- Don't store in bathroom medicine cabinet. Heat and moisture may change the action of the herb.

Safe dosage:
Consult your doctor for the appropriate dose for your condition.

 ## Toxicity

Comparative-toxicity rating is not available from standard references.

For symptoms of toxicity: See *Adverse Reactions, Side Effects or Overdose Symptoms* section below.

 ## Adverse Reactions, Side Effects or Overdose Symptoms

Signs and symptoms	What to do
Diarrhea	Discontinue. Call doctor immediately.
Nausea or vomiting	Discontinue. Call doctor immediately.

Prickly Poppy (Mexican Poppy, Thistle Poppy)

 ## Basic Information

Biological name (genus and species):
Argemone mexicana

Parts used for medicinal purposes:
Seeds

Chemicals this herb contains:
- Berberine
- Dihydrosanguinarine
- Protopine
- Sanguinarine

 ## Known Effects

Mildly depresses central nervous system

Miscellaneous information:
This poppy is not the origin of morphine, codeine or other narcotics.

 ## Possible Additional Effects

Smoking prickly poppy may produce euphoria and reduce pain.

➜

MEDICINAL HERBS

Warnings and Precautions

Don't take if you:

- Are pregnant, think you may be pregnant or plan pregnancy in the near future
- Have any chronic disease of the gastrointestinal tract, such as stomach or duodenal ulcers, reflux esophagitis, ulcerative colitis, spastic colitis, diverticulosis or diverticulitis

Consult your doctor if you:

- Take this herb for any medical problem that doesn't improve in 2 weeks (There may be safer, more effective treatments.)
- Take any medicinal drugs or herbs including aspirin, laxatives, cold and cough remedies, antacids, vitamins, minerals, amino acids, supplements, other prescription or nonprescription drugs

Pregnancy:

Dangers outweigh any possible benefits. Don't use.

Breastfeeding:

Dangers outweigh any possible benefits. Don't use.

Infants and children:

Treating infants and children under 2 with any herbal preparation is hazardous.

Others:

Dangers outweigh any possible benefits. Don't use.

Storage:

- Store in cool, dry area away from direct light, but don't freeze.
- Store safely out of reach of children.
- Don't store in bathroom medicine cabinet. Heat and moisture may change the action of the herb.

Safe dosage:

Consult your doctor for the appropriate dose for your condition.

Toxicity

Rated slightly dangerous, particularly in children, persons over 55 and those who take larger than appropriate quantities for extended periods of time.

For symptoms of toxicity: See *Adverse Reactions, Side Effects or Overdose Symptoms* section below.

Adverse Reactions, Side Effects or Overdose Symptoms

Signs and symptoms	What to do
Diarrhea	Discontinue. Call doctor immediately.
Dizziness	Discontinue. Call doctor immediately.
Fluid retention	Discontinue. Call doctor when convenient.
Loss of consciousness	Seek emergency treatment.
Nausea or vomiting	Discontinue. Call doctor immediately.
Swollen abdomen	Discontinue. Call doctor when convenient.
Vision disturbances	Discontinue. Call doctor immediately.

Prostrate Knotweed (Pigweed)

Basic Information

Biological name (genus and species):
Polygonum aviculare

Parts used for medicinal purposes:
Various parts of the entire plant,
frequently differing by country
and culture

Chemicals this herb contains:
• Avicularin
• Emodin
• Quercetin 3-arabinoside

Known Effects

• Reduces capillary fragility
• Reduces capillary permeability
• Retards destruction of epinephrine

Possible Additional Effects

• May cause watery, explosive bowel
  movements
• May treat kidney and bladder stones

Warnings and Precautions

Don't take if you:
• Are pregnant, think you may be
  pregnant or plan pregnancy in the
  near future
• Have any chronic disease of the
  gastrointestinal tract, such as stomach
  or duodenal ulcers, reflux
  esophagitis, ulcerative colitis, spastic
  colitis, diverticulosis or diverticulitis

Consult your doctor if you:
• Take this herb for any medical
  problem that doesn't improve in
  2 weeks (There may be safer, more
  effective treatments.)
• Take any medicinal drugs or
  herbs including aspirin, laxatives,
  cold and cough remedies, antacids,
  vitamins, minerals, amino acids,
  supplements, other prescription
  or nonprescription drugs

Pregnancy:
Don't use unless prescribed by
your doctor.

Breastfeeding:
Don't use unless prescribed by
your doctor

Infants and children:

Treating infants and children under
2 with any herbal preparation
is hazardous.

Others:
None are expected if you are beyond
childhood, under 45, not pregnant,
basically healthy, take it for only a short
time and do not exceed manufacturer's
recommended dose.

Storage:
• Store in cool, dry area away from
  direct light, but don't freeze.
• Store safely out of reach of children.
• Don't store in bathroom medicine
  cabinet. Heat and moisture may
  change the action of the herb.

Safe dosage:
Consult your doctor for the appropriate dose for your condition.

MEDICINAL HERBS

→

Toxicity

Rated relatively safe when taken in appropriate quantities for short periods of time

For symptoms of toxicity: See *Adverse Reactions, Side Effects or Overdose Symptoms* section below.

Adverse Reactions, Side Effects or Overdose Symptoms

Signs and symptoms	What to do
Abdominal pain	Discontinue. Call doctor when convenient.
Diarrhea	Discontinue. Call doctor immediately.
Nausea or vomiting	Discontinue. Call doctor immediately.
Skin eruptions	Discontinue. Call doctor when convenient.

Rauwolfia (Chandra, Sarpaganda, Snakeroot)

Basic Information

Biological name (genus and species): *Rauwolfia serpentina*

Parts used for medicinal purposes: Roots

Chemicals this herb contains:
- Ajmaline
- Deserpidine
- Rescinnamine
- Reserpine
- Serpentine
- Yohimbine

Known Effects

- Reduces blood pressure
- Depresses activity of central nervous system
- Hypnotic

Miscellaneous information:
- Snakeroot depletes catecholamines and serotonin from nerves in the central nervous system.

- Refined snakeroot has been used extensively in recent years to treat hypertension.
- Animal studies suggest snakeroot may produce cancers.

Possible Additional Effects

- May decrease anxiety
- May decrease fever
- May kill intestinal parasites
- In India, used as antidote for snakebites

Warnings and Precautions

Don't take if you:
- Are pregnant, think you may be pregnant or plan pregnancy in the near future
- Have any chronic disease of the gastrointestinal tract, such as stomach or duodenal ulcers, reflux esophagitis, ulcerative colitis, spastic colitis, diverticulosis or diverticulitis

Consult your doctor if you:

• Take this herb for any medical problem that doesn't improve in 2 weeks (There may be safer, more effective treatments.)
• Take any medicinal drugs or herbs including aspirin, laxatives, cold and cough remedies, antacids, vitamins, minerals, amino acids, supplements, other prescription or nonprescription drugs

Pregnancy

Dangers outweigh any possible benefits. Don't use.

Breastfeeding:

Dangers outweigh any possible benefits. Don't use.

Infants and children:

Treating infants and children under 2 with any herbal preparation is hazardous.

Others:

Dangers outweigh any possible benefits. Don't use.

Storage:

• Store in cool, dry area away from direct light, but don't freeze.
• Store safely out of reach of children.
• Don't store in bathroom medicine cabinet. Heat and moisture may change the action of the herb.

Safe dosage:

At present no "safe" dosage has been established.

Toxicity

Rated slightly dangerous, particularly in children, persons over 55 and those who take larger than appropriate quantities for extended periods of time

For symptoms of toxicity: See *Adverse Reactions, Side Effects or Overdose Symptoms* section below.

Adverse Reactions, Side Effects or Overdose Symptoms

Signs and symptoms	What to do
Bizarre dreams	Discontinue. Call doctor when convenient.
Decreased libido and sexual performance	Discontinue. Call doctor when convenient.
Diarrhea	Discontinue. Call doctor immediately.
Drowsiness	Discontinue. Call doctor when convenient.
Nasal congestion	Discontinue. Call doctor when convenient.
Precipitous blood-pressure drop: symptoms include faintness, cold sweat, paleness, rapid pulse	Seek emergency treatment.
Slow heartbeat	Seek emergency treatment.
Stupor	Seek emergency treatment.
Upper abdominal pain	Discontinue. Call doctor when convenient.

MEDICINAL HERBS

Red Raspberry

Basic Information

Biological name (genus and species):
Rubus strigosus, R. idaeus

Parts used for medicinal purposes:
• Bark
• Leaves
• Roots

Chemicals this herb contains:
• Citric acid
• Tannins (see Glossary)

Known Effects

• Relaxes uterine spasms
• Relaxes intestinal spasms
• Gargle for sore throats

Miscellaneous information:
• Berries are delicious, nutritious and nontoxic.
• When eaten as a common food, no problems are expected for anyone.

Possible Additional Effects

• May increase contractions of labor pains
• May decrease excessive menstrual bleeding
• May relieve morning sickness
• May treat mouth ulcers

Warnings and Precautions

Don't take if you:
Are pregnant, think you may be pregnant or plan pregnancy in the near future.

Consult your doctor if you:
• Take this herb for any medical problem that doesn't improve in 2 weeks (There may be safer, more effective treatments.)
• Take any medicinal drugs or herbs including aspirin, laxatives, cold and cough remedies, antacids, vitamins, minerals, amino acids, supplements, other prescription or nonprescription drugs
• Are pregnant and want to use for morning sickness

Pregnancy:
Don't use unless prescribed by your doctor.

Breastfeeding:
Don't use unless prescribed by your doctor.

Infants and children:
Treating infants and children under 2 with any herbal preparation is hazardous.

Others:
None are expected if you are beyond childhood, under 45, not pregnant, basically healthy, take it for only a short time and do not exceed manufacturer's recommended dose.

Storage:
• Store in cool, dry area away from direct light, but don't freeze.
• Store safely out of reach of children.
• Don't store in bathroom medicine cabinet. Heat and moisture may change the action of the herb.

Safe dosage:
Consult your doctor for the appropriate dose for your condition.

Toxicity

Comparative-toxicity rating is not available from standard references.

For symptoms of toxicity: See *Adverse Reactions, Side Effects or Overdose Symptoms* section below.

 Adverse Reactions, Side Effects or Overdose Symptoms

Signs and symptoms	What to do
Diarrhea	Discontinue. Call doctor immediately.
Nausea	Discontinue. Call doctor immediately.

Rhatany

 Basic Information

Biological name (genus and species): *Krameria triandra*

Parts used for medicinal purposes: Various parts of the entire plant, frequently differing by country and culture

Chemicals this herb contains:
• Calcium oxalate
• Gum (see Glossary)
• Lignin
• N-Methyltyrosine
• Saccharine
• Starch
• Tannins (see Glossary)

 Known Effects
• Anti-inflammatory
• Helps treat canker sores

 Possible Additional Effects
• May treat sore throat
• May treat hemorrhoids
• May treat chronic bowel inflammations
• May treat diarrhea
• Potential mouthwash

MEDICINAL HERBS

→

Warnings and Precautions

Don't take if you:

• Are pregnant, think you may be pregnant or plan pregnancy in the near future
• Have any chronic disease of the gastrointestinal tract, such as stomach or duodenal ulcers, reflux esophagitis, ulcerative colitis, spastic colitis, diverticulosis or diverticulitis

Consult your doctor if you:

• Take this herb for any medical problem that doesn't improve in 2 weeks (There may be safer, more effective treatments.)
• Take any medicinal drugs or herbs including aspirin, laxatives, cold and cough remedies, antacids, vitamins, minerals, amino acids, supplements, other prescription or nonprescription drugs

Pregnancy

Dangers outweigh any possible benefits. Don't use.

Breastfeeding:

Dangers outweigh any possible benefits. Don't use.

Infants and children:

Treating infants and children under 2 with any herbal preparation is hazardous.

Others:

None are expected if you are beyond childhood, under 45, not pregnant, basically healthy, take it for only a short time and do not exceed manufacturer's recommended dose.

Storage:

• Store in cool, dry area away from direct light, but don't freeze.
• Store safely out of reach of children.
• Don't store in bathroom medicine cabinet. Heat and moisture may change the action of the herb.

Safe dosage:

Consult your doctor for the appropriate dose for your condition.

 Toxicity

Comparative-toxicity rating is not available from standard references.

For symptoms of toxicity: See *Adverse Reactions, Side Effects or Overdose Symptoms* section below.

 Adverse Reactions, Side Effects or Overdose Symptoms

Signs and symptoms	What to do
Diarrhea	Discontinue. Call doctor immediately.
Kidney damage characterized by blood in urine, decreased urine flow, swelling of hands and feet	Seek emergency treatment.
Nausea or vomiting	Discontinue. Call doctor immediately.

Rheumatism Root (Wild-yam Root)

Basic Information

Biological name (genus and species):
Dioscorea villosa

Parts used for medicinal purposes:
Roots

Chemicals this herb contains:
- Dioscin
- Diosgenin
- Resin (see Glossary)
- Saponin (see Glossary)

Known Effects

Breaks membranous covering,
destroying red blood cells (toxic to
fish and amoeba)

Miscellaneous information:
Diosgenin is a steroid base used to
synthesize cortisone and progesterone
(hormones).

Possible
Additional Effects

- May treat arthritis by allegedly
  removing accumulated waste in
  joints
- May reduce menopausal symptoms
- May relieve morning sickness
- May treat menstrual cramps

Warnings and
Precautions

Don't take if you:
- Are pregnant, think you may be
  pregnant or plan pregnancy in the
  near future

- Have any chronic disease of the
  gastrointestinal tract, such as stomach
  or duodenal ulcers, reflux
  esophagitis, ulcerative colitis, spastic
  colitis, diverticulosis or diverticulitis
- Are pregnant and want to treat
  morning sickness

Consult your doctor if you:
- Take this herb for any medical
  problem that doesn't improve in
  2 weeks (There may be safer, more
  effective treatments.)
- Take any medicinal drugs or
  herbs including aspirin, laxatives,
  cold and cough remedies, antacids,
  vitamins, minerals, amino acids,
  supplements, other prescription
  or nonprescription drugs

Pregnancy
Dangers outweigh any possible
benefits. Don't use.

Breastfeeding:
Dangers outweigh any possible
benefits. Don't use.

Infants and children:
Treating infants and children under
2 with any herbal preparation
is hazardous.

Others:
None are expected if you are beyond
childhood, under 45, not pregnant,
basically healthy, take it for only a short
time and do not exceed manufacturer's
recommended dose.

Storage:
- Store in cool, dry area away from
  direct light, but don't freeze.
- Store safely out of reach of children.
- Don't store in bathroom medicine
  cabinet. Heat and moisture may
  change the action of the herb.

MEDICINAL HERBS

Safe dosage:
Consult your doctor for the appropriate dose for your condition.

Toxicity

Generally regarded as safe when taken in appropriate quantities for short periods of time

For symptoms of toxicity: See *Adverse Reactions, Side Effects or Overdose Symptoms* section below.

Adverse Reactions, Side Effects or Overdose Symptoms

Signs and symptoms	What to do
Diarrhea	Discontinue. Call doctor immediately.
Nausea or vomiting	Discontinue. Call doctor immediately.

Rose

Basic Information

Biological name (genus and species):
Rosa

Parts used for medicinal purposes:
• Berries/fruits
• Petals/flower

Chemicals this herb contains:
• Ascorbic acid
• Cyanogenic glycoside (see Glossary)
• Quercitrin
• Tannins (see Glossary)
• Vitamins A and C
• Volatile oils (see Glossary)

Known Effects

• Anti-inflammatory
• Calming effects

Miscellaneous information:
• North American Indians formerly used fruit as a food source.
• Leaves are used to make tea or salad and smoked like tobacco.

• Rose hips are used in vitamin-C supplements.
• Rose adds flavor to foods during cooking.

Possible Additional Effects

• May smooth skin
• Potential astringent
• Potential sedative
• May help induce sleep

Warnings and Precautions

Don't take if you:
Are pregnant, think you may be pregnant or plan pregnancy in the near future.

Consult your doctor if you:
Are pregnant, think you may be pregnant or plan pregnancy in the near future.

Pregnancy:
Don't use unless prescribed by your doctor.

Breastfeeding:
Don't use unless prescribed by
your doctor.

Infants and children:
Treating infants and children under
2 with any herbal preparation
is hazardous.

Others:
None are expected if you are beyond
childhood, under 45, not pregnant,
basically healthy, take it for only a short
time and do not exceed manufacturer's
recommended dose.

Storage:
• Store in cool, dry area away from
  direct light, but don't freeze.
• Store safely out of reach of children.

• Don't store in bathroom medicine
  cabinet. Heat and moisture may
  change the action of the herb.

Safe dosage:
Consult your doctor for the appropriate dose for your condition.

Toxicity

Comparative-toxicity rating is not available from standard references.

Adverse Reactions, Side Effects or Overdose Symptoms

None are expected.

Rosemary

Basic Information

Biological name (genus and species):
Rosmarinus officinalis

Parts used for medicinal purposes:
• Berries/fruits
• Leaves

Chemicals this herb contains:
• Bitters (see Glossary)
• Borneol
• Camphene
• Camphor
• Cineole
• Pinene
• Resin (see Glossary)
• Tannins (see Glossary)
• Volatile oils (see Glossary)

Known Effects

• Irritates tissue and kills bacteria
  (volatile oils)
• Astringent
• Increases stomach acidity, helps
  reduce indigestion
• Helps expel gas from intestinal tract

Miscellaneous information:
• Rosemary is used as an ingredient in
  perfumes, hair lotions and soaps.
• No effects are expected on the body,
  either good or bad, when the herb is
  used in very small amounts to
  enhance the flavor of food.

➜

Possible Additional Effects

- May redden skin by increasing blood supply to it
- May stimulate appetite
- May treat skin infections when used externally
- May help treat constipation
- Potential diuretic

Warnings and Precautions

Don't take if you:

- Are pregnant, think you may be pregnant or plan pregnancy in the near future
- Have any chronic disease of the gastrointestinal tract, such as stomach or duodenal ulcers, reflux esophagitis, ulcerative colitis, spastic colitis, diverticulosis or diverticulitis

Consult your doctor if you:

- Take this herb for any medical problem that doesn't improve in 2 weeks (There may be safer, more effective treatments.)
- Take any medicinal drugs or herbs including aspirin, laxatives, cold and cough remedies, antacids, vitamins, minerals, amino acids, supplements, other prescription or nonprescription drugs

Pregnancy:

Don't use unless prescribed by your doctor.

Breastfeeding:

Don't use unless prescribed by your doctor.

Infants and children:

Treating infants and children under 2 with any herbal preparation is hazardous.

Others:

None are expected if you are beyond childhood, under 45, not pregnant, basically healthy, take it for only a short time and do not exceed manufacturer's recommended dose.

Storage:

- Store in cool, dry area away from direct light, but don't freeze.
- Store safely out of reach of children.
- Don't store in bathroom medicine cabinet. Heat and moisture may change the action of the herb.

Safe dosage:

Consult your doctor for the appropriate dose for your condition.

Toxicity

Rated relatively safe when taken in appropriate quantities for short periods of time

For symptoms of toxicity: See *Adverse Reactions, Side Effects or Overdose Symptoms* section below.

Adverse Reactions, Side Effects or Overdose Symptoms

Signs and symptoms	What to do
Diarrhea	Discontinue. Call doctor immediately.
Nausea or vomiting	Discontinue. Call doctor immediately.
Skin eruptions	Discontinue. Call doctor when convenient.

Rue (Garden Rue, German Rue)

 Basic Information

Biological name (genus and species):
Ruta graveolens

Parts used for medicinal purposes:
Entire plant

Chemicals this herb contains:
• Esters
• Methyl-N-nonyl-ketone
• Phenols
• Rutin
• Tannins (see Glossary)
• Volatile oils (see Glossary)

 Known Effects

• Stimulates uterine contractions
• Prolongs action of epinephrine
• Relieves spasm in skeletal or smooth muscle
• Decreases capillary fragility
• Interferes with absorption of iron and other minerals when taken internally

 Possible Additional Effects

• May cause onset of menstruation
• May treat hysteria
• May treat intestinal parasites (worms)
• May treat colic
• May control postpartum bleeding

 Warnings and Precautions

Don't take if you:
• Are pregnant, think you may be pregnant or plan pregnancy in the near future
• Have any chronic disease of the gastrointestinal tract, such as stomach or duodenal ulcers, reflux esophagitis, ulcerative colitis, spastic colitis, diverticulosis or diverticulitis

Consult your doctor if you:
• Take this herb for any medical problem that doesn't improve in 2 weeks (There may be safer, more effective treatments.)
• Take any medicinal drugs or herbs including aspirin, laxatives, cold and cough remedies, antacids, vitamins, minerals, amino acids, supplements, other prescription or nonprescription drugs

Pregnancy
Dangers outweigh any possible benefits. Don't use.

Breastfeeding:
Dangers outweigh any possible benefits. Don't use.

Infants and children:
Treating infants and children under 2 with any herbal preparation is hazardous.

Others:
None are expected if you are beyond childhood, under 45, not pregnant,

MEDICINAL HERBS

basically healthy, take it for only a short time and do not exceed manufacturer's recommended dose.

Storage:
- Store in cool, dry area away from direct light, but don't freeze.
- Store safely out of reach of children.
- Don't store in bathroom medicine cabinet. Heat and moisture may change the action of the herb.

Safe dosage:
Consult your doctor for the appropriate dose for your condition.

 Toxicity

Rated relatively safe when taken in appropriate quantities for short periods of time

For symptoms of toxicity: See *Adverse Reactions, Side Effects or Overdose Symptoms* section below.

 Adverse Reactions, Side Effects or Overdose Symptoms

Signs and symptoms	What to do
Abdominal pain	Discontinue. Call doctor when convenient.
Abortion	Seek emergency treatment.
Confusion	Discontinue. Call doctor immediately.
Diarrhea	Discontinue. Call doctor immediately.
Jaundice (yellow skin and eyes)	Discontinue. Call doctor immediately.
Nausea or vomiting	Discontinue. Call doctor immediately.
Skin rashes	Discontinue. Call doctor when convenient.

Scotch Broom

 Basic Information

Biological name (genus and species): *Cytisus scoparius*

Parts used for medicinal purposes: Leaves

Chemicals this herb contains:
- Cytisine
- Genisteine
- Hydroxytyramine
- Sarothamnine
- Scoparin
- Sparteine

 Known Effects

- Stimulates uterine contractions
- Helps body dispose of excess fluid by increasing amount of urine produced
- Sometimes causes sharp rise in blood pressure

 Possible Additional Effects

- May treat congestive heart failure
- May produce sedative-hypnotic effect when smoked

Warnings and Precautions

Don't take if you:

• Are pregnant, think you may be pregnant or plan pregnancy in the near future
• Have any chronic disease of the gastrointestinal tract, such as stomach or duodenal ulcers, reflux esophagitis, ulcerative colitis, spastic colitis, diverticulosis or diverticulitis

Consult your doctor if you:

• Take this herb for any medical problem that doesn't improve in 2 weeks (There may be safer, more effective treatments.)
• Take any medicinal drugs or herbs including aspirin, laxatives, cold and cough remedies, antacids, vitamins, minerals, amino acids, supplements, other prescription or nonprescription drugs

Pregnancy:
Don't use unless prescribed by your doctor.

Breastfeeding:
Don't use unless prescribed by your doctor.

Infants and children:
Treating infants and children under 2 with any herbal preparation is hazardous.

Others:
None are expected if you are beyond childhood, under 45, not pregnant, basically healthy, take it for only a short time and do not exceed manufacturer's recommended dose.

Storage:
• Store in cool, dry area away from direct light, but don't freeze.
• Store safely out of reach of children.
• Don't store in bathroom medicine cabinet. Heat and moisture may change the action of the herb.

Safe dosage:
Consult your doctor for the appropriate dose for your condition.

 ## Toxicity

Rated slightly dangerous, particularly in children, persons over 55 and those who take larger than appropriate quantities for extended periods of time

For symptoms of toxicity: See *Adverse Reactions, Side Effects or Overdose Symptoms* section below.

 ## Adverse Reactions, Side Effects or Overdose Symptoms

Signs and symptoms	What to do
Diarrhea	Discontinue. Call doctor immediately.
Nausea or vomiting	Discontinue. Call doctor immediately.

MEDICINAL HERBS

→

Silverweed (Goose Tansy)

Basic Information

Biological name (genus and species):
Potentilla anserina

Parts used for medicinal purposes:
Entire plant

Chemicals this herb contains:
• Ellagic acid (see Glossary)
• Kinovic acid
• Tannins (see Glossary)

Known Effects

• Shrinks tissues
• Prevents secretion of fluids
• Causes protein molecules to clump together
• Stimulates uterine contractions
• Interferes with absorption of iron and other minerals when taken internally

Possible Additional Effects

• May treat dysmenorrhea (painful menstruation)
• May treat tetanus in absence of medical help, when used with lobelia

Warnings and Precautions

Don't take if you:
• Are pregnant, think you may be pregnant or plan pregnancy in the near future
• Have any chronic disease of the gastrointestinal tract, such as stomach or duodenal ulcers, reflux esophagitis, ulcerative colitis, spastic colitis, diverticulosis or diverticulitis

Consult your doctor if you:
• Take this herb for any medical problem that doesn't improve in 2 weeks (There may be safer, more effective treatments.)
• Take any medicinal drugs or herbs including aspirin, laxatives, cold and cough remedies, antacids, vitamins, minerals, amino acids, supplements, other prescription or nonprescription drugs

Pregnancy
Dangers outweigh any possible benefits. Don't use.

Breastfeeding:
Dangers outweigh any possible benefits. Don't use.

Infants and children:
Treating infants and children under 2 with any herbal preparation is hazardous.

Others:
None are expected if you are beyond childhood, under 45, not pregnant, basically healthy, take it for only a short time and do not exceed manufacturer's recommended dose.

Storage:
• Store in cool, dry area away from direct light, but don't freeze.
• Store safely out of reach of children.
• Don't store in bathroom medicine cabinet. Heat and moisture may change the action of the herb.

Safe dosage:
Consult your doctor for the appropriate dose for your condition.

Toxicity

Comparative-toxicity rating is not available from standard references.

For symptoms of toxicity: See *Adverse Reactions, Side Effects or Overdose Symptoms* section below.

 Adverse Reactions, Side Effects or Overdose Symptoms

Signs and symptoms	What to do
Diarrhea	Discontinue. Call doctor immediately.
Nausea or vomiting	Discontinue. Call doctor immediately.
Painful urination	Discontinue. Call doctor when convenient.

Snakeplant

 Basic Information

Biological name (genus and species): *Rivea corymbosa*

Parts used for medicinal purposes: Seeds

Chemicals this herb contains: *Five related LSD-like alkaloids*

- Chanoclavine
- D-isolysergic acid amide
- D-lysergic acid amide
- Elymoclavine
- Lysergol

 Known Effects

Depresses central nervous system

Miscellaneous information: Snakeplant is used primarily by Mexican Indians in religious ceremonies. They call it *badah*.

 Possible Additional Effects

- May change mood
- May cause hallucinations

MEDICINAL HERBS

➡

Warnings and Precautions

Don't take if you:
- Are pregnant, think you may be pregnant or plan pregnancy in the near future
- Have any chronic disease of the gastrointestinal tract, such as stomach or duodenal ulcers, reflux esophagitis, ulcerative colitis, spastic colitis, diverticulosis or diverticulitis

Consult your doctor if you:
- Take this herb for any medical problem that doesn't improve in 2 weeks (There may be safer, more effective treatments.)
- Take any medicinal drugs or herbs including aspirin, laxatives, cold and cough remedies, antacids, vitamins, minerals, amino acids, supplements, other prescription or nonprescription drugs

Pregnancy
Dangers outweigh any possible benefits. Don't use.

Breastfeeding:
Dangers outweigh any possible benefits. Don't use.

Infants and children:
Treating infants and children under 2 with any herbal preparation is hazardous.

Others:
Dangers outweigh any possible benefits. Don't use.

Storage:
- Store in cool, dry area away from direct light, but don't freeze.
- Store safely out of reach of children.
- Don't store in bathroom medicine cabinet. Heat and moisture may change the action of the herb.

Safe dosage:
Consult your doctor for the appropriate dose for your condition.

 ## Toxicity

Rated slightly dangerous, particularly in children, persons over 55 and those who take larger than appropriate quantities for extended periods of time

For symptoms of toxicity: See *Adverse Reactions, Side Effects or Overdose Symptoms* section below.

 ## Adverse Reactions, Side Effects or Overdose Symptoms

Signs and symptoms	What to do
Blurred vision	Discontinue. Call doctor immediately.
Coma	Seek emergency treatment.
Confusion	Discontinue. Call doctor immediately.
Hallucinations	Seek emergency treatment.
Nausea or vomiting	Discontinue. Call doctor immediately.
Stupor	Discontinue. Call doctor immediately.

Snakeroot (Serpentaria, Virginia Snakeroot)

Basic Information

Biological name (genus and species):
Aristolochia serpentaria

Parts used for medicinal purposes:
Roots

Chemicals this herb contains:
• Aristolochin
• Borneol
• Terpene (see Glossary)
• Volatile oils (see Glossary)

Known Effects

• Stimulates stomach secretions
• Stimulates smooth-muscle
  contractions of gastrointestinal tract
  and heart

Possible Additional Effects

• May increase circulation
• May stimulate heart action
• May treat dyspepsia
• May reduce fever
• May treat sores on skin

Warnings and Precautions

Don't take if you:
• Are pregnant, think you may be
  pregnant or plan pregnancy in the
  near future
• Have any chronic disease of the
  gastrointestinal tract, such as stomach
  or duodenal ulcers, reflux
  esophagitis, ulcerative colitis, spastic
  colitis, diverticulosis or diverticulitis

Consult your doctor if you:
• Take this herb for any medical
  problem that doesn't improve in
  2 weeks (There may be safer, more
  effective treatments.)
• Take any medicinal drugs or
  herbs including aspirin, laxatives,
  cold and cough remedies, antacids,
  vitamins, minerals, amino acids,
  supplements, other prescription
  or nonprescription drugs

Pregnancy
Dangers outweigh any possible
benefits. Don't use.

Breastfeeding:
Dangers outweigh any possible
benefits. Don't use.

Infants and children:
Treating infants and children under
2 with any herbal preparation
is hazardous.

Others:
None are expected if you are beyond
childhood, under 45, not pregnant,
basically healthy, take it for only a short
time and do not exceed manufacturer's
recommended dose.

Storage:
• Store in cool, dry area away from
  direct light, but don't freeze.
• Store safely out of reach of children.
• Don't store in bathroom medicine
  cabinet. Heat and moisture may
  change the action of the herb.

Safe dosage:
Consult your doctor for the appropriate dose for your condition.

MEDICINAL HERBS

Toxicity

Rated relatively safe when taken in appropriate quantities for short periods of time

For symptoms of toxicity: See *Adverse Reactions, Side Effects or Overdose Symptoms* section below.

Adverse Reactions, Side Effects or Overdose Symptoms

Signs and symptoms	What to do
Diarrhea	Discontinue. Call doctor immediately.
Nausea or vomiting	Discontinue. Call doctor immediately.
Tenesmus (spasm of rectal sphincter)	Discontinue. Call doctor when convenient.

Spanish Broom

Basic Information

Biological name (genus and species): *Spartium junceum*

Parts used for medicinal purposes: Petals/flower

Chemicals this herb contains:
• Anagyrine
• Cytisine
• Methylcytisine

Known Effects

• Stimulates uterine contractions
• Helps body dispose of excess fluid by increasing amount of urine produced
• Stimulates gastrointestinal tract
• Causes vomiting

Possible Additional Effects

• May induce labor
• May cause watery, explosive bowel movements

Warnings and Precautions

Don't take if you:
• Are pregnant, think you may be pregnant or plan pregnancy in the near future
• Have any chronic disease of the gastrointestinal tract, such as stomach or duodenal ulcers, reflux

esophagitis, ulcerative colitis, spastic colitis, diverticulosis or diverticulitis

Consult your doctor if you:

• Take this herb for any medical problem that doesn't improve in 2 weeks (There may be safer, more effective treatments.)
• Take any medicinal drugs or herbs including aspirin, laxatives, cold and cough remedies, antacids, vitamins, minerals, amino acids, supplements, other prescription or nonprescription drugs

Pregnancy:

Dangers outweigh any possible benefits. Don't use.

Breastfeeding:

Dangers outweigh any possible benefits. Don't use.

Infants and children:

Treating infants and children under 2 with any herbal preparation is hazardous.

Others:

None are expected if you are beyond childhood, under 45, not pregnant, basically healthy, take it for only a short time and do not exceed manufacturer's recommended dose.

Storage:

• Store in cool, dry area away from direct light, but don't freeze.
• Store safely out of reach of children.

• Don't store in bathroom medicine cabinet. Heat and moisture may change the action of the herb.

Safe dosage:

Consult your doctor for the appropriate dose for your condition.

 Toxicity

Comparative-toxicity rating is not available from standard references.

For symptoms of toxicity: See *Adverse Reactions, Side Effects or Overdose Symptoms* section below.

 Adverse Reactions, Side Effects or Overdose Symptoms

Signs and symptoms	What to do
Diarrhea	Discontinue. Call doctor immediately.
Kidney damage characterized by blood in urine, decreased urine flow, swelling of hands and feet	Seek emergency treatment.
Muscle weakness	Discontinue. Call doctor immediately.
Nausea or vomiting	Discontinue. Call doctor immediately.

Spearmint

 Basic Information

Biological name (genus and species):
Mentha spicata

Parts used for medicinal purposes:
• Leaves
• Petals/flower

Chemicals this herb contains:
• Carvone
• Resin (see Glossary)
• Volatile oils (see Glossary)

 Known Effects

• Stimulates muscular action of gastrointestinal tract
• Helps treat nausea

Miscellaneous information:
Spearmint is used as a flavoring agent in many foods.

 Possible Additional Effects

• May help expel gas from intestinal tract
• May soothe sore throats
• May treat sinus congestion

 Warnings and Precautions

Don't take if you:
• Are pregnant, think you may be pregnant or plan pregnancy in the near future
• Have any chronic disease of the gastrointestinal tract, such as stomach or duodenal ulcers, reflux esophagitis, ulcerative colitis, spastic colitis, diverticulosis or diverticulitis

Consult your doctor if you:
• Take this herb for any medical problem that doesn't improve in 2 weeks (There may be safer, more effective treatments.)
• Take any medicinal drugs or herbs including aspirin, laxatives, cold and cough remedies, antacids, vitamins, minerals, amino acids, supplements, other prescription or nonprescription drugs
• Want to use for morning sickness

Pregnancy:
Don't use unless prescribed by your doctor.

Breastfeeding:
Don't use unless prescribed by your doctor.

Infants and children:
Treating infants and children under 2 with any herbal preparation is hazardous.

Others:
None are expected if you are beyond childhood, under 45, not pregnant, basically healthy, take it for only a short time and do not exceed manufacturer's recommended dose.

Storage:
• Store in cool, dry area away from direct light, but don't freeze.
• Store safely out of reach of children.
• Don't store in bathroom medicine cabinet. Heat and moisture may change the action of the herb.

Safe dosage:
Consult your doctor for the appropriate dose for your condition.

 Toxicity

Comparative-toxicity rating is not available from standard references.

For symptoms of toxicity: See *Adverse Reactions, Side Effects or Overdose Symptoms* section below.

 Adverse Reactions, Side Effects or Overdose Symptoms

Signs and symptoms	What to do
Convulsions and coma	Seek emergency treatment.
Diarrhea	Discontinue. Call doctor immediately.
Nausea or vomiting	Discontinue. Call doctor immediately.

Strawberry (Earth Mulberry)

 Basic Information

Biological name (genus and species):
Fragaria vesca, F. americana

Parts used for medicinal purposes:
• Berries
• Leaves
• Roots

Chemicals this herb contains:
• Catechins
• Leucoanthocyanin
• Minerals
• Vitamin C

 Known Effects

• Prevents scurvy
• Inhibits production of histamines

Miscellaneous information:
Wild strawberry is a member of the rose family.

 Possible Additional Effects

No additional effects are known.

 Warnings and Precautions

Don't take if you:
Are allergic to strawberries.

Consult your doctor if you:
• Take this herb for any medical problem that doesn't improve in 2 weeks (There may be safer, more effective treatments.)
• Take any medicinal drugs or herbs including aspirin, laxatives, cold and cough remedies, antacids, vitamins, minerals, amino acids, supplements, other prescription or nonprescription drugs

Pregnancy:
Pregnant women should experience no problems taking usual amounts as part of a balanced diet. Other products extracted from this herb have not been proved to cause problems.

Breastfeeding:
Breastfed infants of lactating mothers should experience no problems when mother takes usual amounts as part of a balanced diet. Other products

MEDICINAL HERBS

→

extracted from this herb have not been proved to cause problems.

Infants and children:
Treating infants and children under 2 with any herbal preparation is hazardous.

Others:
None are expected if you are beyond childhood, under 45, not pregnant, basically healthy, take it for only a short time and do not exceed manufacturer's recommended dose.

Storage:
- Store in cool, dry area away from direct light, but don't freeze.
- Store safely out of reach of children.
- Don't store in bathroom medicine cabinet. Heat and moisture may change the action of the herb.

Safe dosage:
Consult your doctor for the appropriate dose for your condition.

 Toxicity

Generally regarded as safe when taken in appropriate quantities for short periods of time

 Adverse Reactions, Side Effects or Overdose Symptoms

None are expected.

Sumac

 Basic Information

Biological name (genus and species): *Rhus glabra*

Parts used for medicinal purposes:
- Bark
- Berries
- Leaves

Chemicals this herb contains:
- Albumin
- Malic acid
- Resin (see Glossary)
- Tannins (see Glossary)
- Volatile oils (see Glossary)

 Known Effects

Bark:
- Shrinks tissues
- Prevents secretion of fluids
- Inhibits growth and development of germs

Berries:
- Helps body dispose of excess fluid by increasing amount of urine produced
- Interferes with absorption of iron and other minerals when taken internally

Miscellaneous information:
Sumac is in the same plant family as poison ivy and poison oak.

Possible Additional Effects

- May treat diarrhea
- May treat rectal bleeding
- May treat asthma when leaves are smoked

Warnings and Precautions

Don't take if you:
Are pregnant, think you may be pregnant or plan pregnancy in the near future.

Consult your doctor if you:
- Take this herb for any medical problem that doesn't improve in 2 weeks (There may be safer, more effective treatments.)
- Take any medicinal drugs or herbs including aspirin, laxatives, cold and cough remedies, antacids, vitamins, minerals, amino acids, supplements, other prescription or nonprescription drugs

Pregnancy:
Don't use unless prescribed by your doctor.

Breastfeeding:
Don't use unless prescribed by your doctor.

Infants and children:
Treating infants and children under 2 with any herbal preparation is hazardous.

Others:
None are expected if you are beyond childhood, under 45, not pregnant, basically healthy, take it for only a short time and do not exceed manufacturer's recommended dose.

Storage:
- Store in cool, dry area away from direct light, but don't freeze.
- Store safely out of reach of children.
- Don't store in bathroom medicine cabinet. Heat and moisture may change the action of the herb.

Safe dosage:
Consult your doctor for the appropriate dose for your condition.

Toxicity

Comparative-toxicity rating is not available from standard references.

Adverse Reactions, Side Effects or Overdose Symptoms

None are expected.

Sundew

Basic Information

Biological name (genus and species):
Drosera rotundifolia

Parts used for medicinal purposes:
Various parts of the entire plant, frequently differing by country and culture

Chemicals this herb contains:
- Citric acid
- Droserone
- Malic acid
- Resin (see Glossary)
- Tannins (see Glossary)

MEDICINAL HERBS

→

Known Effects

- Interferes with absorption of iron and other minerals when taken internally
- Loosens bronchial secretions

Possible Additional Effects

- May treat whooping cough
- May treat laryngitis
- May treat smoker's cough

Warnings and Precautions

Don't take if you:
Are pregnant, think you may be pregnant or plan pregnancy in the near future.

Consult your doctor if you:
- Take this herb for any medical problem that doesn't improve in 2 weeks (There may be safer, more effective treatments.)
- Take any medicinal drugs or herbs including aspirin, laxatives, cold and cough remedies, antacids, vitamins, minerals, amino acids, supplements, other prescription or nonprescription drugs

Pregnancy:
Don't use unless prescribed by your doctor.

Breastfeeding:
Don't use unless prescribed by your doctor.

Infants and children:
Treating infants and children under 2 with any herbal preparation is hazardous.

Others:
None are expected if you are beyond childhood, under 45, not pregnant, basically healthy, take it for only a short time and do not exceed manufacturer's recommended dose.

Storage:
- Store in cool, dry area away from direct light, but don't freeze.
- Store safely out of reach of children.
- Don't store in bathroom medicine cabinet. Heat and moisture may change the action of the herb.

Safe dosage:
Consult your doctor for the appropriate dose for your condition.

Toxicity

Comparative-toxicity rating is not available from standard references.

Adverse Reactions, Side Effects or Overdose Symptoms

None are expected.

Sunflower

 Basic Information

Biological name (genus and species):
Helianthus annuus

Parts used for medicinal purposes:
• Leaves
• Petals/flower
• Seeds

Chemicals this herb contains:
• Arachidic acid
• Behenic acid
• Linoleic acid
• Oleic acid
• Palmitic acid
• Stearic acid
• Vitamin E

 Known Effects

• Antioxidant
• Treats vitamin-E deficiency (seeds)

Miscellaneous information:
Sunflower is a food source.

 Possible Additional Effects

May help reduce pain of arthritis

 Warnings and Precautions

Don't take if you:
Are pregnant, think you may be pregnant or plan pregnancy in the near future.

Consult your doctor if you:
• Take this herb for any medical problem that doesn't improve in

2 weeks (There may be safer, more effective treatments.)
• Take any medicinal drugs or herbs including aspirin, laxatives, cold and cough remedies, antacids, vitamins, minerals, amino acids, supplements, other prescription or nonprescription drugs

Pregnancy:
Don't use unless prescribed by your doctor.

Breastfeeding:
Don't use unless prescribed by your doctor.

Infants and children:
Treating infants and children under 2 with any herbal preparation is hazardous.

Others:
None are expected if you are beyond childhood, under 45, not pregnant, basically healthy, take it for only a short time and do not exceed manufacturer's recommended dose.

Storage:
• Store in cool, dry area away from direct light, but don't freeze.
• Store safely out of reach of children.
• Don't store in bathroom medicine cabinet. Heat and moisture may change the action of the herb.

Safe dosage:
Consult your doctor for the appropriate dose for your condition.

 Toxicity

Comparative-toxicity rating is not available from standard references.

MEDICINAL HERBS

→

For symptoms of toxicity: See
*Adverse Reactions, Side Effects or
Overdose Symptoms* section below.

Adverse Reactions, Side Effects or Overdose Symptoms

Signs and symptoms	What to do
Allergic reaction	Discontinue. Call doctor immediately.

Sweet Violet

Basic Information

Biological name (genus and species):
Viola odorata

Parts used for medicinal purposes:
• Leaves
• Seeds

Chemicals this herb contains:
• Glycosides (see Glossary)
• Myrosin

Known Effects

• Irritates mucous membranes
• Stimulates gastrointestinal tract

Miscellaneous information:
Sweet violet was used to treat cancer
as early as 500 B.C., but evidence of
real benefit is lacking.

Possible Additional Effects

• May treat cancer when used as
  poultice (see Glossary)
• May treat skin disease

• Potential mild laxative
• May cause vomiting
• May decrease thickness and increase
  fluidity of mucus in lungs and
  bronchial tubes
• May treat coughs

Warnings and Precautions

Don't take if you:
• Are pregnant, think you may be
  pregnant or plan pregnancy in the
  near future
• Have any chronic disease of the
  gastrointestinal tract, such as stomach
  or duodenal ulcers, reflux
  esophagitis, ulcerative colitis, spastic
  colitis, diverticulosis or diverticulitis

Consult your doctor if you:
• Take this herb for any medical
  problem that doesn't improve in
  2 weeks (There may be safer, more
  effective treatments.)
• Take any medicinal drugs or
  herbs including aspirin, laxatives,
  cold and cough remedies, antacids,
  vitamins, minerals, amino acids,
  supplements, other prescription
  or nonprescription drugs

Pregnancy:
Don't use unless prescribed by your doctor.

Breastfeeding:
Don't use unless prescribed by your doctor.

Infants and children:
Treating infants and children under 2 with any herbal preparation is hazardous.

Others:
None are expected if you are beyond childhood, under 45, not pregnant, basically healthy, take it for only a short time and do not exceed manufacturer's recommended dose.

Storage:
• Store in cool, dry area away from direct light, but don't freeze.
• Store safely out of reach of children.
• Don't store in bathroom medicine cabinet. Heat and moisture may change the action of the herb.

Safe dosage:
Consult your doctor for the appropriate dose for your condition.

 Toxicity

Comparative-toxicity rating is not available from standard references.

For symptoms of toxicity: See *Adverse Reactions, Side Effects or Overdose Symptoms* section below.

 Adverse Reactions, Side Effects or Overdose Symptoms

Signs and symptoms	What to do
Seeds:	
Diarrhea	Discontinue. Call doctor immediately.
Nausea or vomiting	Discontinue. Call doctor immediately.

Tansy

 Basic Information

Biological name (genus and species):
Tanacetum vulgare

Parts used for medicinal purposes:
Entire plant

Chemicals this herb contains:
• Bitters (see Glossary)
• Borneol
• Camphor
• Resin (see Glossary)
• Tanacetin
• Tanacetol
• Thujone

 Known Effects

• Stimulates uterine contractions
• Stimulates appetite
• Kills intestinal parasites

Miscellaneous information:
Tansy is a powerful herb that should be avoided or used only under strict medical supervision.

 Possible Additional Effects

• May treat pain
• May cause euphoria

→

- May treat roundworms and pinworms
- May treat menstrual difficulties

Warnings and Precautions

Don't take if you:
- Are pregnant, think you may be pregnant or plan pregnancy in the near future
- Have any chronic disease of the gastrointestinal tract, such as stomach or duodenal ulcers, reflux esophagitis, ulcerative colitis, spastic colitis, diverticulosis or diverticulitis

Consult your doctor if you:
- Take this herb for any medical problem that doesn't improve in 2 weeks (There may be safer, more effective treatments.)
- Take any medicinal drugs or herbs including aspirin, laxatives, cold and cough remedies, antacids, vitamins, minerals, amino acids, supplements, other prescription or nonprescription drugs

Pregnancy
Dangers outweigh any possible benefits. Don't use.

Breastfeeding:
Dangers outweigh any possible benefits. Don't use.

Infants and children:
Treating infants and children under 2 with any herbal preparation is hazardous.

Others:
Dangers outweigh any possible benefits. Don't use.

Storage:
- Store in cool, dry area away from direct light, but don't freeze.
- Store safely out of reach of children.
- Don't store in bathroom medicine cabinet. Heat and moisture may change the action of the herb.

Safe dosage:
Consult your doctor for the appropriate dose for your condition.

Toxicity

Rated dangerous, particularly in children, persons over 55 and those who take larger than appropriate quantities for extended periods of time

For symptoms of toxicity: See *Adverse Reactions, Side Effects or Overdose Symptoms* section below.

Adverse Reactions, Side Effects or Overdose Symptoms

Signs and symptoms	What to do
Coma	Seek emergency treatment.
Convulsions	Seek emergency treatment.
Diarrhea	Discontinue. Call doctor immediately.
Dilated pupils	Seek emergency treatment.
Nausea or vomiting	Discontinue. Call doctor immediately.
Weak, rapid pulse	Seek emergency treatment.

Thyme, Common

Basic Information

Biological name (genus and species):
Thymus vulgaris

Parts used for medicinal purposes:
• Berries/fruits
• Leaves

Chemicals this herb contains:
• Gum (see Glossary)
• Tannins (see Glossary)
• Thyme oil

Known Effects

• Inhibits growth and development of germs
• Stimulates gastrointestinal tract
• Decreases thickness of bronchial secretions

Possible Additional Effects

• May reduce flatulence
• May treat coughs
• May treat bronchitis
• May treat bacterial infections
• May reduce menstrual cramps
• May help treat asthma
• Under study for cancer preventive properties

Warnings and Precautions

Don't take if you:
Are pregnant, think you may be pregnant or plan pregnancy in the near future.

Consult your doctor if you:
• Take this herb for any medical problem that doesn't improve in 2 weeks (There may be safer, more effective treatments.)
• Take any medicinal drugs or herbs including aspirin, laxatives, cold and cough remedies, antacids, vitamins, minerals, amino acids, supplements, other prescription or nonprescription drugs
• Have high blood pressure

Pregnancy:
Don't use unless prescribed by your doctor.

Breastfeeding:
Don't use unless prescribed by your doctor.

Infants and children:
Treating infants and children under 2 with any herbal preparation is hazardous.

Others:
None are expected if you are beyond childhood, under 45, not pregnant, basically healthy, take it for only a short time and do not exceed manufacturer's recommended dose.

Storage:
• Store in cool, dry area away from direct light, but don't freeze.
• Store safely out of reach of children.
• Don't store in bathroom medicine cabinet. Heat and moisture may change the action of the herb.

Safe dosage:
Consult your doctor for the appropriate dose for your condition.

MEDICINAL HERBS

→

Toxicity

Rated relatively safe when taken in appropriate quantities for short periods of time

For symptoms of toxicity: See *Adverse Reactions, Side Effects or Overdose Symptoms* section below.

 Adverse Reactions, Side Effects or Overdose Symptoms

Signs and symptoms	What to do
Diarrhea	Discontinue. Call doctor immediately.
Nausea or vomiting	Discontinue. Call doctor immediately.

Tonka Bean (Tonquin Bean)

 Basic Information

Biological name (genus and species): *Coumarouna odorata, Dipteryx odorata*

Parts used for medicinal purposes: Seeds

Chemicals this herb contains:
- Coumarin
- Gum (see Glossary)
- Sitosterin
- Starch
- Stigmasterin
- Sugar

 Known Effects

- Delays or stops blood clotting
- Anticoagulant

Miscellaneous information:
- Coumarin interferes with the synthesis of vitamin K in the human intestines. The absence of adequate vitamin K prevents blood clotting.
- The tonka bean was once a common adulterant of vanilla extracts.
- It's used as flavoring in tobacco.
- The FDA has banned its use as a flavoring agent in foods.

 Possible Additional Effects

- May prevent clotting in deep veins
- May prevent blood clots from breaking away from blood vessels and lodging in vital organs, such as lung or brain (use must be monitored carefully with frequent laboratory studies of prothrombin time)

 Warnings and Precautions

Don't take if you:
Are pregnant, think you may be pregnant or plan pregnancy in the near future.

Consult your doctor if you:
- Take this herb for any medical problem that doesn't improve in 2 weeks (There may be safer, more effective treatments.)
- Take any medicinal drugs or herbs including aspirin, laxatives, cold and cough remedies, antacids, vitamins, minerals, amino acids, supplements, other prescription or nonprescription drugs

Pregnancy:
Dangers outweigh any possible benefits. Don't use.

Breastfeeding:
Dangers outweigh any possible benefits. Don't use.

Infants and children:
Treating infants and children under 2 with any herbal preparation is hazardous.

Others:
Dangers outweigh any possible benefits. Don't use.

Storage:
• Store in cool, dry area away from direct light, but don't freeze.
• Store safely out of reach of children.
• Don't store in bathroom medicine cabinet. Heat and moisture may change the action of the herb.

Safe dosage:
Consult your doctor for the appropriate dose for your condition.

Toxicity

Comparative-toxicity rating is not available from standard references.

For symptoms of toxicity: See *Adverse Reactions, Side Effects or Overdose Symptoms* section below.

Adverse Reactions, Side Effects or Overdose Symptoms

Signs and symptoms	What to do
Growth retardation	Discontinue. Call doctor when convenient.
Jaundice (yellow skin and eyes)	Discontinue. Call doctor when convenient.
Testicle atrophy	Discontinue. Call doctor when convenient.
Uncontrollable internal bleeding	Seek emergency treatment.

Tormentil

Basic Information

Biological name (genus and species):
Potentilla erecta, P. tormentilla

Parts used for medicinal purposes:
Roots

Chemicals this herb contains:
• Ellagic acid (see Glossary)
• Kinovic acid
• Tannins (see Glossary)

Known Effects

• Shrinks tissues
• Prevents secretion of fluids
• Interferes with absorption of iron and other minerals when taken internally

Possible Additional Effects

• May treat diarrhea
• May treat sore throat
• May treat wounds when used as a poultice (see Glossary)

MEDICINAL HERBS

➜

Warnings and Precautions

Don't take if you:

• Are pregnant, think you may be pregnant or plan pregnancy in the near future
• Have any chronic disease of the gastrointestinal tract, such as stomach or duodenal ulcers, reflux esophagitis, ulcerative colitis, spastic colitis, diverticulosis or diverticulitis

Consult your doctor if you:

• Take this herb for any medical problem that doesn't improve in 2 weeks (There may be safer, more effective treatments.)
• Take any medicinal drugs or herbs including aspirin, laxatives, cold and cough remedies, antacids, vitamins, minerals, amino acids, supplements, other prescription or nonprescription drugs

Pregnancy:

Don't use unless prescribed by your doctor.

Breastfeeding:

Don't use unless prescribed by your doctor.

Infants and children:

Treating infants and children under 2 with any herbal preparation is hazardous.

Others:

None are expected if you are beyond childhood, under 45, not pregnant, basically healthy, take it for only a short time and do not exceed manufacturer's recommended dose.

Storage:

• Store in cool, dry area away from direct light, but don't freeze.
• Store safely out of reach of children.
• Don't store in bathroom medicine cabinet. Heat and moisture may change the action of the herb.

Safe dosage:

Consult your doctor for the appropriate dose for your condition.

 ## Toxicity

Comparative-toxicity rating is not available from standard references.

For symptoms of toxicity: See *Adverse Reactions, Side Effects or Overdose Symptoms* section below.

 ## Adverse Reactions, Side Effects or Overdose Symptoms

Signs and symptoms	What to do
Diarrhea	Discontinue. Call doctor immediately.
Kidney damage characterized by blood in urine, decreased urine flow, swelling of hands and feet	Seek emergency treatment.
Nausea or vomiting	Discontinue. Call doctor immediately.

Unicorn Root (Colic Root, Star Grass)

Basic Information

Biological name (genus and species):
Aletris farinosa

Parts used for medicinal purposes:
- Leaves
- Roots

Chemicals this herb contains:
- Diosgenin
- Resin (see Glossary)
- Saponins (see Glossary)
- Volatile oils (see Glossary)

Known Effects

Reduces smooth-muscle spasms

Miscellaneous information:

Serves as a base substance to produce synthetic progesterone (a female hormone).

Possible Additional Effects

- May treat painful menstruation
- May decrease chances of miscarriage
- May soothe sore breasts
- May relieve flatulence
- May relieve arthritis

Warnings and Precautions

Don't take if you:
- Are pregnant, think you may be pregnant or plan pregnancy in the near future
- Have any chronic disease of the gastrointestinal tract, such as stomach or duodenal ulcers, reflux esophagitis, ulcerative colitis, spastic colitis, diverticulosis or diverticulitis

Consult your doctor if you:
- Take this herb for any medical problem that doesn't improve in 2 weeks (There may be safer, more effective treatments.)
- Take any medicinal drugs or herbs including aspirin, laxatives, cold and cough remedies, antacids, vitamins, minerals, amino acids, supplements, other prescription or nonprescription drugs

Pregnancy:
Don't use unless prescribed by your doctor.

Breastfeeding:
Don't use unless prescribed by your doctor.

Infants and children:
Treating infants and children under 2 with any herbal preparation is hazardous.

Others:
None are expected if you are beyond childhood, under 45, not pregnant, basically healthy, take it for only a short time and do not exceed manufacturer's recommended dose.

Storage:
- Store in cool, dry area away from direct light, but don't freeze.
- Store safely out of reach of children.
- Don't store in bathroom medicine cabinet. Heat and moisture may change the action of the herb.

Safe dosage:
Consult your doctor for the appropriate dose for your condition.

MEDICINAL HERBS

→

Toxicity

Rated slightly dangerous, particularly in children, persons over 55 and those who take larger than appropriate quantities for extended periods of time

For symptoms of toxicity: See *Adverse Reactions, Side Effects or Overdose Symptoms* section below.

Adverse Reactions, Side Effects or Overdose Symptoms

Signs and symptoms	What to do
Diarrhea	Discontinue. Call doctor immediately.
Lethargy	Discontinue. Call doctor when convenient.
Vomiting	Discontinue. Call doctor immediately.

Virginian Skullcap

Basic Information

Biological name (genus and species):
Scutellaria lateriflora

Parts used for medicinal purposes:
Entire plant

Chemicals this herb contains:
• Cellulose
• Fat
• Scutellarin
• Sugar
• Tannins (see Glossary)

Known Effects

• Increases stomach acidity
• Irritates mucous membranes
• Relieves spasm in skeletal or smooth muscle
• Interferes with absorption of iron and other minerals when taken internally

Possible Additional Effects

• May stimulate appetite
• May relieve intestinal cramps

Warnings and Precautions

Don't take if you:
Are pregnant, think you may be pregnant or plan pregnancy in the near future.

Consult your doctor if you:
• Take this herb for any medical problem that doesn't improve in 2 weeks (There may be safer, more effective treatments.)
• Take any medicinal drugs or herbs including aspirin, laxatives, cold and cough remedies, antacids, vitamins, minerals, amino acids, supplements, other prescription or nonprescription drugs

Pregnancy:
Don't use unless prescribed by your doctor.

Breastfeeding:
Don't use unless prescribed by
your doctor.

Infants and children:
Treating infants and children under 2
with any herbal preparation
is hazardous.

Others:
None are expected if you are beyond
childhood, under 45, not pregnant,
basically healthy, take it for only a short
time and do not exceed manufacturer's
recommended dose.

Storage:
• Store in cool, dry area away from
  direct light, but don't freeze.
• Store safely out of reach of children.
• Don't store in bathroom medicine
  cabinet. Heat and moisture may
  change the action of the herb.

Safe dosage:
Consult your doctor for the appropriate dose for your condition.

 Toxicity

Rated relatively safe when taken in
appropriate quantities for short
periods of time

For symptoms of toxicity: See
*Adverse Reactions, Side Effects or
Overdose Symptoms* section below.

 Adverse Reactions,
Side Effects or
Overdose Symptoms

Signs and symptoms	What to do
Confusion	Discontinue. Call doctor immediately.
Giddiness	Discontinue. Call doctor when convenient.
Irregular heartbeat	Seek emergency treatment.
Stupor	Seek emergency treatment.

Watercress

 Basic Information

Biological name (genus and species):
Nasturtium officinale

Parts used for medicinal purposes:
Various parts of the entire plant,
frequently differing by country
and culture

Chemicals this herb contains:
• Several trace element minerals, such
  as vanadium and cobalt
• Vitamins A, C, B-1 and B-2

 Known Effects

Provides a good source of vitamins and
minerals to treat or prevent
various deficiencies

Miscellaneous information:
• Watercress is a nutritious food
  source.
• Toxicity is unlikely.

 Possible
Additional Effects

• May treat kidney infections
• May treat urinary bladder stones
• May increase urine flow

MEDICINAL HERBS

→

• May treat heart disease
• May diminish pain during childbirth

 ## Warnings and Precautions

Don't take if you:
Are pregnant, think you may be pregnant or plan pregnancy in the near future.

Consult your doctor if you:
• Take this herb for any medical problem that doesn't improve in 2 weeks (There may be safer, more effective treatments.)
• Take any medicinal drugs or herbs including aspirin, laxatives, cold and cough remedies, antacids, vitamins, minerals, amino acids, supplements, other prescription or nonprescription drugs

Pregnancy:
Don't use unless prescribed by your doctor.

Breastfeeding:
Don't use unless prescribed by your doctor.

Infants and children:
Treating infants and children under 2 with any herbal preparation is hazardous.

Others:
None are expected if you are beyond childhood, under 45, not pregnant, basically healthy, take it for only a short time and do not exceed manufacturer's recommended dose.

Storage:
• Store in cool, dry area away from direct light, but don't freeze.
• Store safely out of reach of children.
• Don't store in bathroom medicine cabinet. Heat and moisture may change the action of the herb.

Safe dosage:
Consult your doctor for the appropriate dose for your condition.

 ## Toxicity

Comparative-toxicity rating is not available from standard references.

 ## Adverse Reactions, Side Effects or Overdose Symptoms

None are expected.

White Pine

 ## Basic Information

Biological name (genus and species):
Pinus strobus, P. alba

Parts used for medicinal purposes:
Inner bark

Chemicals this herb contains:
• Coniferin
• Coniferyl alcohol
• Mucilage (see Glossary)
• Oleoresin
• Tannic acid
• Vanillin
• Volatile oils (see Glossary)

Known Effects

Decreases thickness and increases fluidity of mucus in lungs and bronchial tubes

 Possible Additional Effects

May treat coughs when mixed with other expectorants

 Warnings and Precautions

Don't take if you:
Are pregnant, think you may be pregnant or plan pregnancy in the near future.

Consult your doctor if you:
• Take this herb for any medical problem that doesn't improve in 2 weeks (There may be safer, more effective treatments.)
• Take any medicinal drugs or herbs including aspirin, laxatives, cold and cough remedies, antacids, vitamins, minerals, amino acids, supplements, other prescription or nonprescription drugs

Pregnancy:
Don't use unless prescribed by your doctor.

Breastfeeding:
Don't use unless prescribed by your doctor.

Infants and children:
Treating infants and children under 2 with any herbal preparation is hazardous.

Others:
None are expected if you are beyond childhood, under 45, not pregnant, basically healthy, take it for only a short time and do not exceed manufacturer's recommended dose.

Storage:
• Store in cool, dry area away from direct light, but don't freeze.
• Store safely out of reach of children.
• Don't store in bathroom medicine cabinet. Heat and moisture may change the action of the herb.

Safe dosage:
Consult your doctor for the appropriate dose for your condition.

 Toxicity

Rated slightly dangerous, particularly in children, persons over 55 and those who take larger than appropriate quantities for extended periods of time

For symptoms of toxicity: See *Adverse Reactions, Side Effects or Overdose Symptoms* section below.

 Adverse Reactions, Side Effects or Overdose Symptoms

Signs and symptoms	What to do
Abdominal discomfort	Discontinue. Call doctor immediately.

MEDICINAL HERBS

Willow

Basic Information

Willow is also called black willow, pussy willow, white willow and yellow willow.

Biological name (genus and species): *Salix nigra, S. alba*

Parts used for medicinal purposes: Bark

Chemicals this herb contains:
• Salicin
• Salinigrin
• Tannins (see Glossary)

Known Effects

• Produces puckering
• Reduces fever
• Anti-inflammatory

Possible Additional Effects

• Potential antiseptic for ulcerated surfaces on skin
• May help reduce symptoms of gout, arthritis
• May help treat headaches
• May help heal open wounds because of tannins

Warnings and Precautions

Don't take if you:
Are pregnant, think you may be pregnant or plan pregnancy in the near future.

Consult your doctor if you:
• Take this herb for any medical problem that doesn't improve in 2 weeks (There may be safer, more effective treatments.)
• Take any medicinal drugs or herbs including aspirin, laxatives, cold and cough remedies, antacids, vitamins, minerals, amino acids, supplements, other prescription or nonprescription drugs

Pregnancy:
Don't use unless prescribed by your doctor.

Breastfeeding:
Don't use unless prescribed by your doctor.

Infants and children:
Treating infants and children under 2 with any herbal preparation is hazardous.

Others:
• None are expected if you are beyond childhood, under 45, not pregnant, basically healthy, take it for only a short time and do not exceed manufacturer's recommended dose.
• Salicylate poisoning is possible. Symptoms include dizziness, vomiting, ringing in ears.

Storage:
• Store in cool, dry area away from direct light, but don't freeze.
• Store safely out of reach of children.
• Don't store in bathroom medicine cabinet. Heat and moisture may change the action of the herb.

Safe dosage:
Consult your doctor for the appropriate dose for your condition.

Toxicity

Comparative-toxicity rating is not available from standard references.

For symptoms of toxicity: See *Adverse Reactions, Side Effects or Overdose Symptoms* section below.

Adverse Reactions, Side Effects or Overdose Symptoms

Signs and symptoms	What to do
Dizziness	Discontinue. Call doctor immediately.
Nausea or vomiting	Discontinue. Call doctor immediately.
Ringing in ears	Discontinue. Call doctor immediately.

Wintergreen (Boxberry, Teaberry)

Basic Information

Biological name (genus and species): *Gaultheria procumbens*

Parts used for medicinal purposes:
• Leaves
• Roots
• Stems

Chemicals this herb contains:
• Methyl salicylate
• Monotropitoside

Known Effects

• Blocks impulses to pain center in brain
• Irritates stomach
• Treats pain of sprains and bruises when used externally

Miscellaneous information:
• Toxicity is unlikely unless you consume very large amounts of the entire plant.
• Do not apply after vigorous exercise as it may cause salicylate toxicity.

Possible Additional Effects

• May relieve headache
• May treat toothache

Warnings and Precautions

Don't take if you:
Are pregnant, think you may be pregnant or plan pregnancy in the near future.

Consult your doctor if you:
• Take this herb for any medical problem that doesn't improve in 2 weeks (There may be safer, more effective treatments.)
• Take any medicinal drugs or herbs including aspirin, laxatives, cold and cough remedies, antacids, vitamins, minerals, amino acids, supplements, other prescription or nonprescription drugs

Pregnancy
Dangers outweigh any possible benefits. Don't use.

MEDICINAL HERBS

→

Breastfeeding:
Dangers outweigh any possible benefits. Don't use.

Infants and children:
Treating infants and children under 2 with any herbal preparation is hazardous.

Others:
None are expected if you are beyond childhood, under 45, not pregnant, basically healthy, take it for only a short time and do not exceed manufacturer's recommended dose.

Storage:
• Store in cool, dry area away from direct light, but don't freeze.
• Store safely out of reach of children.
• Don't store in bathroom medicine cabinet. Heat and moisture may change the action of the herb.

Safe dosage:
Consult your doctor for the appropriate dose for your condition.

 Toxicity

Rated slightly dangerous, particularly in children, persons over 55 and those who take larger than appropriate quantities for extended periods of time

 Adverse Reactions, Side Effects or Overdose Symptoms

Signs and symptoms	What to do
Abdominal pain	Discontinue. Call doctor when convenient.

Witch Hazel

 Basic Information

Biological name (genus and species):
Hamamelis virginiana

Parts used for medicinal purposes:
• Bark
• Leaves
• Twigs

Chemicals this herb contains:
• Bitters (see Glossary)
• Calcium oxalate
• Gallic acid
• Hamamelitannin
• Hexose sugar
• Tannins (see Glossary)
• Volatile oils (see Glossary)

 Known Effects

Shrinks tissues (when used as ointment, solution, suppository)

 Possible Additional Effects

• May treat diarrhea
• May soothe irritated skin or hemorrhoids
• Potential astringent (non-distilled form only)

Warnings and Precautions

Don't take if you:

• Are pregnant, think you may be pregnant or plan pregnancy in the near future
• Have any chronic disease of the gastrointestinal tract, such as stomach or duodenal ulcers, reflux esophagitis, ulcerative colitis, spastic colitis, diverticulosis or diverticulitis

Consult your doctor if you:

• Take this herb for any medical problem that doesn't improve in 2 weeks (There may be safer, more effective treatments.)
• Take any medicinal drugs or herbs including aspirin, laxatives, cold and cough remedies, antacids, vitamins, minerals, amino acids, supplements, other prescription or nonprescription drugs

Pregnancy:

Dangers outweigh any possible benefits. Don't use.

Breastfeeding:

Dangers outweigh any possible benefits. Don't use.

Infants and children:

Treating infants and children under 2 with any herbal preparation is hazardous.

Others:

None are expected if you are beyond childhood, under 45, not pregnant, basically healthy, take it for only a short time and do not exceed manufacturer's recommended dose.

Storage:

• Store in cool, dry area away from direct light, but don't freeze.
• Store safely out of reach of children.
• Don't store in bathroom medicine cabinet. Heat and moisture may change the action of the herb.

Safe dosage:

Consult your doctor for the appropriate dose for your condition.

 ## Toxicity

Rated relatively safe when taken in appropriate quantities for short periods of time

For symptoms of toxicity: See *Adverse Reactions, Side Effects or Overdose Symptoms* section below.

 ## Adverse Reactions, Side Effects or Overdose Symptoms

Signs and symptoms	What to do
Constipation	Discontinue. Call doctor when convenient.
Jaundice (yellow skin and eyes)	Discontinue. Call doctor immediately.
Nausea or vomiting	Discontinue. Call doctor immediately.

MEDICINAL HERBS

Woodruff

Basic Information

Biological name (genus and species):
Asperula odorata, Galium odoratum

Parts used for medicinal purposes:
Entire plant

Chemicals this herb contains:
• Asperuloside
• Bitters (see Glossary)
• Coumarin
• Oil
• Tannins (see Glossary)

Known Effects

• Stimulates gastrointestinal tract
• Decreases thickness and increases fluidity of mucus in lungs and bronchial tubes
• Interferes with absorption of iron and other minerals when taken internally

Miscellaneous information:
Woodruff is used as a flavoring agent in May wine and in sachets for its pleasant odor.

Possible Additional Effects

• May treat coughs
• May help expel gas from intestinal tract

Warnings and Precautions

Don't take if you:
Are pregnant, think you may be pregnant or plan pregnancy in the near future.

Consult your doctor if you:
• Take this herb for any medical problem that doesn't improve in 2 weeks (There may be safer, more effective treatments.)
• Take any medicinal drugs or herbs including aspirin, laxatives, cold and cough remedies, antacids, vitamins, minerals, amino acids, supplements, other prescription or nonprescription drugs

Pregnancy:
Don't use unless prescribed by your doctor.

Breastfeeding:
Don't use unless prescribed by your doctor.

Infants and children:
Treating infants and children under 2 with any herbal preparation is hazardous.

Others:
None are expected if you are beyond childhood, under 45, not pregnant, basically healthy, take it for only a short time and do not exceed manufacturer's recommended dose.

Storage:
- Store in cool, dry area away from direct light, but don't freeze.
- Store safely out of reach of children.
- Don't store in bathroom medicine cabinet. Heat and moisture may change the action of the herb.

Safe dosage:
Consult your doctor for the appropriate dose for your condition.

Toxicity

Comparative-toxicity rating is not available from standard references.

Adverse Reactions, Side Effects or Overdose Symptoms

None are expected.

Wormseed (Pigweed)

Basic Information

Biological name (genus and species):
Chenopodium ambrosioides

Parts used for medicinal purposes:
- Berries/fruits
- Roots

Chemicals this herb contains:
- Ascaridol
- Calcium
- Cymene
- D-camphor
- Limonene
- Saponin (see Glossary)
- Terpene (see Glossary)
- Vitamins A and C
- Volatile oils (see Glossary)

Known Effects

- Inhibits growth and development of germs
- Decreases blood pressure
- Decreases heart rate
- Depresses central nervous system
- Decreases stomach contractions

Miscellaneous information:
Wormseed is used externally as a poultice (see Glossary).

Possible Additional Effects

- May treat arthritis
- May kill intestinal parasites

STOP Warnings and Precautions

Don't take if you:
- Are pregnant, think you may be pregnant or plan pregnancy in the near future
- Have any chronic disease of the gastrointestinal tract, such as stomach or duodenal ulcers, reflux esophagitis, ulcerative colitis, spastic colitis, diverticulosis or diverticulitis

Consult your doctor if you:
- Take this herb for any medical problem that doesn't improve in 2 weeks (There may be safer, more effective treatments.)

MEDICINAL HERBS

→

• Take any medicinal drugs or herbs including aspirin, laxatives, cold and cough remedies, antacids, vitamins, minerals, amino acids, supplements, other prescription or nonprescription drugs

Pregnancy:
Dangers outweigh any possible benefits. Don't use.

Breastfeeding:
Dangers outweigh any possible benefits. Don't use.

Infants and children:
Treating infants and children under 2 with any herbal preparation is hazardous.

Others:
None are expected if you are beyond childhood, under 45, not pregnant, basically healthy, take it for only a short time and do not exceed manufacturer's recommended dose.

Storage:
• Store in cool, dry area away from direct light, but don't freeze.
• Store safely out of reach of children.
• Don't store in bathroom medicine cabinet. Heat and moisture may change the action of the herb.

Safe dosage:
Consult your doctor for the appropriate dose for your condition.

Toxicity

Rated slightly dangerous, particularly in children, persons over 55 and those who take larger than appropriate quantities for extended periods of time

For symptoms of toxicity: See *Adverse Reactions, Side Effects or Overdose Symptoms* section below.

Adverse Reactions, Side Effects or Overdose Symptoms

Signs and symptoms	What to do
Breathing difficulties	Seek emergency treatment.
Drowsiness	Discontinue. Call doctor when convenient.
Headache	Discontinue. Call doctor when convenient.
Hearing problems	Discontinue. Call doctor immediately.
Nausea or vomiting	Discontinue. Call doctor immediately.
Ringing in ears	Discontinue. Call doctor when convenient.
Slow heartbeat	Seek emergency treatment.
Stomach ulcers	Discontinue. Call doctor immediately.
Vision problems	Discontinue. Call doctor immediately.

Wormwood (Absinthium)

Basic Information

Biological name (genus and species):
Artemisia absinthium

Parts used for medicinal purposes:
• Berries/fruits
• Leaves

Chemicals this herb contains:
• Thujone (absinthol)
• Volatile oils (see Glossary)

Known Effects

- Depresses central nervous system
- Thujone causes mind-altering changes, may lead to psychosis
- Increases stomach acidity

Miscellaneous information:
Wormwood can be habit-forming, like ethyl alcohol.

Possible Additional Effects

- May treat anxiety
- Potential mild sedative
- May stimulate appetite

Warnings and Precautions

Don't take if you:
Are pregnant, think you may be pregnant or plan pregnancy in the near future.

Consult your doctor if you:
- Take this herb for any medical problem that doesn't improve in 2 weeks (There may be safer, more effective treatments.)
- Take any medicinal drugs or herbs including aspirin, laxatives, cold and cough remedies, antacids, vitamins, minerals, amino acids, supplements, other prescription or nonprescription drugs

Pregnancy:
Dangers outweigh any possible benefits. Don't use.

Breastfeeding:
Dangers outweigh any possible benefits. Don't use.

Infants and children:
Treating infants and children under 2 with any herbal preparation is hazardous.

Others:
This product will not help you and may cause toxic symptoms.

Storage:
- Store in cool, dry area away from direct light, but don't freeze.
- Store safely out of reach of children.
- Don't store in bathroom medicine cabinet. Heat and moisture may change the action of the herb.

Safe dosage:
Consult your doctor for the appropriate dose for your condition.

Toxicity

Rated slightly dangerous, particularly in children, persons over 55 and those who take larger than appropriate quantities for extended periods of time

For symptoms of toxicity: See *Adverse Reactions, Side Effects or Overdose Symptoms* section below.

Adverse Reactions, Side Effects or Overdose Symptoms

Signs and symptoms	What to do
Convulsions	Seek emergency treatment.
Stupor	Seek emergency treatment.
Trembling	Discontinue. Call doctor when convenient.

MEDICINAL HERBS

Yarrow

 Basic Information

Biological name (genus and species):
Achillea millefolium

Parts used for medicinal purposes:
• Berries/fruits
• Leaves

Chemicals this herb contains:
• Achilleine
• Coumarins
• Polyacetylenes
• Salicylic acid
• Tannins
• Triterpenes
• Volatile oils (see Glossary)

 Known Effects

• Reduces blood-clotting time
• Reduces pain
• Anti-inflammatory

 Possible Additional Effects

• Potential mild sedative
• May help reduce menstrual cramps
• May help reduce blood pressure

 Warnings and Precautions

Don't take if you:
Are pregnant, think you may be pregnant or plan pregnancy in the near future.

Consult your doctor if you:
• Take this herb for any medical problem that doesn't improve in 2 weeks (There may be safer, more effective treatments.)
• Take any medicinal drugs or herbs including aspirin, laxatives, cold and cough remedies, antacids, vitamins, minerals, amino acids, supplements, other prescription or nonprescription drugs
• Have ragweed allergy—a rash may occur

Pregnancy:
Don't use unless prescribed by your doctor.

Breastfeeding:
Don't use unless prescribed by your doctor.

Infants and children:
Treating infants and children under 2 with any herbal preparation is hazardous.

Others:
None are expected if you are beyond childhood, under 45, not pregnant, basically healthy, take it for only a short time and do not exceed manufacturer's recommended dose.

Storage:
• Store in cool, dry area away from direct light, but don't freeze.
• Store safely out of reach of children.
• Don't store in bathroom medicine cabinet. Heat and moisture may change the action of the herb.

Safe dosage:
Consult your doctor for the appropriate dose for your condition.

 Toxicity

Generally regarded as safe when taken in appropriate quantities for short periods of time

For symptoms of toxicity: See
*Adverse Reactions, Side Effects or
Overdose Symptoms* section below.

Adverse Reactions, Side Effects or Overdose Symptoms

Signs and symptoms	What to do
Diarrhea	Discontinue. Call doctor immediately.

Yellow Cedar (Arbor Vitae)

Basic Information

Biological name (genus and species):
Thuja occidentalis

Parts used for medicinal purposes:
Leaves

Chemicals this herb contains:
- Fenchone
- Pinopicrin
- Tannins (see Glossary)
- Thujone
- Volatile oils (see Glossary)

Known Effects

- Stimulates central nervous system
- Stimulates heart muscle to contract more efficiently
- Destroys intestinal worms
- Causes uterine contractions
- Interferes with absorption of iron and other minerals when taken internally

Miscellaneous information:
Yellow cedar has caused deaths when misused to induce abortions.

Possible Additional Effects

- May relieve muscular aches and pains
- May treat warts
- May cause abortions (miscarriages)

Warnings and Precautions

Don't take if you:
Are pregnant, think you may be pregnant or plan pregnancy in the near future.

Consult your doctor if you:
- Take this herb for any medical problem that doesn't improve in 2 weeks (There may be safer, more effective treatments.)

MEDICINAL HERBS

→

- Take any medicinal drugs or herbs including aspirin, laxatives, cold and cough remedies, antacids, vitamins, minerals, amino acids, supplements, other prescription or nonprescription drugs

Pregnancy:
Dangers outweigh any possible benefits. Don't use.

Breastfeeding:
Dangers outweigh any possible benefits. Don't use.

Infants and children:
Treating infants and children under 2 with any herbal preparation is hazardous.

Others:
Dangers outweigh any possible benefits. Don't use.

Storage:
- Store in cool, dry area away from direct light, but don't freeze.
- Store safely out of reach of children.
- Don't store in bathroom medicine cabinet. Heat and moisture may change the action of the herb.

Safe dosage:
Consult your doctor for the appropriate dose for your condition.

 Toxicity

Comparative-toxicity rating is not available from standard references.

For symptoms of toxicity: See *Adverse Reactions, Side Effects or Overdose Symptoms* section below.

 Adverse Reactions, Side Effects or Overdose Symptoms

Signs and symptoms	What to do
Abortion	Seek emergency treatment.
Coma	Seek emergency treatment.
Convulsions	Seek emergency treatment.
Precipitous blood-pressure drop: symptoms include faintness, cold sweat, paleness, rapid pulse	Seek emergency treatment.

Yellow Dock

 Basic Information

Biological name (genus and species):
Rumex crispus

Parts used for medicinal purposes:
- Leaves
- Rhizomes
- Roots

Chemicals this herb contains:
- Oxalic acid
- Potassium oxalate
- Vitamins A and C

 Known Effects

- Irritates skin when handled
- Stimulates gastrointestinal tract as a mild laxative
- Stimulates bile production

Miscellaneous information:
Yellow dock is used as food in salads.

Possible
Additional Effects

May temporarily relieve constipation

 Warnings and
Precautions

Don't take if you:
- Are pregnant, think you may be pregnant or plan pregnancy in the near future
- Have any chronic disease of the gastrointestinal tract, such as stomach or duodenal ulcers, reflux esophagitis, ulcerative colitis, spastic colitis, diverticulosis or diverticulitis

Consult your doctor if you:
- Take this herb for any medical problem that doesn't improve in 2 weeks (There may be safer, more effective treatments.)
- Take any medicinal drugs or herbs including aspirin, laxatives, cold and cough remedies, antacids, vitamins, minerals, amino acids, supplements, other prescription or nonprescription drugs

Pregnancy:
Dangers outweigh any possible benefits. Don't use.

Breastfeeding:
Dangers outweigh any possible benefits. Don't use.

Infants and children:
Treating infants and children under 2 with any herbal preparation is hazardous.

Others:
Dangers outweigh any possible benefits. Don't use.

Storage:
- Store in cool, dry area away from direct light, but don't freeze.
- Store safely out of reach of children.
- Don't store in bathroom medicine cabinet. Heat and moisture may change the action of the herb.

Safe dosage:
Consult your doctor for the appropriate dose for your condition.

 Toxicity

Rated slightly dangerous, particularly in children, persons over 55 and those who take larger than appropriate quantities for extended periods of time

For symptoms of toxicity: See *Adverse Reactions, Side Effects or Overdose Symptoms* section below.

 Adverse Reactions,
Side Effects or
Overdose Symptoms

Signs and symptoms	What to do
Diarrhea	Discontinue. Call doctor immediately.
Kidney damage characterized by blood in urine, decreased urine flow, swelling of hands and feet	Seek emergency treatment.
Nausea or vomiting	Discontinue. Call doctor immediately.
Skin eruptions	Discontinue. Call doctor when convenient.

MEDICINAL HERBS

Yellow Lady's Slipper

 Basic Information

Biological name (genus and species):
Cypripedium pubescens

Parts used for medicinal purposes:
Roots

Chemicals this herb contains:
• Resin (see Glossary)
• Tannins (see Glossary)
• Volatile acid
• Volatile oils (see Glossary)

 Known Effects

• Irritates mucous membranes
• Stimulates gastrointestinal tract
• Increases perspiration

Miscellaneous information:
• Hairs on stems and leaves irritate body when touched.
• May produce skin eruptions similar to those caused by poison ivy.

 Possible Additional Effects

• Potential sedative to treat anxiety or restlessness
• May increase perspiration
• May help expel gas from intestinal tract
• May relieve spasm in skeletal or smooth muscle

 Warnings and Precautions

Don't take if you:
• Are pregnant, think you may be pregnant or plan pregnancy in the near future

• Have any chronic disease of the gastrointestinal tract, such as stomach or duodenal ulcers, reflux esophagitis, ulcerative colitis, spastic colitis, diverticulosis or diverticulitis

Consult your doctor if you:
• Take this herb for any medical problem that doesn't improve in 2 weeks (There may be safer, more effective treatments.)
• Take any medicinal drugs or herbs including aspirin, laxatives, cold and cough remedies, antacids, vitamins, minerals, amino acids, supplements, other prescription or nonprescription drugs

Pregnancy:
Don't use unless prescribed by your doctor.

Breastfeeding:
Don't use unless prescribed by your doctor.

Infants and children:
Treating infants and children under 2 with any herbal preparation is hazardous.

Others:
None are expected if you are beyond childhood, under 45, not pregnant, basically healthy, take it for only a short time and do not exceed manufacturer's recommended dose.

Storage:
• Store in cool, dry area away from direct light, but don't freeze.
• Store safely out of reach of children.
• Don't store in bathroom medicine cabinet. Heat and moisture may change the action of the herb.

Safe dosage:
Consult your doctor for the appropriate dose for your condition.

Toxicity

Rated relatively safe when taken in appropriate quantities for short periods of time

For symptoms of toxicity: See *Adverse Reactions, Side Effects or Overdose Symptoms* section below.

 Adverse Reactions, Side Effects or Overdose Symptoms

Signs and symptoms	What to do
Drowsiness	Discontinue. Call doctor when convenient.
Nausea or vomiting	Discontinue. Call doctor immediately.

Yerba Maté (Paraguay Tea, South American Holly)

 Basic Information

Biological name (genus and species):
Ilex paraguariensis

Parts used for medicinal purposes:
Leaves

Chemicals this herb contains:
Caffeine

 Known Effects

• Stimulates central nervous system
• Helps body dispose of excess fluid by increasing amount of urine produced
• Causes hallucinations

 Possible Additional Effects

• Potential laxative
• May increase perspiration

 Warnings and Precautions

Don't take if you:
• Are pregnant, think you may be pregnant or plan pregnancy in the near future
• Have any chronic disease of the gastrointestinal tract, such as stomach or duodenal ulcers, reflux esophagitis, ulcerative colitis, spastic colitis, diverticulosis or diverticulitis

Consult your doctor if you:
• Take this herb for any medical problem that doesn't improve in 2 weeks (There may be safer, more effective treatments.)
• Take any medicinal drugs or herbs including aspirin, laxatives, cold and cough remedies, antacids, vitamins, minerals, amino acids, supplements, other prescription or nonprescription drugs

Pregnancy:
Dangers outweigh any possible benefits. Don't use.

Breastfeeding:
Dangers outweigh any possible benefits. Don't use.

MEDICINAL HERBS

Infants and children:

Treating infants and children under
2 with any herbal preparation
is hazardous.

Others:

None are expected if you are beyond
childhood, under 45, not pregnant,
basically healthy, take it for only a short
time and do not exceed manufacturer's
recommended dose.

Storage:

• Store in cool, dry area away from
  direct light, but don't freeze.
• Store safely out of reach of children.
• Don't store in bathroom medicine
  cabinet. Heat and moisture may
  change the action of the herb.

Safe dosage:

Consult your doctor for the appropriate dose for your condition.

Toxicity

Rated relatively safe when taken in
appropriate quantities for short
periods of time

For symptoms of toxicity: See
*Adverse Reactions, Side Effects or
Overdose Symptoms* section below.

Adverse Reactions, Side Effects or Overdose Symptoms

Signs and symptoms	What to do
Confusion	Seek emergency treatment.
Excessive urination	Discontinue. Call doctor when convenient.
Hallucinations	Seek emergency treatment.
Heartburn	Discontinue. Call doctor when convenient.
Insomnia	Discontinue. Call doctor when convenient.
Irritability	Discontinue. Call doctor when convenient.
Nausea	Discontinue. Call doctor immediately.
Nervousness	Discontinue. Call doctor when convenient.
Rapid heartbeat	Seek emergency treatment.

Yerba Santa (Bear's Weed)

Basic Information

Biological name (genus and species):
Eriodictyon californicum

Parts used for medicinal purposes:
Leaves

Chemicals this herb contains:
• Formic acid
• Pentatriacontane eriodictyol
• Resin (see Glossary)
• Tannic acid
• Tannins (see Glossary)

Known Effects

• Masks taste of bitter medicines
• Decreases thickness and increases
  fluidity of mucus in lungs and
  bronchial tubes
• Interferes with absorption of iron
  and other minerals when
  taken internally

Possible Additional Effects

- May treat hay fever and other nasal allergies
- May treat hemorrhoids

Warnings and Precautions

Don't take if you:

- Are pregnant, think you may be pregnant or plan pregnancy in the near future
- Have any chronic disease of the gastrointestinal tract, such as stomach or duodenal ulcers, reflux esophagitis, ulcerative colitis, spastic colitis, diverticulosis or diverticulitis

Consult your doctor if you:

- Take this herb for any medical problem that doesn't improve in 2 weeks (There may be safer, more effective treatments.)
- Take any medicinal drugs or herbs including aspirin, laxatives, cold and cough remedies, antacids, vitamins, minerals, amino acids, supplements, other prescription or nonprescription drugs

Pregnancy:

Dangers outweigh any possible benefits. Don't use.

Breastfeeding:

Dangers outweigh any possible benefits. Don't use.

Infants and children:

Treating infants and children under 2 with any herbal preparation is hazardous.

Others:

None are expected if you are beyond childhood, under 45, not pregnant, basically healthy, take it for only a short time and do not exceed manufacturer's recommended dose.

Storage:

- Store in cool, dry area away from direct light, but don't freeze.
- Store safely out of reach of children.
- Don't store in bathroom medicine cabinet. Heat and moisture may change the action of the herb.

Safe dosage:

Consult your doctor for the appropriate dose for your condition.

Toxicity

Comparative-toxicity rating is not available from standard references.

For symptoms of toxicity: See *Adverse Reactions, Side Effects or Overdose Symptoms* section below.

Adverse Reactions, Side Effects or Overdose Symptoms

Signs and symptoms	What to do
Diarrhea	Discontinue. Call doctor immediately.
Nausea or vomiting	Discontinue. Call doctor immediately.

Optimal Daily Intake Information

Vitamin or Mineral	Daily Value (DV)	Recommended Dietary Allowances	Dietary Reference Intakes	Tolerable Upper Intake	Probable Optimal Intake for Disease
A	5,000IU	Men 1,000mcg Women 800mcg			5,000IU
B-12	6mcg	2mcg 60mg	2.4mcg 60mg		2.4–10mcgC 150–1,000mg
Calcium	1,000mg	800–1,200mg	1,000–1,200mg	2,500mg	1,200–1,500mg
Choline			Men 550mg Women 425mg	3,500mg	375–550mg
Chromium					50–150mcg
Copper	2mg				2–3mg
D	400IU	5–10mcg	5–10mcg	50mcg	400–600IU
E	30IU	Men 10mg Women 8mg			400IU
Fluoride			Men 4mg Women 3mg	10mg	2–10mg
Folic Acid/ Folate	400mcg	Men 200mcg Women 180mcg	400mcg	1,000mcg (synthetic folic acid)	400–800mcg
Iodine	150mcg	150mcg			150mcg
Iron	18mg	Men 10mg Women 15mg			Supplement only if a deficiency exists
K		Men 70–80mcg Women 60–65mcg			Supplement not required in healthy diet

About This Chart:

The amounts listed in this chart are recommended for healthy adults.

Dietary Value (DV) is a standard set forth by the Food and Drug Administration (FDA). It combines Reference Daily Intakes (RDI) and Daily Recommended Values (DRV). DRVs were developed to cover nutrients that are not included in RDIs. The term DV is used in food labeling. You should use it as a reference for determining how much of your nutrient needs are being met through the consumption of a specific food.

Recommended Dietary Allowances (RDA), Dietary Reference Intakes (DRI) and Tolerable Upper Intake Level (UL) are determined by the Food and Nutrition Board of the Institute of Medicine, National Academy of Sciences.

RDAs determine the minimum amount of a nutrient needed to prevent deficiency.

Vitamin or Mineral	Daily Value (DV)	Recommended Dietary Allowances	Dietary Reference Intakes	Tolerable Upper Intake	Probable Optimal Intake for Disease
Magnesium	400mg	Men 350mg Women 280mg	Men 400–420mg Women 310–320mg	350mg (from pharmacological source only)	500–1,000mg
Manganese					2–5mg
Molybdenum					75–250mcg
Niacin (B-3)	20mg	Men 15–19mg Women 13–15mg	Men 16mg Women 14mg	35mg	15–35mg
Pantothenic Acid (B-5)	10mg		5mg		5–20mg
Phosphorus	1,000mg	800–1,200mg	700mg	4,000mg	1,200–1,500mg
Potassium	3,500mg				4,000mg
Pyridoxine (B-6)	2mg	Men 2mg Women 1.6mg	1.3–1.7mg	100 mg	1.5–50mg
Riboflavin (B-2)	1.7mg	Men 1.4–1.7mg Women 1.2–1.3mg	Men 1.3mg Women 1.1mg		1.3–50mg
Selenium		Men 70mcg Women 55mcg			100mcg
Sodium	2,400mg				2,400mg
Thiamine (B-1)	1.5mg	Men 1.2–1.5mg Women 1–1.1mg	Men 1.2mg Women 1.1mg		1.2–50mg
Zinc	15mg	Men 15mg Women 12mg			15–25mg

Reprinted with permission from *Dietary Reference Intakes.* Copyright 1998 by the National Academy of Sciences. Courtesy of the National Academy Press, Washington, D.C.

DRIs will expand upon RDAs by focusing on optimal health and the use of nutrients in promoting long-term health.

UL determines the maximum nutrient intake without risk of side effects, when the scientific evidence is available.

DRI guidelines are being announced in phases. The project is expected to be complete by 2000.

Sources:

DV information was taken from the U.S. Food and Drug Administration website: http://www.fda.gov

RDA, DRI and UL information was taken from the Food and Nutrition Board, Institute of Medicine, National Academy of Sciences—Dietary Reference Intakes: recommended levels for individual intake.

Phytochemicals and Health

Phytochemicals are chemicals found in or derived from plants.

Phytochemicals and Disease Prevention		
Phytochemical	Food source(s)	Clinical significance
Alpha-linolenic acid	flaxseed, soy, walnuts	reduces inflammation, lowers blood cholesterol, may protect against breast cancer, enhances immunity
Beta-carotene	green and yellow fruits and vegetables	reduces risk of cataracts, coronary artery disease, lung and breast cancers; enhances immunity (elderly)
Capsaicin	chili peppers	reduces risk for colon, gastric and rectal cancer; inhibits tumor promotion
Carotenoid lycopene	tomato sauce, catsup, red grapefruit, guava, dried apricots, watermelon, fresh tomatoes	antioxidant, reduces risk of prostate cancer, may reduce cardiovascular disease
Curcumin	turmeric, curry, cumin	may lower cholesterol, reduces risk of skin cancer
Cynarin	artichokes	decreases cholesterol levels
Ellagic acid	wine, grapes, currants, nuts (pecans), berries (strawberries, blackberries, raspberries), seeds	reduces cancer risk, inhibits carcinogen binding to DNA, reduces LDL cholesterol while increasing HDL cholesterol
Flavonols, polyphenols: catechin (theaflavins, thearubigins), theogallin, EGCG	green and black tea, berries	reduces risk of gastric cancer, antioxidant, increases immune function, decreases cholesterol production, protects against chemically induced cancers and skin cancer, may protect against esophageal cancer, antitumor promoter, inhibits nitrosamine formation, inhibits phase I and enhances phase II enzyme activity
Genistein	soybeans	reduces risk of hormone-dependent cancers; alters hormone levels; inhibits angiogenesis; promotes cell differentiation; reduces cholesterol levels; reduces thrombi formation, osteoporosis, menopausal symptoms
Indoles	cabbage, broccoli, brussels sprouts, spinach, watercress, cauliflower, turnips, kohlrabi, kale, rutabaga, horseradish, mustard greens	reduces risk of hormone-related cancers, may "inactivate" estrogen, increases glutathione-S-transferase activity, inhibits growth of transformed cells

Phytochemical	Food source(s)	Clinical significance
Isothiocyanates sulforaphane	cabbage, cauliflower, broccoli and broccoli sprouts, brussels sprouts, mustard greens, horseradish, radishes	reduces risk of tobacco-induced tumors, inhibits tobacco-related carcinogens from damaging DNA, induces phase II enzymes, inhibits cP450 activation of carcinogens
Lignans	high fiber foods, especially seeds	reduces cancer risk (colon), reduces blood glucose and cholesterol
Monterpene limonene	citrus (peel, membrane), mint, caraway, thyme, coriander	antioxidant, reduces cancer risk (skin, breast), inhibits p21ras (G protein), suppresses HMG-CoA, induces apoptosis, reduces cholesterol production, reduces premenstrual symptoms
Organosulfur compounds allylic acid	garlic, onion, watercress, cruciferous vegetables, leeks	decreases lipid peroxidation; reduces risk of gastric, colon and lung cancers; inhibits tumor promotion by inhibiting DNA adduct formation; induces phase II enzymes; antithrombotic; reduces cholesterol; reduces blood pressure; antimicrobial
Polyacetylene	parsley, carrots, celery	decreases risk of tobacco-induced tumors, alters prostaglandin formation
Quercetin	pear skin, apple skin, bell pepper, kohlrabi, tomato leaves, onion, wine, grape juice	flavonoid, anticancer, antioxidant, associated with reduced coronary heart disease, decreases platelet aggregation
Phenolic acid	cruciferous vegetables, eggplant, peppers, tomatoes, celery, parsley, soy, licorice root, flaxseed, citrus, whole grains, berries	inhibits cancer by inhibiting nitrosamine formation, reduces risk for lung and skin cancers

Glossary

abortifacient. Induces abortions (miscarriages).

absorption. Process by which nutrients are absorbed through the lining of the intestinal tract into capillaries and into the bloodstream. Nutrients must be absorbed to affect the body.

acids. Compounds often found in plant tissues, especially fruits, that shrink tissues and prevent secretion of fluids. They taste sour or tart.

active principle. Chemical component of a plant or compound that has a therapeutic effect.

acute. Short, relatively severe. Usually referred to in connection with an illness. Opposite of acute is *chronic*.

addiction. Psychological or physiological dependence on a drug. With true addictions, severe symptoms appear when the addicted person stops taking the drug on which he or she is dependent.

adrenal gland. Gland located immediately adjacent to the kidney that produces epinephrine (adrenaline) and several steroid hormones, including cortisone and hydrocortisone.

adulterant. Substance that makes another substance impure when the two are mixed together.

allergen. Capable of producing an allergic response.

allergy. Excessive sensitivity to a substance.

alpha linolenic acid. An essential fatty acid important for healing and maintaining good health.

alumina. Another term for aluminum oxide or hydrated aluminum oxide.

amenorrhea. Absence of menstruation.

amino acid. Chemical building blocks that help produce proteins in the body.

anabolic. Building up of tissues in the body, or constructive metabolism.

analog. Employing measurement along scales rather than by numerical counting.

anaphylaxis. Severe allergic response to a substance. Symptoms include wheezing, itching, nasal congestion, hives, immediate intense burning of hands and feet, collapse with severe drop in blood pressure, loss of consciousness and cardiac arrest. Symptoms of anaphylaxis appear within a few seconds or minutes after exposure to the substance causing reaction—this can be medication or herbs taken by injection, by mouth, vaginally, rectally, through a breathing apparatus or applied to skin. Anaphylaxis is an uncommon occurrence, but when it occurs, it is a *severe medical emergency!* Without appropriate immediate treatment, it can cause death. Yell for help. Don't leave victim. Begin CPR (cardiopulmonary resuscitation), mouth-to-mouth breathing and external cardiac massage. Have someone dial "0" or 911. Don't stop CPR until help arrives.

anemia. Too few healthy red blood cells in the bloodstream or too little hemoglobin in the red blood cells. Anemia is usually caused by excessive blood loss, such as excessive bleeding or menstruation, increased blood destruction, such as hemolytic anemia or leukemia, or decreased blood production, such as iron-deficiency anemia.

anemia, pernicious. Anemia caused by vitamin-B-12 deficiency. Symptoms include easy fatigue, weakness, lemon-colored skin, numbness and tingling of hands and feet, and symptoms of degeneration of the central nervous system, such as irritability, emotional problems, personality changes and paralysis of extremities.

anesthetic. Used to abolish pain.

angina (angina pectoris). Chest pain, with sensation of impending death. Pain may radiate into jaw, ear lobes, between shoulder blades or down shoulder and arm on either side, most frequently the left side. Pain is caused by a temporary reduction in the amount of oxygen to the heart muscle through narrowed, diseased coronary arteries.

antacid. Neutralizes acid. In medical terms, the neutralized acid is located in the stomach, esophagus or first part of the duodenum.

antagonist. A drug that blocks or reverses the effect of another drug.

antibacterial. Destroys bacteria (germs) or suppresses their growth or reproduction.

antibiotic. Inhibits growth of germs or kills germs. When it inhibits growth, it is called *bacteriostatic*. When it kills germs, it is called *bacteriocidal*.

anticholinergic. Reduces nerve impulses through the part of the autonomic nervous system called *parasympathetic*.

anticoagulant. Delays or stops blood clotting.

antiemetic. Prevents or stops nausea and vomiting.

antihelmintic. Destroys intestinal worms.

antihistamine. Reduces histamine, the chemical in body tissues that dilates smallest blood vessels, constricts smooth muscle surrounding bronchial tubes and stimulates stomach secretions by acting on tissues of the body.

antihypertensive. Reduces blood pressure.

antimicrobial. Destroys or inhibits growth of microorganisms.

antimitotic. Inhibits or prevents cell division.

antineoplastic. Inhibits or prevents growth of neoplasms (cancers).

antioxidant. Prevents or delays the process of *oxidation*. Antioxidant substances include superoxide dismutase, selenium, vitamins C and E, and zinc.

antipyretic. Reduces fevers.

antiseptic. Prevents or retards growth of germs.

antispasmodic. Relieves spasm in skeletal or smooth muscle.

aperitive. Stimulates the appetite.

aphrodisiac. Arouses or enhances instinctive sexual desire.

aromatic. Chemical with a spicy fragrance and stimulant characteristics used to relieve various symptoms.

artery. Blood vessel that carries blood away from the heart.

asthma. Disease with recurrent attacks of breathing difficulty characterized by wheezing. It is caused by spasms of the bronchial tubes, which can be caused by many factors including adverse reactions to drugs, vitamins, minerals or medicinal herbs.

astringent. Shrinks tissues and prevents secretion of fluids.

bacteria. Microscopic germs. Some bacteria contribute to health; others cause disease.

bioavailability. The degree to which a drug becomes available to the target tissue after administration.

bitters. Medicine with a bitter taste. Used as a tonic or appetizer.

blepharitis. Inflammation of the eyelid.

blood sugar (blood glucose). Necessary element in blood to sustain life. The blood level of glucose is determined by insulin, a hormone secreted by the pancreas. When the pancreas no longer satisfies this function, the disease *diabetes mellitus* results.

bronchitis. Inflammation of the breathing tubes.

bulb. Modified plant bulb with scaly leaves that grows beneath the soil.

carcinogen. Chemical or substance that can cause cancer.

cardiac. Pertaining to the heart.

cardiac arrhythmias. Abnormal heart rate or rhythm.

cardiomyopathy. Chronic disorder of the heart muscle of unknown association.

carminative. Aids in expelling gas from the intestinal tract.

cathartic. Very strong laxative that produces explosive, watery bowel movements.

cell. Unit of protoplasm, the essential living matter of all plants and animals.

central nervous system. Brain and spinal cord and their nerve endings.

central-nervous-system depressant. Causes changes in the body, including changes in consciousness, lethargy, loss of judgment or coma.

chronic. Disease of long standing. Opposite of *acute.*

coenzyme. Heat-stable molecule that must be loosely associated with an *enzyme* for the enzyme to perform its function.

cofactor. Element with which another must unite to function.

colic. Abdominal pain that recurs in a pattern every few seconds or minutes.

collagen. Gelatinous protein used to make body tissues.

congestive. Excess accumulation of blood. Congestive heart failure is the result of blood congregating in lungs, liver, kidney and other parts to cause shortness of breath, swelling of ankles, sleep disturbances, rapid heartbeat and easy fatigue.

conjunctivitis. Inflammation of the outer membrane of the eye.

constriction. Tightness or pressure.

contraceptive. Prevents pregnancy.

contraindication. Inadvisability of using a substance that may cause harm under specific circumstances. For example, high-caloric intake in someone who is overweight is contraindicated.

convulsion. Violent, uncontrollable contraction of the voluntary muscles.

corticosteroid (adrenocorticosteroid). Hormones produced by the body or manufactured synthetically.

counterirritant. Process of applying an irritating substance to the skin to produce increased blood circulation to the area. Classic example (now considered an outdated treatment) is mustard plaster applied to the chest to relieve bronchial congestion or cough.

cyanogenic glycosides. Sugars capable of producing cyanide.

cynarin. Acid that stimulates bile secretion.

cystitis. Inflammation of the urinary bladder.

decoction. Extract of a crude drug obtained by boiling the substance in water.

dehiscent. Fruit that splits open when ripe.

delirium. Temporary mental disturbance accompanied by hallucinations, agitation, incoherence.

demineralization. Excessive elimination of mineral or inorganic salts.

demulcent. Mucilaginous or oily substance capable of protecting scraped tissues.

dermatitis. Skin inflammation or irritation.

diaphoretic. Increases perspiration.

diuretic. Increases urine flow. Most diuretics force kidneys to excrete more than the usual amount of sodium. Sodium forces more water and urine to be excreted.

DNA (deoxyribonucleic acid). Complex protein chemical in genes that determines the type of life form into which a cell will develop.

dosage. The amount of medicine to be taken for a specific problem. Dosages may be listed as liquids (ml or milliliters, cc or cubic centimeters, teaspoons, tablespoons), dry weight (kg or kilograms, mg or milligrams, g or grams) or by biological assay (retinol units, international units).

drupe. Fleshy fruit with a hard stone, such as an apricot or peach.

duodenum. First 12 inches of small intestine.

dysentery. Disorder with inflammation of the intestines, especially the colon, accompanied by pain, a feeling of urgent need to have bowel movements, and frequent stools containing blood or mucus.

dysmenorrhea. Painful or difficult menstruation.

dyspepsia. Digestion impairment causing uncomfortable feeling of indigestion.

eczema. Noncontagious disease of skin characterized by redness, itching, scaling and lesions with discharge. Frequently becomes encrusted. Eczema primarily affects young children. The underlying cause is usually an allergy to many things, including foods, wool, skin lotions. The disorder may begin in month-old babies. It usually subsides by age 3 but may flare again at age 10 to 12 and last through puberty.

electrolyte. Chemical substance with an available electron in its atomic structure that can transmit electrical impulses when dissolved in fluids.

ellagic acid. A crystalline phenolic lactone obtained from oak bark.

emetic. Causes vomiting.

emmenagogue. Triggers onset of menstrual period.

emollient. Softens or soothes.

emphysema. Lung disease characterized by loss of elasticity of muscles surrounding air sacs. Lungs cannot supply adequate oxygen to body cells for normal function.

endometriosis. Medical condition in which uterine tissue is found outside the uterus. Symptoms include pain, abnormal menstruation, infertility.

enzyme. Protein chemical that accelerates a chemical reaction in the body without being consumed in the process.

GLOSSARY

epilepsy. Symptom or disease characterized by episodes of brain disturbance that cause convulsions and loss of consciousness.

essential oils. Same as volatile oils. Oils evaporate at room temperature.

estrogens. Female sex hormones that must be present for secondary sexual characteristics of the female to develop. Estrogens serve many functions in the body, including preparation of the uterus to receive a fertilized egg.

eupeptic. Promotes optimum digestion.

expectorant. Decreases thickness and increases fluidity of mucus in the lungs and bronchial tubes.

extract. Solution prepared by soaking plant in solvent, then allowing solution to evaporate.

extremity. Arm, hand, leg, foot.

fat soluble. Dissolves in fat.

fatty acids. Nutritional substances found in nature that are fats or lipids. These include triglycerides, cholesterol, fatty acids and prostaglandins. Fatty acids include stearic, palmitic, linoleic, linolenic, eicosapentaenoic (EPA), docosahexaenoic acid (DHA). Other lipids of nutritional importance include lecithin, choline, gamma-linoleic acid and inositol.

fixed oil(s). Lipids, fats or waxes often made from seeds of plants.

flatulence. Swelling of the stomach or other parts of the intestinal tract with air or other gases.

flavonoids. A category of powerful antioxidants.

fluid extract. Alcoholic solution of a chemical or drug of plant origin. Fluid extracts usually contain 1 gram of dry drug in each milliliter.

free radicals. Highly reactive molecules with an unpaired free electron that combines with any other molecule that accepts it. Free radicals are usually toxic oxygen molecules that damage cell membranes and fat molecules. To protect against possible damage from free radicals, the body has several defenses. The most important appear at present to be antioxidant substances, such as superoxide dismutase, selenium, vitamin C, vitamin E, zinc and others.

G6PD. Deficiency of glucose-6-phosphate, a chemical necessary for glucose metabolism. Some people have inherited deficiencies of this substance and have added risks when taking some drugs.

GABA (gamma-aminobutyric acid). An amino acid that functions as a neurotransmitter in the *central nervous system.*

gastritis. Inflammation of the lining of the stomach.

gastroenteritis. Inflammation of stomach and intestines characterized by pain, nausea and diarrhea.

gastrointestinal. Pertaining to stomach, small intestine, large intestine, colon, rectum and sometimes the liver, pancreas and gallbladder.

generic. Relating to or descriptive of an entire group or class.

genistein. A component of soybeans thought to be an anticarcinogen.

genitourinary. Relating to the genital and urinary organs and functions.

gingivitis. Inflammation of the gums surrounding teeth.

gland. Cells that manufacture and excrete materials not required for their own metabolic needs.

glossitis. Inflammation of the tongue.

gluten. Mixture of plant proteins occurring in grains, chiefly corn and wheat. People who are sensitive to gluten develop gastrointestinal symptoms that can be controlled only by eating a gluten-free diet.

glycoside(s). Plant substance that produces a sugar and other substances when combined with oxygen and hydrogen.

griping. Intestinal cramps.

gums. Translucent substances without form. Usually a decomposition product of cellulose. Gums dissolve in water.

hallucinogen. Produces hallucintions—apparent sights, sounds or other sensual experiences that do not actually exist.

HDL (high density lipoprotein). "Good cholesterol" that scavenges excess cholesterol from the bloodstream and carries it to the liver for excretion.

heart block. An electrical disturbance in the controlling system of the heartbeat. Heart block can cause unconsciousness and in its worst form can lead to cardiac arrest.

hematuria. Blood in the urine.

hemoglobin. Pigment necessary for red blood cells to transport oxygen. Iron is a necessary component of hemoglobin.

hemolysis. Breaking a membranous covering or destroying red blood cells.

hemorrhage. Extensive bleeding.

hemostatic. Prevents bleeding and promotes clotting of blood.

hepatitis. Inflammation of liver cells, usually accompanied by *jaundice.*

herb. Plant or plant part valued for its medicinal qualities, pleasant aroma or pleasing taste.

histamine. Chemical in the body tissues that constricts the smooth muscle surrounding bronchial tubes, dilates small blood vessels, allows leakage of fluid to form itching skin and hives and increases secretion of acid in stomach.

hives. Elevated patches on skin usually caused by an allergic reaction accompanied by a release of histamine into the body tissues. Patches are redder or paler than the surrounding skin and itch intensely.

homeopathy. Practice of using extremely small doses of medicines and herbs that would, in a healthy person, cause the same symptoms the disease causes. Homeopaths (practitioners of homeopathy) acknowledge no diseases, only symptoms.

hormone. Chemical substance produced by endocrine glands—thymus, pituitary, thyroid, parathyroid, adrenal, ovaries, testicles, pancreas—that regulates many body functions to maintain homeostasis (a steady state).

humectant. Moistens or dilutes.

hypercalcemia. Abnormally high level of calcium in the blood.

hypercholesterolemia Excess cholesterol in the blood.

hyperplasia An unusual increase in the elements composing a part (such as cells composing tissue).

hypertension. High blood pressure.

hypocalcemia. Abnormally low level of calcium in the blood.

hypoglycemia. Abnormally low blood sugar.

impotence. Inability of a male to achieve and maintain an erection of the penis to allow satisfying sexual intercourse.

indehiscent. Fruit that remains closed upon reaching maturity.

indoles. A chemical compound in plants that has been used in drugs to combat a variety of illnesses.

inflorescence. Flower head of a plant.

infusion. Product that results when a drug or herb is steeped to extract its medicinal properties.

insomnia. Inability to sleep.

interaction. Change in body's response to one substance when another is taken. Interactions may increase the response, decrease the response, cause toxicity or completely change the response expected from either substance. Interactions may occur between drugs and drugs, drugs and vitamins, drugs and herbs, drugs and foods, vitamins and vitamins, minerals and minerals, vitamins and foods, minerals and foods, vitamins and herbs, herbs and herbs, and so forth.

international units. Measurement of biological activity. In the case of vitamin E, for example, 1 international unit (IU) equals 1 milligram (mg). International units are measured differently for different substances.

invert sugar. A mixture of dextrose and levulose found in fruits or produced artificially by the inversion of sucrose.

ischemia. Localized tissue anemia caused by obstructed blood flow in the arteries.

isothiocyanide. A phytochemical that stimulates the manufacture of *enzymes*.

I.U. or IU. International units (see above).

jaundice. Symptom of liver damage, bile obstruction or excessive red-blood-cell destruction. Jaundice is characterized by yellowing of the whites of the eyes, yellow skin, dark urine and light stool.

kidney stones. Small, solid stones made from calcium, cysteine, cholesterol and other chemicals in the bloodstream. They are produced in the kidneys.

lactagogue. Increases the flow of breast milk in a woman.

lactase. *Enzyme* that helps body convert lactose to glucose and galactose.

lactase deficiency. Lack of adequate supply of the enzyme *lactase*. People with lactase deficiency have difficulty digesting milk and milk products.

larvacide. Kills larvae.

latex. Milky juice produced by plants.

laxative. Stimulates bowel movements.

LDH (lactic dehydrogenase). A blood test to measure liver function and to detect damage to the heart muscle.

LDL (low density lipoprotein). "Bad cholesterol" protein that contains large amounts of fats and triglycerides.

libido. Sex drive.

lignans. A type of *phytochemical.*

lipid. Fat or fatty substance.

lycopene. An antioxidant pigment that gives tomatoes, guava and pink grapefruit their characteristic colors.

lymph glands. Glands located in the lymph vessels of the body that trap foreign material, including infectious material, and protect the bloodstream from becoming infected.

maceration. Softening of a plant by soaking.

magnesia. Another term for magnesium hydroxide.

malabsorption. Poor absorption of nutrients from the intestinal tract into the bloodstream.

mcg. Abbreviation for microgram, which is 1/1,000,000th (1/1-millionth) of a gram or 1/1,000th of a milligram.

megadose. Very large dose. In terms of Recommended Dietary Allowance (RDA), anything 10 or more times the RDA is considered a megadose. Nutritionists urge no one take megadoses of *any* substance because these doses may be toxic, cause an imbalance of other nutrients, cause damage to an unborn child and do not provide benefits beyond rational doses.

menopause. End of menstruation in the female caused by decreased production of female hormones. Symptoms include hot flashes, irritability, vaginal dryness, changes in the skin and bones.

metabolism. Chemical and physical processes in the maintenance of life.

mg. Abbreviation for milligram, which is 1/1,000th of a gram.

migraine. Periodic headaches caused by constriction of arteries in the skull. Symptoms include visual disturbances, nausea, vomiting, light sensitivity and severe pain.

milk sickness. Intolerance to milk and milk products due to a deficiency of an enzyme called *lactase*.

mitochondria. Components of cells, found outside the nucleus, that produce energy for the cell and are rich in fats, proteins, and *enzymes*.

mitogen. Causes nucleus of cell to divide; leads to a new cell.

mucilage. Gelatinous substance that contains proteins and polysaccharides.

narcotic. Depresses the central nervous system, reduces pain and causes drowsiness and euphoria. Narcotics are addictive substances.

naturopathy. Medical practice that uses herbs and various methods to return body to healthy state by stimulating innate defenses—never supplanting them—with drugs. In early years, many naturopathic physicians were ill-prepared to practice a healing profession. Many received mail-order degrees and had little training. However, by the 1950s, some degree of academic acceptability returned. Several accredited schools award degrees for training, and many states now require examinations and licensure to ensure competence.

neuropathy. Group of symptoms caused by abnormalities in sensory or motor nerves. Symptoms include tingling and numbness in hands or feet, followed by gradually progressive muscular weakness.

neurotransmitter. A substance that transmits nerve impulses across a synapse.

occlusion. Obstruction.

oleoresin. Resins and *volatile oils* in a homogenous mixture.

osteoporosis. Softening of bones.

oxidation. Combining a substance with oxygen.

oxidation-reduction. A chemical reaction that involves the transfer of an electron from one molecule or atom to another.

oxygenation. Saturation of a substance (particularly blood) with oxygen.

parasympathetic. Division of the autonomic nervous system. Parasympathetic nerves control functions of digestion, heart and lung activity, constriction of eye pupils and many other normal functions of the body.

Parkinson's disease. Disease of the central nervous system characterized by a fixed, emotionless expression of the face, slower-than-normal muscle movements, tremor (particularly when attempting to reach or hold objects), weakness, changed gait and a forward-leaning posture.

paronychia. Infection around a finger-nail bed.

peduncle. Stalk attached to a flower.

pellagra. Disease caused by a deficiency of niacin (vitamin B-3). Symptoms include diarrhea, skin inflammation and dementia (brain disturbance).

peristalsis. Wave of contractions of the intestinal tract.

pernicious anemia. See *Anemia, pernicious.*

pharyngitis. Inflammation of the throat.

phenylketonuria. Inherited disease caused by lack of an *enzyme* neces-sary for converting phenylalanine into a form the body can use. Accumulation of too much phenylalanine can cause poor mental and physical develop-ment in a newborn. Most states require a test at birth to detect the disease. When detected early and treated, phenylketonuria symptoms can be prevented by dietary control.

phosphates. Salts of phosphoric acid. Important part of the body system that controls acid-base balance. Other chemicals involved in acid-base balance include sodium, potassium, bicarbonate and proteins.

photosensitization. Process by which a substance or organism becomes sensitive to light.

photosensitizing pigment. Pigment that makes a substance sensitive to light.

phytochemical. Any one of many substances present in fruits and vegetables that have various health-promoting properties.

platelet aggregation. A collective of individual blood platelets.

potassium. Important element found in body tissue that plays a critical role in electrolyte and fluid balance in the body.

poultice. Applied to a body surface to provide heat and moisture. Material is held between layers of muslin or other cloth. Poultices contain an active substance and a base. They are placed on any part of the body and changed when cool. Purpose is to relieve pain and reduce congestion or inflammation.

prostate. Gland in the male that surrounds the neck of the bladder and urethra. In older men, it may become infected (prostatitis) or obstructed (prostatic hypertrophy), cause urinary difficulties or become cancerous.

psoriasis. Chronic, recurrent skin disease characterized by patches of flaking skin with discoloration.

psychosis. Mental disorder character-ized by deranged personality, loss of contact with reality, delusions and hallucinations.

purgative. Powerful laxative usually leading to explosive, watery diarrhea.

purine base. A crystalline base that is the parent of uric-acid compounds. Also a constituent of *DNA* and *RNA.*

purine foods. Foods metabolized into uric acid; these include anchovies, brains, liver, sweetbreads, sardines, meat extracts, oysters, lobster and other shellfish.

pyrimidine base. An organic base. Also a constituent of *DNA* and *RNA.*

quercetin. A pharmacologically active *flavonoid* that inhibits the synthesis of *enzymes* necessary for the release of histamines.

RDA (Recommended Dietary Allowance). Recommendations based on data derived from different popula-tion groups and ages. The quoted RDA figures represent the *average* amount of a particular nutrient needed per day to maintain good health in the average healthy person. Data for these recommendations have been collected and analyzed by the Food and Nutrition Board of the National Research Council. These figures serve as a reference point for comparison. The latest revised amounts were published in 1980, with a new revision promised soon. It is only within the framework of statistical probability that RDA can be used legitimately and meaningfully.

renal. Pertaining to the kidneys.

resin. Complex chemicals, usually hard, transparent or translucent, that frequently cause adverse effects in the body.

retina. Inner covering of the eyeball on which images form to be perceived in the brain via the optic nerve.

rhizome. Root-like, horizontal-growing stem just below the surface of the soil.

rickets. Bone disease caused by vitamin-D deficiency. Bones become bent and distorted during infancy or childhood if there is insufficient vitamin D for normal growth and development.

RNA (ribonucleic acid). Complex protein chemical in genes that determines the type of life form into which a cell will develop.

rubefacient. Reddens skin by increasing blood supply to it.

saponins. Chemicals from plants, frequently associated with adverse or toxic reactions. They uniformly produce soapy lathers.

sedative. Reduces excitement or anxiety.

sensory neuropathy. See *neuropathy.*

SGOT. Abbreviation for *serum glutamic oxaloacetic transaminase,* a blood test to measure liver function or detect damage to the heart muscle.

spasmolytic. Decreases spasm of smooth muscle or skeletal (striated) muscle.

steroidal chemicals. Group of chemicals with same properties as steroids. Steroids are fat-soluble compounds with carbon and acid components. They are found in nature in the form of hormones and bile acids, and in plants as naturally occurring drugs, such as digitalis.

stimulant. Stimulates; temporarily arouses or accelerates physiological activity of an organ or organ system.

stomachic. Promotes increased contraction of stomach muscles.

stomatitis. Inflammation of the mouth.

stroke. Sudden, severe attack that results in brain damage. Usually sudden paralysis or speech difficulty results from injury to the brain or spinal cord by a blood clot, hemorrhage or occlusion of blood supply to the brain from a narrowed or blocked artery.

tannins. Complex acidic mixtures of chemicals.

tenesmus. Urgent feeling of having to have a bowel movement or to urinate.

terpenes. Complex hydrocarbons. Most *volatile oils* contain terpenes.

thrombophlebitis. Inflammation of a vein, usually caused by a blood clot. If the clot becomes detached and travels to the lung, the condition is called thromboembolism.

tincture. Solution of chemicals in a highly alcoholic solvent made by simple solution or by methods described in the United States Pharmacopoeia or the National Formulary.

tonic. Medicinal preparations used to restore normal tone to tissues or to stimulate the appetite.

GLOSSARY

toxicity. Poisonous reaction that impairs body functions or damages cells.

toxin. Poison in dead or live organism.

tranquilizer. Calms a person without clouding mental function.

tremor. Involuntary trembling.

tyramine. Chemical component of the body. In normal quantities, without interference from other chemicals, tyramine helps sustain normal blood pressure. In the presence of some drugs—monoamine-oxidase inhibitors and some rauwolfia compounds—tyramine levels can rise and cause toxic or fatal levels in the blood.

urethra. Hollow tube through which urine is transported from the bladder to outside the body. In men, semen is also transported through the urethra from the testicles.

uterus. Hollow, muscular organ in the female in which an embryo develops into a fetus. Menstruation occurs when the lining sloughs periodically.

vein. Blood vessel that returns blood to the heart.

virus. Infectious organism that reproduces in the cells of an infected host.

volatile oils. Chemicals that evaporate at room temperature. Same as *essential oils.*

water soluble. Dissolves in water.

wax. High-molecular-weight hydrocarbons; they are insoluble in water.

yeast. Single-cell organism that can cause infection of the skin, mouth, vagina, rectum and other parts of the gastrointestinal system. The terms *yeast fungus* and *monilia* are used interchangeably.

Metric Chart

The following units of measurement and weight are commonly used in establishing doses of vitamins, minerals, supplements and medicinal herbs.

Unit	Abbreviation	Volume	Approximate U.S. Equivalent
Cubic centimeter	cc	0.000001 cubic meter	0.061 cubic inch
Liter	l	1 liter	1.057 quarts
Deciliter	dl	0.10 liter	0.21 quart
Centiliter	cl	0.01 liter	0.338 fluid ounce
Milliliter	ml	0.001 liter	0.27 fluid dram
Kilogram	kg	1,000 grams	2.2046 pounds
Gram	g or gm	1 gram	0.035 ounce
Milligram	mg	0.001 gram	0.015 grain
Microgram	mcg	0.000001 gram	0.0000154 grain

Bibliography

Adams, Ruth. *Health Foods*. New York: Larchmont Books, 1975.

Aloe Vera: the Miracle Plant. Mountain View, Calif.: Anderson World Books, 1983.

American Dietetic Association. *Handbook of Clinical Dietetics*. New Haven, Conn.: Yale University Press, 1981.

American Medical Association. *Drug Evaluations*. 6th ed. Chicago: American Medical Association, 1986.

Balch, James F., M.D., and Phyllis A. Balch, C.N.C. *Prescription for Nutritional Healing*. 2d ed. Garden City Park, N.Y.: Avery Publishing Group, 1997.

Benowicz, Robert J. *Vitamins and You*. New York: Grosset & Dunlap, 1979.

Blumenthal, Mark, and Chance W. Riggins. *Popular Herbs in the U.S. Market: Therapeutic Monographs*. Austin, Texas: American Botanical Council, 1997.

Bricklin, Mark. *The Practical Encyclopedia of Natural Healing*. Emmaus, Pa.: Rodale Press, 1976.

Britton, Jade, and Tamara Kircher. *The Complete Book of Herbal Remedies*. Buffalo, N.Y.: Firefly Books, 1998.

Brown, Donald J. *Herbal Prescriptions for Better Health*. Rocklin, Calif.: Prima Publishing, 1996.

Butler, Kurt, and Lynn Rayner. *The Best Medicine: The Complete Health and Preventive Medicine Handbook*. San Francisco: Harper & Row, 1985.

Chevallier, Andrew. *The Encyclopedia of Medicinal Plants*. New York: DK Publishing, 1996.

Clayman, Charles B., M.D., ed. *American Medical Association Encyclopedia of Medicine*. New York: Random House, 1989.

The Complete Book of Vitamins. Emmaus, Pa: Rodale Press, 1984.

Consumer Guide. *Herbs for Health and Healing*. Lincolnwood, IL: Publications International, Ltd., 1997.

Duke, James A., Ph.D. *CRC Handbook of Medicinal Herbs*. Boca Raton, Fla.: CRC Press, 1985.

——*The Green Pharmacy*. Emmaus, Pa.: Rodale Press, 1997.

Eades, Mary Dan, M.D. *The Doctor's Complete Guide to Vitamins and Minerals*. New York: Dell, 1994.

Edmunds, Marilyn W., ed. *Nursing Drug Reference: A Practitioner's Guide.* Bowie, Md.: Brady Communications Company, 1985.

Eisenhauer, Laurel A. *The Nurse's 1984-85 Guide to Drug Therapy: Drug Profiles for Patient Care.* Englewood Cliffs, N.J.: Prentice-Hall, 1984.

Fischer, William L. *Miracle Healing Power Through Nature's Pharmacy.* Canfield, Ohio: Fischer Publishing Corporation, 1986.

Garrison, Robert, Jr., and Elizabeth Somer. *Nutrition Desk Reference.* New Canaan, Conn.: Keats Publishing, 1985.

Harris, Ben Charles. *The Compleat Herbal.* Barre, Mass.: Barre Publishers, 1972.

Harris, Lloyd J. *The Book of Garlic.* rev. ed. New York: Simon & Schuster, 1979.

Heinerman, John. *Aloe Vera, Jojoba and Yucca.* New Canaan, Conn.: Keats Publishing, 1982.

—*Heinerman's Encyclopedia of Healing Herbs and Spices* Englewood Cliffs, NJ: Prentice-Hall, 1996.

Hemphill, John, and Rosemary Hemphill. *Hemphills' Herbs for Health.* Dorset, U.K.: Blandford Press, 1985.

Hendler, Sheldon Saul. *The Complete Guide to Anti-Aging Nutrients.* New York: Simon & Schuster, 1985.

Herbert, Victor. *Nutrition Cultism: Facts and Fictions.* Philadelphia: George F. Stickley Company, 1981.

Holford, Patrick. *Vitamin Vitality.* New York: Bantam Books, 1986.

"How to Use Herbal Medicines Safely." *Medical Self-Care* (March-April 1987): 40-51.

Kay, Margarita Artschwager. *Healing with Plants in the American and Mexican West.* Tucson: The University of Arizona Press, 1996.

Kirschmann, John D. *Nutrition Almanac.* 2d ed. New York: McGraw-Hill, 1984.

Lasswell, Anita B., et. al. *Nutrition for Family and Primary Care Practitioners.* Philadelphia: George F. Stickley Company, 1986.

Lee, William H. *Kelp, Dulse and Other Sea Supplements.* New Canaan, Conn.: Keats Publishing, 1983.

Lieberman, Shari, Ph.D., and Nancy Bruning. *The Real Vitamin & Mineral Book.* 2d ed. Garden City Park, N.Y.: Avery Publishing Group, 1997.

Lust, John. *The Herb Book.* New York: Bantam Books, 1974.

Magic and Medicine of Plants. Pleasantville, N.Y.: Reader's Digest Association, 1986.

Marshall, Charles W. *Vitamins and Minerals: Help or Harm?* Philadelphia: George F. Stickley Company, 1983.

McDonald, Arline, Ph.D., R.D., Annette Natow, Ph.D., R.D., JoAnn Heslin, M.A., R.D., and Susan Male Smith, M.A., R.D. *Complete Book of Vitamins & Minerals.* Lincolnwood, Ill.: Publications International, Ltd., 1996.

Merriam-Webster's Collegiate Dictionary. 10th ed. Springfield, Mass.: Merriam-Webster, Inc., 1997.

Mervyn, Leonard. *The Dictionary of Vitamins: The Complete Guide to Vitamins and Vitamin Therapy.* New York: Thorsons Publishers, 1984.

Mindell, Earl. *Earl Mindell's Herb Bible.* New York: Fireside Books, 1992

——*Earl Mindell's New and Revised Vitamin Bible.* New York: Warner Books, 1985.

Mosby's Complete Drug Reference: Physicians GenRx. 7th ed. St. Louis, Mo.: Mosby Year Book, Inc., 1997.

Murray, Michael T. *The Healing Power of Herbs.* 2d ed. Rocklin, Calif.: Prima Publishing, 1995.

Nutritional Labeling, How It Can Work for You. Bethesda, Md.: National Nutrition Consortium, 1975.

Pressman, Alan H., D.C., Ph.D., C.C.N., and Sheila Buff. *The Complete Idiot's Guide to Vitamins and Minerals.* New York: Alpha Books, 1997.

Silverman, Harold. *The Vitamin Book.* New York: Bantam Books, 1985.

Somer, Elizabeth, M.A., R.D., and Health Media of America. *The Essential Guide to Vitamins and Minerals.* New York: Harper Perennial, 1995.

Spoerke, David G., Jr. *Herbal Medications.* Santa Barbara, Calif.: Woodbridge Press Publishing Company, 1980.

Switzer, Larry. *Spirulina, the Whole Food Revolution.* New York: Bantam Books, 1982.

Tierra, Michael. *The Way of Herbs.* New York: Washington Square Press, 1983.

Time-Life Books. *The Drug & Natural Medicine Advisor.* Alexandria, Va.: Time-Life Inc., 1997.

Tyler, Varro E., Ph.D., Sc.D. *Herbs of Choice: The Therapeutic Use of Phytomedicinals.* New York: Pharmaceutical Products Press, 1994.

Understanding Vitamins and Minerals. Emmaus, Pa.: Rodale Press, 1984.

United States Department of Agriculture. "Dietary Guidelines for Americans." Nutrition and Your Health. *Home and Garden Bulletin* No. 232 (1985).

United States Pharmacopeial Convention, Inc. *USP DI, Volume I, Drug Information for the Health Care Professional.* 17th ed. Taunton, Mass.: Rand McNally, 1997.

University of California at Berkeley Wellness Newsletter. New York, NY: Health Letter Associates, 1984–

Webb, Marcus A. *The Herbal Companion: The Essential Guide to Using Herbs for Your Health and Well-Being.* London: Quintet Publishing Limited, 1997.

Weiss, Gaea and Shandor Weiss. *Growing & Using the Healing Herbs.* Emmaus, Pa.: Rodale Press, 1985.

Willard, Mervyn D. *Nutrition for the Practicing Physician.* Menlo Park, Calif: Addison-Wesley Publishing Company, 1982.

Index

Note: Entries in **bold** refer to main headings

A

Abortion, may cause, 256, 469
Abrin. *See* Jequirity Bean
Absinthium. *See* Wormwood
Absorption diseases, 65
Acetylcholine, negates activity of, 365
Acid-base balance, regulates, 77, 103, 113
Acidophilus, 148-149
Acne, aids in treating, 189, 248, 283
Aconite, 254-255
Acquired Immune Deficiency Syndrome.
  See AIDS
Adrenal glands, 158, 480
  aids in function of, 32
African Rue. *See* Harmel
Agar, similar to, 358
Agave, 255-256
Ague Weed. *See* Boneset
AIDS, 187, 192
Alcoholism, 65, 79, 103
Alder, Black, 257-258
Alder Buckthorn. *See* Alder, Black
Alfalfa, 258-259
Algae. *See* Spirulina
Allergy symptoms, decreases, 149
Allspice, 259-260
Aloe, 261-262
Aloe Vera. *See* Aloe
Alphatocopherol. *See* Vitamin E
Altamisa. *See* Feverfew
Alum Root, 262-263
Alzheimer's disease, may treat, 35, 40, 164,
  217
Amebiasis, may treat, 357
Amenorrhea. *See* Menstruation, absence
  of
American Boxwood. *See* American
  Dogwood
American Dogwood, 264
American Hellebore. *See* Hellebore
American Mandrake. *See* Mayapple
American Sanicle. *See* Alum Root
Amino Acids, 123-145
  aids metabolism of, 49
  defined, 123, 480

Anemia, 32, 49, 60, 81, 83
  defined, 481
  iron-deficiency, 92
  pernicious, 35, 36, 81, 481
Angelica, 265-266
Anise, 266-267
Anorexia Nervosa, 81
Antacid, acts as, 73, 96
Anti-aging remedy, 158
Antianxiety, 226
Antiarrhythmic, 224
Antibacterial, 214, 242, 247, 261, 273, 285,
  326, 431. *See also* Bacteria
Antibiotic, 207, 220, 234
Antibodies, promotes production of, 130,
  137
Anticoagulant, 214, 345, 452
Antifungal, 234, 247, 258
Anti-inflammatory, 162, 189, 191, 194, 201,
  208, 212, 221, 223, 254, 285, 314, 331,
  399, 427, 430, 460, 468
Antioxidant, 46, 98, 109, 118, 128, 188,
  193, 214, 218, 223, 228, 419, 447
Anti-parasitic, 234
Antispasmodic, 211
Antiviral, 214, 261
Anxiety, relieves, 242
Aphrodisiac, possible use as, 203, 218,
  251, 276, 281, 304
Appetite
  improves, 218, 306, 449
  suppresses, 302
Arginine, 124-125
Aromatic, 296
Arsenic, 70-71
Arteriosclerosis, protects against, 171, 252
Arthritis, may treat, 293, 304, 314, 315,
  321, 335, 386, 388, 420, 447, 455, 460,
  465
Asafetida, 267-268
Ascorbic Acid, 31-34, 196
Aspidium. *See* Male Fern
Asthma, may treat, 299, 334, 341, 365,
  445, 451
  bronchial, 391
Asthma Weed. *See* Indian Tobacco
Astragalus, 187